I0065788

Recent Progress in Pharmaceutical Research

Recent Progress in Pharmaceutical Research

Edited by John Jensen

hayle
medical

New York

Hayle Medical,
750 Third Avenue, 9th Floor,
New York, NY 10017, USA

Visit us on the World Wide Web at:
www.haylemedical.com

© Hayle Medical, 2019

This book contains information obtained from authentic and highly regarded sources. Copyright for all individual chapters remain with the respective authors as indicated. All chapters are published with permission under the Creative Commons Attribution License or equivalent. A wide variety of references are listed. Permission and sources are indicated; for detailed attributions, please refer to the permissions page and list of contributors. Reasonable efforts have been made to publish reliable data and information, but the authors, editors and publisher cannot assume any responsibility for the validity of all materials or the consequences of their use.

ISBN: 978-1-63241-791-6

Trademark Notice: Registered trademark of products or corporate names are used only for explanation and identification without intent to infringe.

Cataloging-in-Publication Data

Recent progress in pharmaceutical research / edited by John Jensen.
    p. cm.
Includes bibliographical references and index.
ISBN 978-1-63241-791-6
1. Pharmacy. 2. Pharmacy--Research. 3. Pharmacology. 4. Drugs.
5. Pharmaceutical industry. I. Jensen, John.
RS122 .R43 2019
615--dc23

Table of Contents

Preface

This book aims to highlight the current researches and provides a platform to further the scope of innovations in this area. This book is a product of the combined efforts of many researchers and scientists, after going through thorough studies and analysis from different parts of the world. The objective of this book is to provide the readers with the latest information of the field.

Pharmaceutical science is concerned with the study and design of drug formulation, disposition and delivery. It also studies the biochemical and physiological effects of drugs on human beings, and encompasses the study of toxic effects, the factors that control the concentration of drugs in different areas of the body, the cellular and molecular interactions of drugs with their receptors, etc. New candidate medications are discovered by screening of chemical libraries of synthetic molecules, natural products or extracts in organisms to identify substances that have the desired therapeutic effect. Such screening hits are optimized for increasing the affinity, efficacy, selectivity, metabolic stability and oral bioavailability. Based on the knowledge of a biological target, molecules that are complementary in charge and shape to the biomolecular target are designed. For a designed molecule to be safe and effective, properties such as bioavailability, side effects and metabolic half-life need to be optimized. Drug delivery is another important aspect of pharmaceutical research. Techniques of drug delivery modify drug release profile, distribution, absorption and elimination. This book contains some path-breaking studies in the field of pharmaceutical science. It will also provide interesting topics for research, which interested readers can take up. Scientists and students actively engaged in this field will find this book full of crucial and unexplored concepts.

I would like to express my sincere thanks to the authors for their dedicated efforts in the completion of this book. I acknowledge the efforts of the publisher for providing constant support. Lastly, I would like to thank my family for their support in all academic endeavors.

Editor

1

Gastroprotective Effects of Sulphated Polysaccharides from the Alga *Caulerpa mexicana* Reducing Ethanol-Induced Gastric Damage

José Gerardo Carneiro [1,2], Ticiana de Brito Lima Holanda [1], Ana Luíza Gomes Quinderé [1], Annyta Fernandes Frota [1], Vitória Virgínia Magalhães Soares [1], Rayane Siqueira de Sousa [1], Manuela Araújo Carneiro [1], Dainesy Santos Martins [3], Antoniella Souza Gomes Duarte [3] and Norma Maria Barros Benevides [1,*]

[1] Department of Biochemistry and Molecular Biology, Federal University of Ceará, s/n Humberto Monte Avenue, Pici Campus, 60455-760 Fortaleza, Brazil; gerardo@ifce.edu.br (J.G.C.); ticipesca@yahoo.com.br (T.d.B.L.H.); aninhaquindere@gmail.com (A.L.G.Q.); annyta.frota@gmail.com (A.F.F.); vitoriabio8@gmail.com (V.V.M.S.); gerardoifce@hotmail.com (R.S.d.S.); manuela.carneiro@hotmail.com (M.A.C.)
[2] Federal Institute of Education, Science and Technology of Ceará, Armando Sales Louzada Street, 62580-000 Acaraú, Brazil
[3] Department of Morphoology, Faculty of Medicine, Federal University of Ceará, s/n Delmiro de Farias Street, Porangabuçu Campus, 60416-030 Fortaleza, Brazil; dainy.santos@gmail.com (D.S.M.); asouzagomes@yahoo.com.br (A.S.G.D.)
* Correspondence: nmbb@ufc.br

Abstract: The development of the gastric lesion is complex and the result of the imbalance between aggressive and protective factors, involving the generation of free radicals and disturbance in nitric oxide (NO) production. Sulphated polysaccharides (SP), from marine algae, are widely used in biotechnological and pharmaceutical areas. In this study, we evaluated the effects of SP from the green marine alga *Caulerpa mexicana* (Cm-SP) in ethanol-induced gastric damage models in mice. Cm-SP (2, 20, or 200 mg/kg), administered p.o., significantly reduced gastric damage, and these effects were inhibited through pretreatment with indomethacin. Cm-SP (200 mg/kg) prevented the ethanol-induced decline in glutathione and restored its normal level. Moreover, it was able to normalize the elevated thiobarbituric acid reactive substance levels. However, Cm-SP did not show any significant effects on NO_2/NO_3 level, when compared to the ethanol group. The pretreatment with L- NAME induced gastric mucosal damage and did not inhibit the gastroprotective effect of Cm-SP (200 mg/kg). In conclusion, the gastroprotective effects of Cm-SP in mice involve prostaglandins and reduction in the oxidative stress and are independent of NO.

Keywords: marine alga; gastric ulcer; gastroprotection; cytoprotection

1. Introduction

Gastrointestinal diseases are an important public health problem affecting many people worldwide. Stress, nutritional disorders, alcohol consumption, prolonged use of non-steroidal anti-inflammatory drugs (NSAID), and glucocorticoids are followed by gastric complications, including stomach ulcers [1–4]. Their development is complex and the result of the imbalance between aggressive and protective factors, involving the generation of free radicals and disturbance in nitric oxide (NO) production [5–7]. In the model of ethanol-induced gastric damage, the administration of absolute ethanol caused macroscopic and microscopic mucosa gastric damage, which is characterized by intense hemorrhage, necrosis, mucosal oedema, and inflammatory infiltrate. Therefore, it is widely used to study gastroprotective effects of new bioactive compounds [1,6].

The discovery of new bioactive compounds with potential pharmaceutical activity, presenting minimal adverse effects, is of great importance. Thus, study groups are currently researching new natural compounds and their wide range of applications. Seaweeds are sources of sulphated polysaccharides, and the chemical structure of these polymers varies according to the species [8–10]. Sulfated polysaccharides (SP) comprise a group of heterogeneous macromolecules (as alginates, agar, agarose, carrageenans, fucoidan, laminaran, ulvan) presenting various biological effects, with biotechnical potential, and already in use in the food, cosmetics, and pharmaceutical industries [8–11]. Our group has demonstrated various biological activities of SP, such as anticoagulant [12], antithrombotic [13], neuroprotective [14], antinociceptive, and anti-inflammatory [15–18].

Caulerpa mexicana Sonder ex Kützing is a marine green alga of the Cauleparceae family, which is widely encountered along the coast of Brazil. SP obtained from this alga species have presented antinociceptive and anti-inflammatory effects in a model of ulcerative colitis [19], in oedema caused by histamine and neutrophils migration [18]. However, no study has described the effects of SP from *C. mexicanain* in gastric lesions models. In the present study, we investigated the effects of SP from the green seaweed *C. mexicana* on ethanol-induced gastric damage in mice and the involvement of endogenous prostaglandins (PG) and NO pathway.

2. Results

2.1. Effect of Cm-SP on Ethanol-Induced Gastric Damage

Oral administration of ethanol absolute (0.2 mL) induced gastric mucosal damage in mice (24.57 ± 2.23 mm^2). Administration of Cm-SP (2, 20 or 200 mg/kg, p.o.) reduced, in a dose-dependent manner, the gastric damage by 49% (12.41 ± 1.71 mm^2), 87% (3.09 ± 0.82 mm^2) and 92% (2.03 ± 0.54 mm^2), respectively, when compared with the ethanol group ($p < 0.05$). Moreover, the groups that received Cm-SP (20 and 200 mg/kg) did not show any significant difference when compared to the control group saline. The treatment with indomethacin reversed the gastroprotective effects that are promoted by Cm-SP (200 mg/kg). Furthermore, the pretreatment with L-NAME induced gastric mucosal damage (29.12 ± 3.48) and did not inhibit the gastroprotective effect of Cm-SP (200 mg/kg; 85%; 4.34 ± 0.93) (Figure 1).

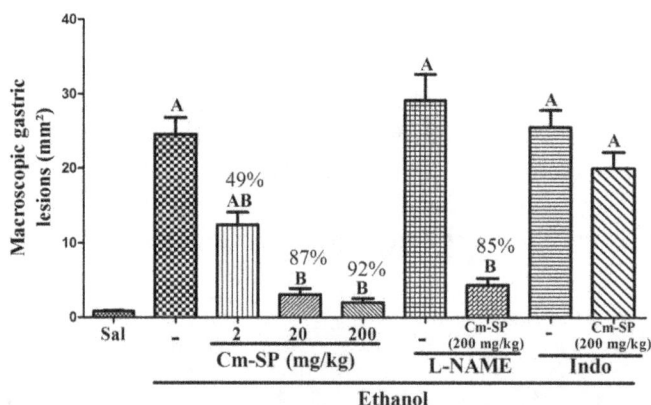

Figure 1. Effect of *Caulerpa mexicana* (Cm-SP) on ethanol-induced gastric damage. Mice were treated with Cm-SP (2, 20, or 200 mg/kg) or saline (sal) by gavage. Another groups received L-NAME (20 mg/kg) or indomethacin (10 mg/kg) (indo). After 1 h, groups were treated with saline (sal) or Cm-SP (200 mg/kg). After 1 h, the gastric damage was induced by administration of ethanol absolute (0.2 mL, p.o.). After 1 h, mice were sacrificed and the total area of macroscopic gastric lesions was determined. The results are expressed as mean $\pm$ SEM of a minimum of 6 animals per group. (**A**) $p < 0.05$ vs. saline group; (**B**) $p < 0.05$ vs. group ethanol; ANOVA and Newman-Keuls test.

2.2. Histological Assessment

Administration of ethanol causes mucosal epithelium damage with disrupted glandular structure, oedema of submucosa, and excessive inflammatory infiltrate (Figure 2).

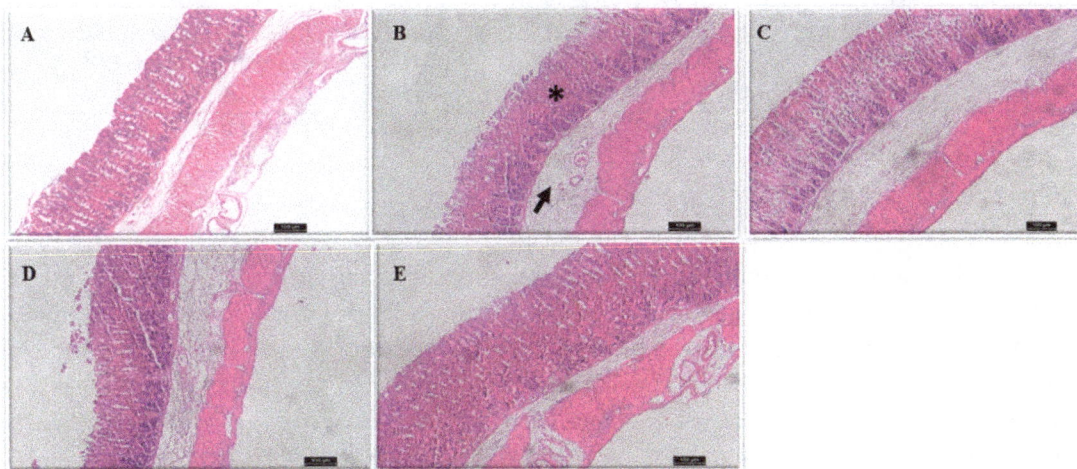

Figure 2. Histological evaluation of the ethanol-induced gastric damage in mice. (**A**) Control stomach: intact gastric epithelium with organized glandular structure and normal submucosa could be seen; (**B–E**) ethanol-induced damage; (**B**) mice pre-treated with vehicle: * indicates damaged mucosal epithelium with disrupted glandular structure and arrow depicts oedema of submucosa and inflammatory infiltrate of mucosa; (**C**) Cm-SP 2 mg/kg; (**D**) Cm-SP 20 mg/kg; (**E**) Cm-SP 200 mg/kg. (**C–E**) depict a recovery in mucosa epithelium and reorganized glandular structure, as well as improvement of oedema by Cm-SP. (H&E staining; magnification 100×).

However, the administration of Cm-SP (2, 20, and 200 mg/kg) maintained the integrity of the mucosa with uninjured epithelium and organized glandular structure, as well as an improvement of oedema of submucosa and of inflammatory infiltrate, suggesting that Cm-SP exerts a gastroprotective effect. Histological analyses showed that Cm-SP (200 mg/kg) decreased hemorrhagic lesion, oedema, and erosion (loss of epithelial cell architecture), induced by ethanol (Table 1).

Table 1. Protective effect of Cm-SP in ethanol-induced microscopic gastric damage.

Experimental Group (N = 6)	Hemorrhagic Lesion (Score 0–4)	Oedema (Score 0–4)	Erosion (Loss of Cell Architecture) (Score 0–3)	Cell Infiltrate (Score 0–3)	Total (Scores 14)
Saline	0	0	0	0	0
Ethanol	4 (3–4) [A]	2 (2–4) [A]	2.5 (2–3) [A]	2 (2–3) [A]	10.5 (9–14) [A]
Cm-SP (2 mg/kg)	1 (0–1) [B]	2 (0–3)	1 (0–2)	0 (0–1) [B]	4 (0–7)
Cm-SP (20 mg/kg)	0 (0–1) [B]	0 (0–3)	0 (0–3)	0 (0–2)	0 (0–9)
Cm-SP (200 kg/mg)	0 (0–0) [B]	0 (0–2) [B]	0 (0–1) [B]	0 (0–2)	0 (0–5) [B]

Values denote median with minimum and maximum, respectively. Test of Kruskal-Wallis. [A] $p < 0.05$ vs. group Saline; [B] $p < 0.05$ vs. group Ethanol.

2.3. Effect of Cm-SP on Malondialdehyde (MDA), Glutathione (GSH), and NO_2/NO_3 Levels

Administration of ethanol decreased GSH levels (20.96 ± 1.87), and elevated lipid peroxidation (TBARS content) (391.42 ± 23.06) in gastric tissues when compared to the saline group. Cm-SP (200 mg/kg) prevented the ethanol-induced decline in GSH content and restored its normal level (38.26 ± 0.57). Moreover, Cm-SP (200 mg/kg) normalized the elevated TBARS levels (153.3 ± 8.28). However, the administration of Cm-SP (200 mg/kg) did not show any significant effects on NO_2/NO_3 level, as compared to the ethanol group (Table 2).

Table 2. Effect of Cm-SP on Malondialdehyde (MDA), Glutathione (GSH), and NO_2/NO_3 levels.

Experimental Groups	MDA	GSH	NO_2/NO_3
Saline	152.30 ± 9.91	31.81 ± 8.48	16.05 ± 3.24
Ethanol	391.42 ± 23.06 [A]	20.96 ± 1.87 [A]	28.02 ± 2.74 [A]
Cm-SP (200 mg/kg)	153.30 ± 8.28 [B]	38.26 ± 0.57 [B]	23.14 ± 3.52
L-NAME	541.60 ± 49.02	19.28 ± 3.74	7.52 ± 1.68
L-NAME + Cm-SP (200 mg/kg)	383.0 ± 23.97 [C]	32.35 ± 1.56 [C]	8.66 ± 1.62

Data are expressed as the mean $\pm$ SEM (n = 6). ANOVA and Newman-Keuls test. [A] $p < 0.05$ vs. group Saline; [B] $p < 0.05$ vs. group Ethanol; [C] $p < 0.05$ vs. group L-NAME.

3. Discussion

The gastric mucosa is continuously exposed to noxious agents and the maintenance of its integrity is ensured by a complex defense system, involving mucus and bicarbonate secretions, modulation of pH, gastric microcirculation, antioxidant factors, PG generation, NO and H_2S release, and HO-1 pathway induction [5,6,20–22]. The pathogenesis of ethanol-induced gastric damage involves direct necrotizing action, mitigation of defensive factors, such as the secretion of bicarbonate and production of mucus, depletion of antioxidant defense, increased oxidative stress, such as free radicals formation and lipid peroxidation, and changes in permeability of mitochondrial membrane prior the increased cell death by apoptosis [1,6,23].

Studies have shown that SP that is extracted from seaweeds exhibit a potential therapeutic effect for several diseases, mainly gastrointestinal tract disorders [9,11,24]. However, studies correlating the gastroprotective action of this polysaccharide are scarce in the literature. Recently, our research group showed that SP enzymatically extracted from the green alga *C. mexicana*, characterized as a mixture rich in sulphated galactan, have presented interesting anti-inflammatory actions with involvement the HO-1 pathway, reduced oedema that is caused by histamine, and inhibited inflammatory cell infiltrate [18].

The administration of absolute ethanol caused macroscopic and microscopic mucosa gastric damage characterized by intense hemorrhage, loss of epithelial structure, oedema of submucosa, and inflammatory infiltrate. The results of the present study showed that Cm-SP (20 and 200 mg/kg, p.o.) presented gastroprotective activities, reducing the gastric damage in 87% and 92% of Cm-SP, respectively, when compared with the ethanol group ($p < 0.05$). Furthermore, there was the preservation the integrity of the structure of the epithelium, reduction of oedema of submucosa, and the inhibition of inflammatory cell infiltrate, as verified by histopathological analysis. This data corroborate previous studies on the gastroprotective effects of other SP extracted from marine algae in experimental models of ethanol-induced gastric damage [25–28].

Several studies show that PG play important roles in modulating the gastric mucosal integrity, mainly against the damaging actions of ethanol. PG are produced from the arachidonic acid by two isozymes of COX, and are main mediators of the inflammatory process [4,7,29]. PG have been implicated in the regulation of various functions of defense gastric mucosal after barrier disruption, including decreased acid secretion, mucus production, mucin release, increased bicarbonate secretion, and mucosal blood flow [4,5,7,22,29,30]. NO is another important mediator of gastric mucosal integrity maintenance. NO's role has been extensively studied, especially by the use of chemical inhibitors, such as L-NAME. A variety of substances dependent on the NO pathway possess cytoprotective actions [21,31]. Therefore, the inhibition of NO synthesis exacerbates gastric mucosal damage induced by ethanol [21]. However, several studies have shown the gastroprotective action of substances without the involvement of the NO pathway [20,32].

To elucidate the possible mechanism of the gastroprotective action of Cm-SP, we investigated the involvement of PG and NO pathway in the ethanol-induced gastric damage in mice. Our results showed that treatment with indomethacin, a COX inhibitor, reversed the gastroprotective effects promoted by Cm-SP (200 mg/kg), indicating the involvement of PG in the Cm-SP protective effects, showed for the first time that endogenous PG can mediate the SP of seaweeds protection against ethanol-induced damage gastric. Which corroborates with the observations reported in other studies on the gastroprotective action in models of gastric injury [33]. Additionally, the administration of L-NAME, a non-selective inhibitor of NOS, did not inhibit the gastroprotective effect of Cm-SP (200 mg/kg). Since the response to Cm-SP was not affected by L-NAME, it is assumed that the gastroprotective effect of SP is independent of the NO pathway. Therefore, Cm-SP is the first marine algal SP that is reported to present gastroprotective effect independent of the NO pathway.

Several mechanisms are involved in the cytoprotection of the gastric mucosa against damage caused by oxidative stress, including vasoactive metabolites, gaseous mediators (H_2S, NO, CO), proteins (GSH, HO-1), and appetite peptides (ghrelin, obestatin) [20,32,34–36]. Oxidative stress is involved in the pathogenesis of ethanol-induced gastric damage through the formation of free radicals and lipid peroxidation, which is demonstrated by the decrease of GSH and increase of MDA levels in stomach tissue [6,34]. We analyzed two important markers of oxidative stress: GSH, a tripeptide that presents great affinity to H_2O_2 and acts mainly as an endogenous antioxidant, being consumed during oxidative metabolism; and MDA, a metabolite of lipid peroxidation. Our findings show that the administration of ethanol induced the generation of free radicals and of lipid peroxidation and that gastroprotective effects of Cm-SP were accompanied by a decrease in oxidative stress in the gastric mucosal, namely, decreased MDA and increased GSH. Our results are consistent with previous reports that demonstrate the involvement of decreased oxidative stress in the action gastroprotective of several SP [25,26,28].

In conclusion, our results indicate that Cm-SP have a gastroprotective activity against ethanol-induced gastric damage, through mechanisms mediated by prostaglandins, independent of the NO pathway and oxidative stress reducer. Thus, we suggest that Cm-SP exhibit potential applications in the development of novel drugs against gastric injury and that further study is needed to explain the mechanism of gastroprotection of Cm-SP.

4. Materials and Methods

4.1. Animals

Mice (35–40 g) from the Animal Care Unit of the Federal University of Ceará, Fortaleza, Brazil, were used throughout the experiments. For each experiment, groups of six animals were segregated and handled separately. This study was conducted in accordance with the guidelines set forth by the U.S. Department of Health and Human Services, and with the approval of the Ethics Committee of the Federal University of Ceará, Fortaleza, Brazil (CEPA n°. 60/13).

4.2. Marine Alga and Extraction of SP

Specimens of *C. mexicana* were collected at Flecheiras Beach, Brazil. A voucher specimen (n°. 47304) was deposited in the Herbarium Prisco Bezerra (EAC) in the Department of Biology, Federal University of Ceará. The SP from *C. mexicana* (Cm-SP) were extracted by the enzymatic method, according to Farias et al. [37], as mentioned in our earlier report [18].

Essentially, 5 g of the dehydrated algal at 25 °C was macerated and subjected to digestion with papain solution (30 mg/mL) in 100 mM sodium acetate buffer (pH 5.0) containing 5 mM cysteine and 5 mM EDTA at 60 °C for 6 h. After, material was centrifuged ($2295 \times g$, 30 min, 10 °C), the SP in solution were precipitated with 16 mL of 10% cetylpyridinium chloride (CPC) solution. After 24 h at room temperature, the mixture was centrifuged at $2560 \times g$ for 20 min at 5 °C. The SP in the pellet were washed with 200 mL of 0.05% CPC solution, dissolved with 100 mL of a 2 M NaCl-ethanol (100:15, v/v) mixture, and precipitated with 100 mL of absolute ethanol. After 24 h at 4 °C, the precipitate was collected by centrifugation (2560 g for 20 min at 5 °C), washed twice with 100 mL of 80% ethanol, and washed once with 100 mL of absolute ethanol. The final precipitate was dialyzed, and freeze-dried. After these procedures, the total SP from *C. mexicana* were obtained [18].

4.3. Effect of Cm-SP on Ethanol-Induced Gastric Damage

This assay was performed as described by Damasceno et al. [25], with modifications. Groups of the mice (n = 6) were treated with Cm-SP (2, 20, or 200 mg/kg) or saline (0.2 mL) by gavage. After 1 h, the gastric damage was induced by administration of ethanol absolute (0.2 mL, p.o.). To evaluate the involvement of endogenous PG and NO pathway in the Cm-SP action, groups were pretreated with indomethacin (10 mg/kg, p.o.), a cyclooxygenase (COX) inhibitor, or N-nitro-L-arginine methyl ester (L-NAME 20 mg/kg, i.p.), a non-selective inhibitor of nitric oxide synthase (NOS). After 1 h, animals were treated, by gavage, with saline (0.2 mL) or Cm-SP (200 mg/kg), and 1 h after the treatment gastric damage was induced by the administration of ethanol absolute (0.2 mL, p.o.). All of the mice were euthanized 1 h after the administration ethanol, and their stomachs were immediately removed and opened via an incision along the greater curvature.

Gastric damage (hemorrhagic or ulcerative lesions) was measured using a computer planimetry program (ImageJ, National Institute of Health, Bethesda, MD, USA). A sample of the corpus region of each stomach was fixed in 10% formalin immediately after removal for subsequent histological assessment. Further, gastric corpus samples were also weighed, frozen, and stored at -80 °C until they were used to determine glutathione (GSH), NO, and malondialdehyde (MDA) levels.

4.4. Histological Assessment

Fixed samples of the stomach were dehydrated by increasing concentrations of ethanol and processed for inclusion in paraffin, sliced in 5-μm-thick sections, stained with hematoxylin–eosin (H&E), and then examined under a light microscope by an experienced pathologist. Specimens were evaluated according to Laine and Weinstein [38]. In summary, a 1-cm length of each histological section was assessed for hemorrhagic lesion (a score of 0 to 4), oedema of submucosa (a score of 0 to 4), erosion with loss of epithelial cell architecture (a score of 0 to 3), and presence of inflammatory cells (a score of 0 to 3), with 14 being the maximum score.

4.5. Determination of GSH Level

GSH levels in the gastric tissue were measured using the method described by Sedlak and Lindsay [39]. Part of the stomach was used to prepare 10% homogenates (w/v). Then, the samples were precipitated with 50% trichloroethanoic acid and were centrifuged at $1000 \times g$ for 5 min. The reaction mixture contained 0.5 mL of supernatant, 2.0 mL of Tris-EDTA buffer (0.2 M, pH 8.9), and 0.1 mL of 10 mM dithiobis (2-nitrobenzoic acid). The solution was kept at room temperature for 5 min, and the absorbance was then read at 412 nm. The results were expressed as micrograms of GSH per gram of tissue (μg/g).

4.6. Determination of MDA Level

Lipid peroxidation was estimated by the measurement of the concentration of MDA in the homogenate from each gastric sample according to Draper and Hadley [40], which is based on a reaction with thiobarbituric acid. Samples were mixed with 1 mL of 10% trichloroacetic acid and 1 mL of 0.6% thiobarbituric acid. The reaction medium was heated in a boiling water bath for 15 min, and then n-butanol (2:1 v/v) was added. After centrifugation ($800 \times g$, 5 min), thiobarbituric acid reactive substances (TBARS) contents were determined at 535 nm. MDA concentrations were expressed as micromoles per gram of tissue (μmol/g).

4.7. Determination of NO_2/NO_3 Level

NO level in the gastric mucosa was evaluated as total NO_2/NO_3 levels, as described by Souza [14]. Part of the stomach was used to prepare 10% homogenates (w/v). After centrifugation ($800 \times g$, 10 min), supernatants were collected, and the NO_2/NO_3 production was determined by the Griess reaction [41]. Briefly, 100 μL of the supernatant was incubated with 100 μL of the Griess reagent [1% sulphanilamide in

1% H_3PO_4/0.1% N-(1-naphthyl)-ethylenediaminedihydrochloride/1% H_3PO_4/distilled water (1:1:1:1)] at room temperature for 10 min. The absorbance was measured at 550 nm. The NO_2/NO_3 concentration (μM) was determined using $NaNO_2$/NO_3 as standard. The results were expressed as micromols of NO_2/NO_3 per gram of tissue (μmol/g).

4.8. Statistical Analyses

All data were analyzed using the program GraphPad Prism 7 (GraphPad Software Inc., La Jolla, CA, USA). Differences between means were determined by One-Way Analysis of Variance (ANOVA) and Newman-Keuls test or Kruskal-Wallis test, when appropriate. All data were presented as the means $\pm$ standard errors (SEM). Values of $p < 0.05$ were considered to be statistically significant.

Acknowledgments: This research was supported by Conselho Nacional de Desenvolvimento Científico e Tecnológico–CNPq, Coordenação de Aperfeiçoamento de Pessoal de Nível Superior–CAPES, Fundação Cearense de Apoio ao Desenvolvimento Científico e Tecnológico–FUNCAP, Rede Nordeste de Biotecnologia–RENORBIO and Instituto Federal de Educação, Ciência e Tecnologia do Ceará–IFCE. We thank Microscopy and Image Processing Core (NEMPI) at Federal University of Ceará and Biotechnology Laboratory of IFCE-Campus Sobral. N.M.B. Benevides is a senior investigator of CNPq/Brazil.

Author Contributions: J.G.C., A.F.F. and N.M.B.B. conceived and designed the experiments; J.G.C., T.d.B.L.H., A.F.F., A.L.G.Q., V.V.M.S., R.S.d.S., M.A.C. and D.S.M. performed the experiments; J.G.C., T.d.B.L.H., A.L.G.Q., M.A.C., D.S.M., A.S.G.D. and N.M.B.B. analyzed the data; J.G.C., T.d.B.L.H., A.L.G.Q. and N.M.B.B. wrote the paper.

Conflicts of Interest: The authors declare no conflict of interest.

References

1.   Amandeep, K.; Robin, S.; Ramica, S.; Sunil, K. Peptic ulcer: A review on etiology and pathogenesis. *Int. Res. J. Pharm.* **2012**, *3*, 34–38.

2.   Kwiecien, S.; Brzozowski, T.; Konturek, S.J. Effects of reactive oxygen species action on gastric mucosa in various models of mucosal injury. *J. Physiol. Pharmacol.* **2002**, *53*, 39–50. [PubMed]

3.   Nayeb-Hashemia, H.; Kaunitz, J.D. Gastroduodenal mucosal defense. *Curr. Opin. Gastroenterol.* **2009**, *25*, 537–543. [CrossRef] [PubMed]

4.   Takeuchi, K. Gastric cytoprotection by prostaglandin E2 and prostacyclin: Relationship to EP1 and IP receptors. *J. Physiol. Pharmacol.* **2014**, *65*, 3–14. [PubMed]

5.   Szabo, S. Gastric cytoprotection is still relevant. *J. Gastroenterol. Hepatol.* **2014**, *29*, 124–132. [CrossRef] [PubMed]

6.   Bhattacharyya, A.; Chattopadhyay, R.; Mitra, S.; Crowe, S.E. Oxidative stress: An essential factor in the pathogenesis of gastrointestinal mucosal diseases. *Physiol. Rev.* **2014**, *94*, 329–354. [CrossRef] [PubMed]

7.   Peskar, B.M. Role of cyclooxygenase isoforms in gastric mucosal defence. *J. Physiol.* **2001**, *95*, 3–9. [CrossRef]

8.   Wijesinghe, W.A.J.P.; Jeon, Y.-J. Biological activities and potential industrial applications of fucose rich sulfated polysaccharides and fucoidans isolated from brown seaweeds: A review. *Carbohydr. Polym.* **2012**, *88*, 13–20. [CrossRef]

9.   Sun, H.; Mao, W.; Fang, F.; Li, H. Polysaccharides from marine green seaweed Ulva species and their characteristics. *Agro Food Ind. Hi Tech* **2007**, *18*, 28–29.

10. Carneiro, J.G.; Rodrigues, J.A.G.; Teles, F.B.; Cavalcante, A.B.D.; Benevides, N.M.B. Analysis of some chemical nutrients in four Brazilian tropical seaweeds. *Acta Sci. Biol. Sci.* **2014**, *36*, 137–145. [CrossRef]

11. Wijesinghe, W.A.J.P.; Jeon, Y.-J. Biological activities and potential cosmeceutical applications of bioactive components from brown seaweeds: A review. *Phytochem. Rev.* **2011**, *10*, 431–443. [CrossRef]

12. Rodrigues, J.A.G.; Vanderlei, E.D.S.O.; Quinderé, A.L.G.; Fontes, B.P.; Queiroz, I.N.L.de.; Benevides, N.M.B. Extraction and anticoagulant activity of sulfated polysaccharides from Caulerpa cupressoides var. lycopodium (Vahl) C. Agardh (Chlorophyceae). *Acta Sci. BioLog. Sci.* **2011**, *33*, 133–140.

13. Quinderé, A.L.G.; Santos, G.R.C.; Oliveira, S.N.M.C.G.; Glauser, B.F.; Fontes, B.P.; Queiroz, I.N.L.; Benevides, N.M.; Pomin, V.H.; Mourão, P.A. Is the antithrombotic effect of sulfated galactans independent of serpin? *J. Thromb. Haemost.* **2014**, *12*, 43–53. [CrossRef] [PubMed]

14. Souza, R.B.; Frota, A.F.; Sousa, R.S.; Cezario, N.A.; Santos, T.B.; Souza, L.M.F.; Coura, C.O.; Monteiro, V.S.; Cristino Filho, G.; Vasconcelos, S.M.; et al. Neuroprotective effects of sulphated agaran from marine alga gracilaria cornea in rat 6-hydroxydopamine parkinson's disease model: Behavioural, neurochemical and transcriptional alterations. *Basic Clin. Pharmacol. Toxicol.* **2017**, *120*, 159–170. [CrossRef] [PubMed]

15. Coura, C.O.; de Araújo, I.W.F.; Vanderlei, E.S.O.; Rodrigues, J.A.G.; Quinderé, A.L.G.; Fontes, B.P.; de Queiroz, I.N.L.; de Menezes, D.B.; Bezerra, M.M.; e Silva, A.A.R.; et al. Antinociceptive and anti-inflammatory activities of sulphated polysaccharides from the red seaweed gracilaria cornea. *Basic Clin. Pharmacol. Toxicol.* **2011**, *110*, 335–341. [CrossRef] [PubMed]

16. Rodrigues, J.A.G.; Vanderlei, E.S.; Silva, L.M.; de Araújo, I.W.F.; de Queiroz, I.N.L.; de Paula, G.A.; Abreu, T.M.; Ribeiro, N.A.; Bezerra, M.M.; Chaves, H.V.; et al. Antinociceptive and anti-inflammatory activities of a sulfated polysaccharide isolated from the green seaweed Caulerpa cupressoides. *Pharmacol. Rep.* **2012**, *64*, 282–292. [CrossRef]

17. Ribeiro, N.A.; Abreu, T.M.; Chaves, H.V.; Bezerra, M.M.; Monteiro, H.S.A.; Jorge, R.J.B.; Benevides, N.M.B. Sulfated polysaccharides isolated from the green seaweed Caulerpa racemosa plays antinociceptive and anti-inflammatory activities in a way dependent on HO-1 pathway activation. *Inflamm. Res.* **2014**, *63*, 569–580. [CrossRef] [PubMed]

18. Carneiro, J.G.; Rodrigues, J.A.G.; de Sousa Oliveira Vanderlei, E.; Souza, R.B.; Quinderé, A.L.G.; Coura, C.O.; de Araújo, I.W.F.; Chaves, H.V.; Bezerra, M.M.; Benevides, N.M.B. Peripheral antinociception and anti-inflammatory effects of sulphated polysaccharides from the alga caulerpa mexicana. *Basic Clin. Pharmacol. Toxicol.* **2014**, *115*, 335–342. [CrossRef] [PubMed]

19. Bitencourt, M.A.O.; Silva, H.M.D.; Abílio, G.M.F.; Miranda, G.E.C.; Moura, A.M.A.; de Araújo-Júnior, J.X.; Silveira, E.J.D.; Santos, B.V.O.; Souto, J.T. Anti-inflammatory effects of methanolic extract of green algae Caulerpa mexicana in a murine model of ulcerative colitis. *Rev. Bras. Farm.* **2015**, *25*, 677–682. [CrossRef]

20. Gomes, A.S.; Gadelha, G.G.; Lima, S.J.; Garcia, J.A.; Medeiros, J.V.R.; Havt, A.; Lima, A.A.; Ribeiro, R.A.; Brito, G.A.C.; Cunha, F.Q.; et al. Gastroprotective effect of heme-oxygenase 1/biliverdin/CO pathway in ethanol-induced gastric damage in mice. *Eur. J. Pharmacol.* **2010**, *642*, 140–145. [CrossRef] [PubMed]

21. Barrachina, M.D.; Panés, J.; Esplugues, J.V. Role of nitric oxide in gastrointestinal inflammatory and ulcerative diseases: Perspective for drugs development. *Curr. Pharm. Des.* **2001**, *7*, 31–48. [CrossRef] [PubMed]

22. Tarnawski, A.; Ahluwalia, A.K.; Jones, M. Gastric cytoprotection beyond prostaglandins: Cellular and molecular mechanisms of gastroprotective and ulcer healing actions of antacids. *Curr. Pharm. Des.* **2012**, *19*, 126–132.

23. Kwiecien, S.; Jasnos, K.; Magierowski, M.; Sliwowski, Z.; Pajdo, R.; Brzozowski, B.; Mach, T.; Wojcik, D.; Brzozowski, T. Lipid peroxidation, reactive oxygen species and antioxidative factors in the pathogenesis of gastric mucosal lesions and mechanism of protection against oxidative stress-induced gastric injury. *J. Physiol. Pharmacol.* **2014**, *65*, 613–622. [PubMed]

24. Mohamed, S.; Hashim, S.N.; Rahman, H.A. Seaweeds: A sustainable functional food for complementary and alternative therapy. *Trends Food Sci. Technol.* **2012**, *23*, 83–96. [CrossRef]

25. Damasceno, S.R.B.; Rodrigues, J.C.; Silva, R.O.; Nicolau, L.A.D.; Chaves, L.S.; Freitas, A.L.P.; Souza, M.H.L.P.; Barbosa, A.L.R.; Medeiros, J.-V.R. Role of the NO/KATP pathway in the protective effect of a sulfated-polysaccharide fraction from the algae Hypnea musciformis against ethanol-induced gastric damage in mice. *Rev. Bras. Farm.* **2013**, *23*, 320–328. [CrossRef]

26. Silva, R.O.; Santos, G.M.P.D.; Nicolau, L.A.D.; Lucetti, L.T.; Santana, A.P.M.; Chaves, L.D.S.; Barros, F.C.N.; Freitas, A.L.P.; Medeiros, J. V. R. Sulfated-Polysaccharide fraction from red algae gracilaria caudata protects mice gut against ethanol-induced damage. *Mar Drugs.* **2011**, *9*, 2188–2200. [CrossRef] [PubMed]

27. Hwang, H.-J.; Kwon, M.-J.; Kim, I.-H.; Nam, T.-J. The effect of polysaccharide extracted from the marine alga capsosiphon fulvescens on ethanol administration. *Food Chem. Toxicol.* **2008**, *46*, 2653–2657. [CrossRef] [PubMed]

28. Choi, E.-Y.; Hwang, H.-J.; Kim, I.-H.; Nam, T.-J. Protective effects of a polysaccharide from Hizikia fusiformis against ethanol toxicity in rats. *Food Chem. Toxicol.* **2009**, *47*, 134–139. [CrossRef] [PubMed]

29. Takeuchi, K.; Hase, S.; Takeeda, M.; Nakashima, M.; Yokota, A. Prostaglandin EP receptor subtypes and gastric cytoprotection. *InflammoPharmacology* **2002**, *10*, 303–312. [CrossRef]

30. Brzozowski, T.; Konturek, P.C.; Konturek, S.J.; Brzozowska, I.; Pawlik, T. Role of prostaglandins in gastroprotection and gastric adaptation. *J. Physiol. Pharmacol.* **2005**, *56*, 33–55. [PubMed]

31. Wiley, J.W. The many faces of nitric oxide: Cytotoxic, cytoprotective or both. *Neurogastroenterol. Motil.* **2007**, *19*, 541–544. [CrossRef] [PubMed]

32. Magierowska, K.; Magierowski, M.; Surmiak, M.; Adamski, J.; Mazur-Bialy, A.; Pajdo, R.; Sliwowski, Z.; Kwiecien, S.; Brzozowski, T. The protective role of carbon monoxide (CO) produced by heme oxygenases and derived from the CO-releasing molecule CORM-2 in the pathogenesis of stress-induced gastric lesions: Evidence for non-involvement of nitric oxide (NO). *Int. J. Mol. Sci.* **2016**, *17*, 442. [CrossRef] [PubMed]

33. Magierowska, K.; Magierowski, M.; Hubalewska-Mazgaj, M.; Adamski, J.; Surmiak, M.; Sliwowski, Z.; Kwiecien, S.; Brzozowski, T. Carbon monoxide (CO) released from tricarbonyldichlororuthenium (II) dimer (CORM-2) in gastroprotection against experimental ethanol-induced gastric damage. *PLoS ONE* **2015**, *10*, e0140493. [CrossRef] [PubMed]

34. Hernández-Muñoz, R.; Montiel-Ruíz, C.; Vázquez-Martínez, O. Gastric mucosal cell proliferation in ethanol-induced chronic mucosal injury is related to oxidative stress and lipid peroxidation in rats. *Lab. Investig.* **2000**, *80*, 1161–1169. [CrossRef] [PubMed]

35. Kalayci, M.; Kocdor, M.A.; Kuloglu, T.; Sahin, I.; Sarac, M.; Aksoy, A.; Yardim, M.; Dalkilic, S.; Gursu, O.; Aydin, S.; et al. Comparison of the therapeutic effects of sildenafil citrate, heparin and neuropeptides in a rat model of acetic acid-induced gastric ulcer. *Life Sci.* **2017**, *186*, 102–110. [CrossRef] [PubMed]

36. Brzozowski, T.; Magierowska, K.; Magierowski, M.; Ptak-Belowska, A.; Pajdo, R.; Kwiecien, S.; Olszanecki, R.; Korbut, R. Recent advances in the gastric mucosal protection against stress-induced gastric lesions. Importance of renin-angiotensin vasoactive metabolites, gaseous mediators and appetite peptides. *Curr. Pharm. Des.* **2017**, *23*, 1.

37. Farias, W.R.L.; Valente, A.-P.; Pereira, M.S.; Mourao, P.A.S. Structure and anticoagulant activity of sulfated galactans: Isolation of a unique sulfated galactan from the red algaebotryocladia occidentalis and comparison of its anticoagulant action with that of sulfated galactans from invertebrates. *J. BioLog. Chem.* **2000**, *275*, 29299–29307. [CrossRef] [PubMed]

38. Laine, L.; Weinstein, W.M. Histology of alcoholic hemorrhagic gastritis: A prospective evaluation. *Gastroenterology* **1988**, *94*, 1254–1262. [CrossRef]

39. Sedlak, J.; Lindsay, R.H. Estimation of total, protein-bound, and nonprotein sulfhydryl groups in tissue with Ellman's reagent. *Anal. Biochem.* **1968**, *25*, 192–205. [CrossRef]

40. Draper, H.H.; Hadley, M. Malondialdehyde determination as index of lipid Peroxidation. *Methods Enzymol.* **1990**, *186*, 421–431. [PubMed]

41. Green, L.C.; Tannenbaum, S.R.; Goldman, P. Nitrate synthesis in the germfree and conventional rat. *Science* **1981**, *212*, 56. [CrossRef] [PubMed]

2

Bacterial Lipopolysaccharide Increases Serotonin Metabolism in Both Medial Prefrontal Cortex and Nucleus Accumbens in Male Wild Type Rats, but Not in Serotonin Transporter Knockout Rats

Gerdien A. H. Korte-Bouws [1,*], Floor van Heesch [1], Koen G. C. Westphal [1], Lisa M. J. Ankersmit [1], Edwin M. van Oosten [1], Onur Güntürkün [2] and S. Mechiel Korte [1,2] 🆔

[1] Division of Pharmacology, Utrecht Institute for Pharmaceutical Sciences (UIPS), Utrecht University, Faculty of Science, Universiteitsweg 99, 3584 CG Utrecht, The Netherlands; floorvheesch@hotmail.com (F.v.H.); K.G.C.Westphal@uu.nl (K.G.C.W.); l.m.j.ankersmit@students.uu.nl (L.M.J.A.); e.m.vanoosten@students.uu.nl (E.M.v.O.); s.m.korte@uu.nl (S.M.K.)

[2] Department of Biopsychology, Faculty of Psychology, Ruhr-Universität Bochum, Universitätsstraße 150, D-44780 Bochum, Germany; onur.guentuerkuen@ruhr-uni-bochum.de

* Correspondence: g.a.h.korte@uu.nl

Abstract: It is well known that bacterial lipopolysaccharides (LPS) both increases proinflammatory cytokines and produces sickness behavior, including fatigue and anhedonia (i.e., the inability to experience pleasure). Previously, we have shown that intraperitoneally (i.p.) administered LPS increased extracellular monoamine metabolite levels in the nucleus accumbens (NAc) and medial prefrontal cortex (mPFC), which was completely, or at least partly, prevented by pretreatment with a triple reuptake inhibitor that also blocks the serotonin (5-HT) transporter (SERT). This suggests indirectly, that LPS may enhance SERT transporter activity, and consequently, increase removal of 5-HT from the synaptic cleft, and increase metabolism of 5-HT. In the present study, we focus more specifically on the role of SERT in this increased metabolism by using rats, that differ in SERT expression. Therefore, the effects of an intraperitoneal LPS injection on extracellular concentrations of 5-HT and its metabolite 5-hydroxyindoleacetic acid (5-HIAA) were investigated by in vivo microdialysis in the NAc and mPFC of wild type (SERT$^{+/+}$), heterozygous (SERT$^{+/-}$) and knockout (SERT$^{-/-}$) rats. Here, we show that LPS-induced 5-HIAA formation in male rats, is significantly increased in SERT$^{+/+}$ rats in both the NAc and mPFC, whereas this increase is partly or totally abolished in SERT$^{+/-}$ and SERT$^{-/-}$ rats, respectively. Thus, the present study supports the hypothesis that systemic LPS in male rats increases SERT function and consequently enhances 5-HT uptake and metabolism in both the NAc and mPFC.

Keywords: lipopolysaccharide; proinflammatory cytokines; serotonin transporter; Slc6a41; metabolism; microdialysis; medial prefrontal cortex; nucleus accumbens

---

1. Introduction

An increasing amount of evidence suggests that alterations in proinflammatory cytokines play an important role in major depression, particularly in depression due to a medical condition [1–4]. For example, patients with chronic inflammatory diseases, such as rheumatoid arthritis, inflammatory bowel disease or psoriasis, have an increased risk of developing sickness behavior, which has a large overlap with depression-like symptoms, such as fatigue, disturbed cognition and anhedonia [5–8].

Anhedonia, i.e., the inability to experience pleasure, is a core symptom of major depression that can be assessed in rodents with the intracranial self-stimulation procedure [9]. Previously, it has been reported that systemic bacterial lipopolysaccharides (LPS) strongly activates the immune system to release proinflammatory cytokines, that induces anhedonia in rats [10–12]. Interestingly, previously we have shown that LPS-induced anhedonia is not observed in serotonin (5-HT) transporter knockout (SERT$^{-/-}$) rats, while LPS-induced anhedonia was decreased in heterozygous rats (SERT$^{+/-}$) compared to wild type animals (SERT$^{+/+}$) [11]. As was previously reported, SERT is completely absent in SERT knockout rats, while heterozygous rats have been shown to have 48–80% SERT activity compared to wild type animals [13]. This indirectly suggests that absence of SERT protects the animals from LPS-induced anhedonia.

The exact mechanism why SERT knockout rats are not susceptible to LPS-induced anhedonia is still unknown. However, since selective serotonin reuptake inhibitors (SSRIs) are expected to alleviate depression by increasing 5-HT availability through inhibition of SERT, differences in 5-HT availability could be responsible for the resistance to LPS-induced anhedonia in SERT knockout rats [14].

Previously, we have shown that i.p. administered LPS increased extracellular 5-HT metabolite (5-HIAA) levels in the nucleus accumbens (NAc) and medial prefrontal cortex (mPFC), which was, completely or at least partly, prevented by pre-treatment with the reuptake inhibitor DOV 216,303, that also blocks SERT. This suggests indirectly, that LPS-induced increased SERT activity does not only lead to increasing removal of 5-HT from the synaptic cleft, but it consequently also leads to increase metabolism of 5-HT.

Therefore, specifically the role of SERT was examined by using heterozygous and knockout SERT male rats. In the present microdialysis experiments, systemic LPS was administered to study serotonergic metabolism (i.e., breakdown of 5-HT to 5-HIAA) in the NAc and mPFC of SERT$^{+/-}$, and $^{SERT-/-}$ male rats in comparison to SERT$^{+/+}$ male rats.

2. Results

2.1. Microdialysis

2.1.1. The Effect of Peripheral LPS on 5-HT and 5-HIAA Levels in the NAc and mPFC of Wild Type Rats and SERT (Partial and Total) Knockout Rats

LPS did not produce significant overall effects on 5-HT levels in the NAc and mPFC of SERT$^{+/+}$ (Figures 1a and 2a, respectively), SERT$^{+/-}$ rats (Figures 1b and 2b, respectively) and SERT$^{-/-}$ rats (Figures 1c and 2c, respectively). Neither did post hoc analyses reveal a significant difference at any time point.

For the serotonergic metabolite 5-HIAA in the NAc of SERT$^{+/+}$ rats, however, significant LPS effects were found, as indicated by a significant time × treatment interaction: $F(1.8,20.0) = 6.0$, $p = 0.011$, $\varepsilon = 0.260$ (Figure 1d), while the overall LPS treatment effect was almost significant: $F(1.0,11) = 4.8$, $p = 0.051$, $\varepsilon = 0.260$. Post hoc t-tests showed that accumbal 5-HIAA levels increased significantly at 150 min, 180 min and 210 min after exposure to LPS (Figure 1d).

LPS also increased 5-HIAA levels in the mPFC of SERT$^{+/+}$ rats, as indicated by an overall treatment effect: $F(1.0,12) = 6.2$, $p = 0.029$, $\varepsilon = 0.281$, together with a time × treatment interaction: $F(2.0,23.6) = 6.3$, $p = 0.007$, $\varepsilon = 0.281$ (Figure 2d). Post hoc t-tests showed that 5-HIAA levels in the mPFC were significantly increased at 120 min, 150 min, 180 min, 210 min and 240 min after exposure to LPS (Figure 2d). LPS induced a significant small increase in 5-HIAA levels in mPFC of SERT$^{+/-}$ rats, as indicated by a significant time × treatment interaction ($F(3.0,39.3) = 5.7$, $p = 0.002$, $\varepsilon = 0.432$ (Figure 2e)), although there was no overall LPS treatment effect. Post hoc analysis revealed that 5-HIAA levels in the mPFC were significantly increased at 240 min after exposure to LPS. In contrast, LPS did not significantly affect 5-HIAA levels in SERT$^{-/-}$ rats at any time point, neither in the mPFC nor in the NAc. As a consequence, neither time × treatment interactions in the NAc (Figure 1f) and in the mPFC were found (Figure 2f), nor a significant effect at any time point.

Microdialysis in NAc

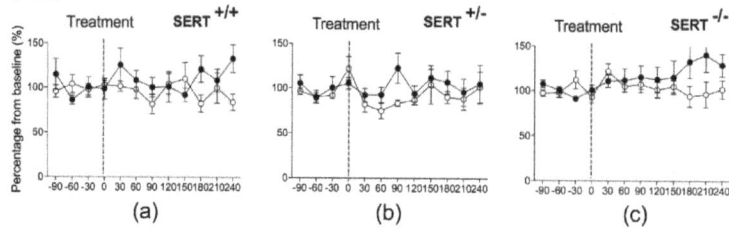

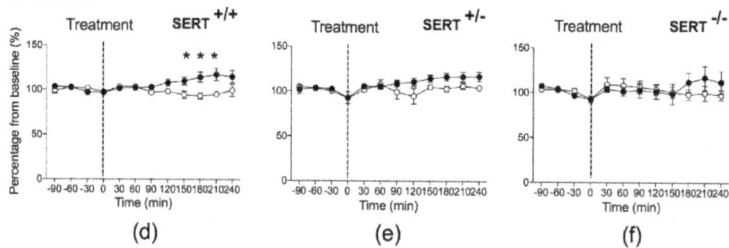

Figure 1. Microdialysis in the Nucleus Accumbens (NAc). At $t = 0$ min, rats received Saline or lipopolysaccharides (LPS). Graph represents percentage from baseline (%) of 5-HT and 5-HIAA from each time point (min). Animals (n) per group were as follows: $n = 6$ for Saline-SERT$^{+/+}$ rats (**a,d**) and $n = 7$ for LPS-SERT$^{+/+}$ rats (**a,d**); $n = 3$ for Saline-SERT$^{+/-}$ rats (**b,e**) and $n = 7$ for LPS-SERT$^{+/-}$ rats (**b,e**); $n = 5$ for Saline-SERT$^{-/-}$ rats (**c,f**) and $n = 5$ for LPS-SERT$^{-/-}$ rats (**c,f**). Significance: * $p < 0.05$.

Microdialysis in mPFC

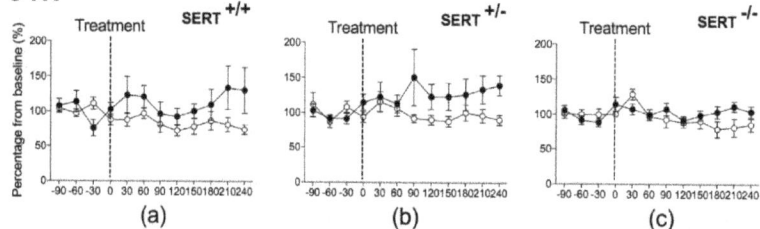

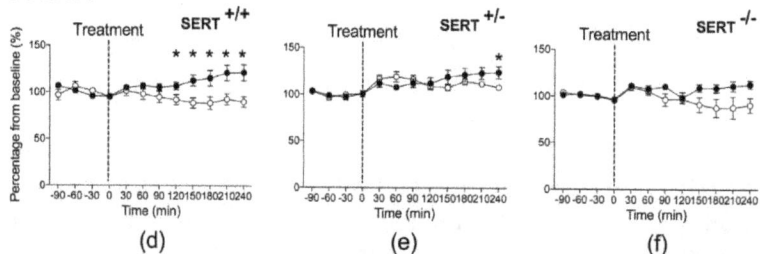

Figure 2. Microdialysis in the medial Prefrontal Cortex (mPFC). At $t = 0$ min, rats received Saline or LPS. Graph represents percentage from baseline (%) of 5-HT and 5-HIAA from each time point (min). Animals (n) per group were as follows: $n = 7$ for Saline-SERT$^{+/+}$ rats (**a,d**) and $n = 7$ for LPS-SERT$^{+/+}$ rats (**a,d**); $n = 7$ for Saline-SERT$^{+/-}$ rats (**b,e**) and $n = 8$ for LPS-SERT$^{+/-}$ rats (**b,e**); $n = 8$ for Saline-SERT$^{-/-}$ rats (**c,f**) and $n = 7$ for LPS-SERT$^{-/-}$ rats (**c,f**). Significance: * $p < 0.05$.

2.1.2. Baseline 5-HT and 5-HIAA Levels in the NAc and mPFC of Wild Type Rats and SERT (Partial and Total) Knockout Rats

Under the baseline conditions, 5-HT levels in the NAc, as well as in the mPFC, were significantly higher in SERT$^{-/-}$ rats compared to SERT$^{+/+}$ (NAc: $p < 0.001$ and mPFC: $p < 0.001$) and SERT$^{+/-}$ rats (NAc: $p < 0.001$ and mPFC: $p < 0.001$) (see Table 1). Remarkably, SERT$^{+/+}$ and SERT$^{+/-}$ rats did not differ from each other in respect to extracellular 5-HT levels in both brain areas. Also, extracellular 5-HIAA levels differed significantly between genotypes in both brain structures. As expected, in the NAc as well as in the mPFC, SERT$^{-/-}$ rats had significantly lower extracellular 5-HIAA levels as compared to SERT$^{+/+}$ (NAc: $p < 0.001$ and mPFC: $p < 0.001$) and SERT$^{+/-}$ rats (NAc: $p = 0.008$ and mPFC: $p < 0.001$). Furthermore, extracellular 5-HIAA level of SERT$^{+/-}$ rats was significantly lower than 5-HIAA levels of SERT$^{+/+}$ rats in both brain areas (NAc: $p = 0.016$ and mPFC: $p = 0.001$).

Table 1. Baseline levels of 5-HT and 5-HIAA (nM) in the NAc and mPFC. The groups SERT$^{-/-}$ and SERT$^{-/+}$ were compared to SERT$^{+/+}$. Significance is described as * $p < 0.05$ and ** $p < 0.01$.

Brain Area	Genotype	5-HT (nM)	5-HIAA (nM)
NAc	SERT$^{+/+}$	0.11	154.25
	SERT$^{+/-}$	0.15	122.51 *
	SERT$^{-/-}$	0.64 **	86.375 **
mPFC	SERT$^{+/+}$	0.16	65.67
	SERT$^{+/-}$	0.22	51.34 **
	SERT$^{-/-}$	0.71 **	34.91 **

3. Discussion

The present microdialysis study shows that LPS-induced 5-HT metabolism (i.e., 5-HIAA formation) is significantly increased in both the NAc and mPFC of homozygous (SERT$^{+/+}$) male rats, whereas this increase is partly or completely abolished in heterozygous (SERT$^{+/-}$) or knockout (SERT$^{-/-}$) male rats, respectively. These results support the hypothesis that systemic LPS administration increases SERT activity in CNS of male rats (possibly in neurons and/or astrocytes located in raphe nuclei, NAc or mPFC).

3.1. LPS Increases SERT Activity in Both NAc and mPFC

The observed LPS-induced increase in extracellular 5-HIAA levels in the mPFC and NAc of normal (SERT$^{+/+}$) rats is in agreement with in vitro, ex vivo and in vivo studies, showing that LPS increases SERT activity in neurons and thereby the reuptake of 5-HT, enabling more metabolism of 5-HT into 5-HIAA [10,15–24]. The partly or completely abolished LPS-induced increase in 5-HIAA in heterozygous (SERT$^{+/-}$) or knockout (SERT$^{-/-}$) rats, suggests a specific role of SERT in this process.

The somewhat larger effect of LPS on serotonergic activity in the mPFC may be explained by the fact that the mPFC is highly innervated by 5-HT neurons, whereas the NAc is not [25].

Previously, different research groups reported that LPS treatment increased both 5-HT release and 5-HIAA levels in hippocampus [26–28] and preoptic area, whereas only 5-HIAA was increased in the NAc [28]. In the present study, LPS did not significantly increase 5-HT in mPFC or NAc in male SERT$^{+/+}$. Whether this is a discrepancy to these previous studies, or because it is the consequence of the measurement of 5-HT in different brain areas, needs more investigation.

The present data support the hypothesis that LPS enhances SERT activity, and thereby the reuptake of 5-HT. However, this is not reflected in a decrease of extracellular 5-HT concentrations below its baseline. Since SERT activity is neurotransmitter concentration dependent, it could be speculated that there is less reuptake of 5-HT when extracellular concentrations are below a certain baseline concentration. However, it is speculated, in contrast to acute infection, that chronic inflammation due to a lower set point is able to shift the baseline to lower concentrations. Therefore, at this moment, we are studying the effects of SERT activity and 5-HT reuptake in an animal model of chronic inflammation.

3.2. Underlying Mechanisms of Increased SERT Activity

It is a known fact that LPS binds to toll-like receptor 4 (TLR4) on macrophages, astrocytes, and microglia to produce proinflammatory cytokines, such as IL-1, IL-6 and TNF-α [12,29,30]. It has been demonstrated that both LPS and proinflammatory cytokines increase monoamine transporter trafficking and function [16,24,31–33] (see Figure 3). There is growing body of evidence that this process is p38 MAPK-dependent [16,17,34–37]. Although, also other mechanisms than p38 MAPK have been proposed in the PFC [24]. In addition, other kinases may be associated with SERT regulation, such as Protein Kinase C, ERK1/2, phosphatidylinositol 3-Kinase/Akt and adenosine [31,34,38].

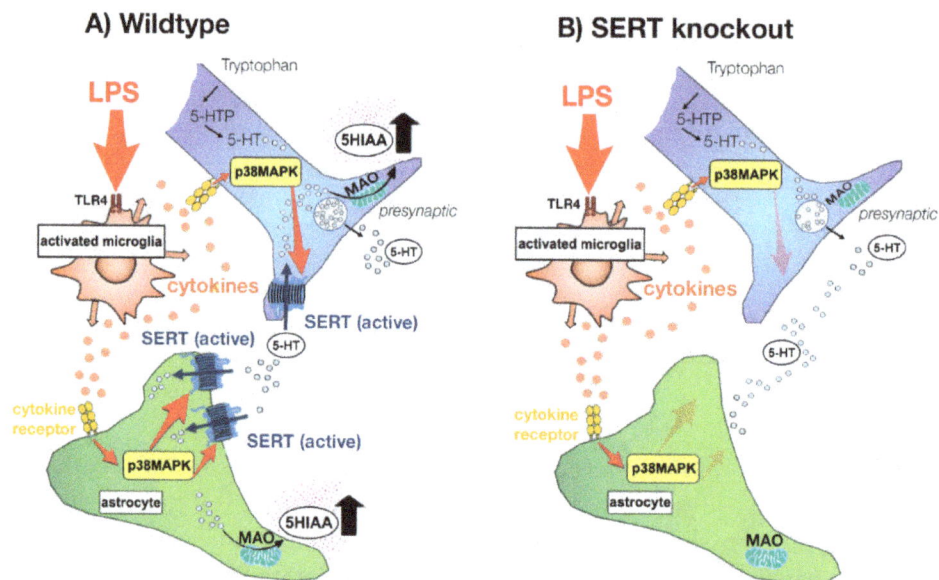

Figure 3. Model of regulation of serotonin (5-HT) transporter (SERT) activity after LPS challenge in SERT Wildtype (SERT$^{+/+}$) rats and SERT Knockout (SERT$^{-/-}$) rats. LPS via the binding to toll-like receptor 4 (TLR-4) on microglia produce its' activation and consequently increase in the release of pro-inflammatory cytokines (e.g., IL-1, IL-6 and TNF-α). This increase in pro-inflammatory cytokines enhance SERT activity in neurons, as well as increase SERT gene expression in astrocytes. Both processes may be mediated by p38 MAPK-dependent pathways, despite the fact that also independent pathways have been suggested. After reuptake by SERT, 5-HT is packed in storage vesicles or metabolized by monoamine oxidase (MAO). In serotonergic neurons and astrocytes, MAO metabolizes 5-HT to 5-hydroxyindole acetaldehyde and thereafter aldehyde dehydrogenase rapidly metabolizes 5-hydroxyindole acetaldehyde to 5-hydroxyindolacetic acid (5-HIAA). Thereafter, 5-HIAA diffuses outside the cells. Thus, SERT plays, besides controlling the length of the cellular actions of 5-HT, an important role in the formation of its' metabolite 5-HIAA. As a consequence, LPS-induced SERT activity results in enhanced 5-HT uptake into astrocytes and neurons and thereby promote 5-HT degradation to 5-HIAA in wildtype animals (**A**). Since SERT does not come to expression in SERT knockout animals, LPS cannot increase SERT activity and associated 5-HT metabolism in these animals (**B**), indicating that the SERT is involved in LPS-induced enhancement of 5-HT metabolism in male rats. (Figure adapted after Haase and Brown, 2015 [33]).

3.3. Baseline Differences in 5-HT and 5-HIAA Levels

Under baseline conditions (see Table 1), we and others have found that extracellular 5-HT levels are significantly increased in hippocampus, NAc and mPFC of SERT$^{-/-}$ rats compared to SERT$^{+/+}$ and/or SERT$^{+/-}$ rats and mice [13,39,40], whereas extracellular levels of 5-HIAA are significantly decreased [34]. These results can be explained by the fact that due to the absence of 5-HT transporters in SERT$^{-/-}$ rats, there is no reuptake of 5-HT into the serotonergic neuron, and consequently no breakdown of 5-HT into 5-HIAA by MAO (monoamine oxidase). This explains why SERT$^{-/-}$ rats have lower 5-HIAA levels and higher levels of 5-HT in the extracellular space.

Although SERT activity is completely absent in SERT$^{-/-}$ rats, limited formation of 5-HIAA is still present, possibly because alternative routes can lead to reuptake of 5-HT and corresponding 5-HIAA formation as well. Indeed, it has been demonstrated that the maximum rate (Vmax) of 5-HT uptake in the hippocampus is reduced by 13.4% in SERT$^{+/-}$ rats and by 72.2% in SERT$^{-/-}$ rats [13]. Interestingly, inhibition of noradrenaline transporters (NET), but not dopamine transporters (DAT), attenuated the reuptake of the remaining 5-HT in the hippocampus of SERT$^{-/-}$ rats [13,38]. Furthermore, dopaminergic neurons in the ventral tegmental area and substantia nigra have been shown to take up 5-HT by DAT in SERT$^{-/-}$ mice [41]. Moreover, it has been demonstrated that NET and DAT concentrations were not different from genotypes throughout the brain [13].

Previously, it has been shown that SERT wild type male rats and SERT knockout male rats do not differ in tryptophan levels, tryptophan (TRP)/total long neutral amino acids ($\sum$LNAA) ratios, tryptophan hydroxylase activity and MAO-A activity [13,42]. In addition, in mice, baseline tryptophan levels were not different between SERT wild type and SERT knockout animals, but tryptophan levels were shown to be higher in female mice as compared to male mice [23]. Furthermore, it has been shown that LPS treatment caused an increase in brain tryptophan levels [22]. In addition, serotonin synthesis is increased in SERT knockout mice, in particular in females [23].

Because the NAc is a smaller brain region than the mPFC in which to insert a microdialysis probe, a probe length of 2 mm was used in the NAc, in contrast to a 3 mm probe length in the mPFC. This may partly explain the higher baseline neurotransmitter concentrations in the mPFC as compared to NAc, although it cannot be excluded that a possibly lower SERT expression in the mPFC than in the NAc, plays a role too [43], which is in agreement with the higher 5-HIAA levels in NAc as compared to mPFC (see Table 1).

3.4. Consequences of LPS- and Cytokine-Induced Increases in SERT Activity

There are strong indications that LPS- and proinflammatory cytokine-induced increase in SERT function are necessary for the development of depression-like behavior, including fatigue and anhedonia.

Further, indications for an important role for increased SERT activity in LPS-induced anhedonia arises from clinical research showing that LPS-induced depressive symptoms could be reduced by 5-day pre-treatment with the SSRI citalopram [44]. Besides, prophylactic administration of SSRIs can be successfully used in a subgroup of patients who are at risk of developing major depression during IFN-α treatment [45]. Previously, it was shown that LPS-induced depression-like behavior (despair and anhedonia, i.e., the inability to experience pleasure probably caused by reduced ability to experience reward), as measured in the tail-suspension test [17] and in the intracranial self-stimulation (ICSS) paradigm, respectively, was abolished in knockout (SERT$^{-/-}$) animals [10,11,46].

In addition, it has been shown in mice, albeit not in rats, that the midline raphe nuclei express in IL-1 receptors [47] and that IL-1β- and LPS-induced increase SERT activity and LPS-induced immobility in the tail suspension test, a measure of behavioral despair, were abolished in IL-1R knockout mice [17]. Moreover, inhibition of the p38 MAPK signaling pathway with SB203580 blocked IL-1β-induced stimulation of SERT [16]. In addition, the IL-1 signaling pathway is pivotally involved in the development of LPS-induced anxiolytic-like behavior in elevated-plus maze test and immobility behavior in both forced-swim test and tail suspension test via a p38 MAPK-dependent pathway in serotonergic dorsal raphe neurons [48], whereas p38 MAPK does not seem to be involved in increased SERT function in the PFC [24].

Interestingly, mice that are more susceptible to develop anhedonia have increased microglial activation, increased TNF-α and SERT expression in the PFC [49].

Remarkably, sex differences in compensatory mechanisms have been reported in SERT knockout mice [43]. Therefore, in the future, more experiments are needed to investigate to what extent sex differences play a role in the suggested mechanisms.

4. Materials and Methods

4.1. Animals

Male serotonin transporter (Slc6a41Hubr) knockout rats generated by N-ethyl-N-nitrosourea (ENU)-induced mutagenesis [50] were bred and reared in the animal facilities of the Utrecht University. Animals were bred by crossing serotonin transporter heterozygous rats (SERT$^{+/-}$). At the age of 21 days, pups were weaned and ear cuts were taken for genotyping. Animals were placed on a 12 h light-dark cycle with lights on at 6:00 a.m. and of at 6:00 p.m. Food and water were available ad libitum. Animals were housed 4 per cage. Each animal was housed with litter mates having the same genotype (SERT$^{+/+}$, SERT$^{+/-}$ or SERT$^{-/-}$) and undergoing the same treatment (saline or LPS). Experiments started once animals were weighing 290–350 g. The study was conducted in accordance with the European and Dutch governmental guidelines and approved by the Ethical Committee for Animal Research of Utrecht University, The Netherlands (license no. DEC 2011.I.01.005).

4.2. Drugs

E. coli derived lipopolysaccharide (LPS) (art no. 0127:B8 Sigma-Aldrich Chemie N.V., Zwijndrecht, The Netherlands) was dissolved in saline (0.9% NaCl in demi water) and prepared freshly on test days from the stock solution (0.5 mg/mL dissolved in saline). LPS (250 µg/kg) was administered intraperitoneally (i.p.) in a volume of 2 mL/kg. Control animals received i.p. injections of saline in a volume of 2 mL/kg.

4.3. Microdialysis

4.3.1. Microdialysis Surgery

All rats ($n = 48$) were anesthetized by inhalation of a mixture of isoflurane gas (2%) and oxygen and were placed in a stereotaxic instrument. Two cuprophane microdialysis probes were implanted per rat. One probe was implanted in the NAc, the other in the mPFC (MAB 4.6.2 CU and MAB 4.7.3 CU, for NAc and mPFC, respectively (Microbiotech/se AB, Stockholm, Sweden)). The coordinates of the NAc and mPFC were anteroposterior +1.6 mm; mediolateral +1.8 mm (under a 0° angle) from bregma; dorsoventral −8.2 mm from skull surface and anteroposterior +3.2 mm; mediolateral +1.0 mm (under a 0° angle) from bregma; dorsoventral −4.0 mm from skull surface, respectively [51]. Probes were anchored with non-acrylic dental cement on the skull. After implantation of the microdialysis probes, rats were housed individually and placed in the microdialysis room until the end of the experiment.

4.3.2. Microdialysis Experiment

The microdialysis experiment was performed in conscious freely moving rats, one day after implantation of the microdialysis probes. A pump (KdScientific Pump 220 series, KD Scientific Inc., Holliston, MA, USA) perfused the system with Ringer solution (147 mM NaCl, 2.3 mM KCl, 2.3 mM CaCl$_2$ and 1 mM MgCl$_2$) at a constant flow rate of 0.02 mL/h. During microdialysis, the flow rate was set at 0.09 mL/h. At 8:00 a.m. rats were connected to a dual channel swivel (type 375/D/22QM, Microbiotech) which allowed them to move freely. Three hours after connection, samples were manually collected every 30 min in vials containing 15 µL of 0.1 M acetic acid and frozen at −80 °C until analysis with HPLC. From 11:00 a.m. until 1:00 p.m. four baseline samples were collected. Subsequently, the animals were injected i.p. with saline (SERT$^{+/+}$ $n = 8$; SERT$^{+/-}$ $n = 8$ and SERT$^{-/-}$ $n = 8$) or LPS (SERT$^{+/+}$ $n = 8$; SERT$^{+/-}$ $n = 8$ and SERT$^{-/-}$ $n = 8$). During the whole experiment, 12 samples were collected per rat. At the end of the microdialysis experiment all animals were sacrificed immediately. The brains were dissected and stored in formaldehyde 30% to verify probe localization later on.

4.3.3. HPLC

Microdialysis samples were stored at $-80\ °C$ until analysis. 5-HT and its metabolite 5-HIAA were detected simultaneously by HPLC with electrochemical detection using an Alexys 100 LC-EC system (Antec Scientific, Zoeterwoude, The Netherlands). The system consisted of two pumps, one auto sampler with a 10-port injection valve, two columns and two detector cells. Column 1 (NeuroSep105 C18 1×50 mm, 3 µm particle size) in combination with detector cell 1, separated and detected 5-HT, whereas column 2 (NeuroSep 115 C18 1×150 mm, 3 µm particle size) in combination with detector cell 2, separated and detected 5-HIAA. The mobile phase for column 1 consisted of 50 mM phosphoric acid, 8 mM KCl, 0.1 mM EDTA (pH 6.0), 18.5 % methanol and 400 mg/L OSA. The mobile phase for column 2 consisted of 50 mM phosphoric acid, 50 mM citric acid, 8 mM KCl, 0.1 mM EDTA (pH 3.25), 19.5 % methanol and 700 mg/L OSA. Both mobile phases were pumped at 50 µL/min. Samples were kept at 8 °C during analysis. From each microdialysis sample 5 µL was injected simultaneously onto each column. 5-HT and 5-HIAA were detected electrochemically using µVT-03 flow cells (Antec) with glassy carbon working electrodes. Potential settings were for 5-HT + 0.30 V versus Ag/AgCl and for 5-HIAA + 0.59 V versus Ag/AgCl. The columns and detector cells were kept at 35 °C in a column oven. The chromatogram was recorded and analyzed using the Alexys data system (Antec). The limit of detection was 0.05 nM (S/N ratio 3:1).

4.3.4. Histology

Two days before brain slicing, the brains were passed from formaldehyde to a 30% sucrose solution. Probe placements were verified on 60 µm cresyl violet stained sections that were cut on a cryostat (Leica CM3050, Leica Biosystems Inc., Buffalo Grove, IL, USA). Data were discarded when the microdialysis probe was outside the NAc or mPFC. In Figure 4, the correct probe localizations are shown of which data were used.

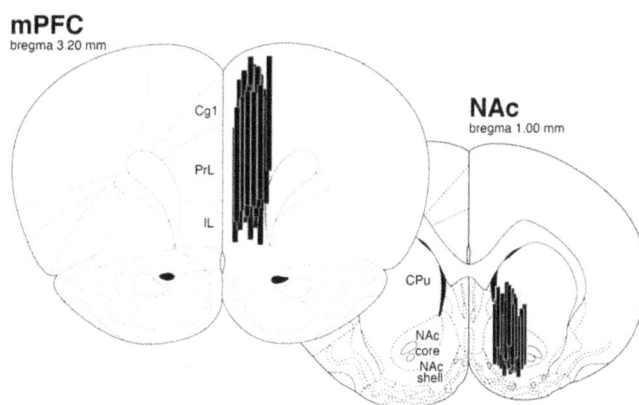

Figure 4. Localization of microdialysis probes in mPFC (3 mm length) and NAc (2 mm length). Cg1 = cingulate cortex, area 1; PrL = prelimbic cortex; IL = infralimbic cortex; CPu = caudate putamen; NAc core and shell = nucleus accumbens core and nucleus accumbens shell.

Some data could not be used due to obstruction of the microdialysis probe, or breaking of the outlet of the probe due to scratching and grooming from seven rats of the NAc study and from three rats of the mPFC study. Wrong probe localization caused eight dropouts in the NAc group, while this caused only one dropout in the mPFC group.

4.4. Statistics

Mean NAc and mPFC baseline 5-HT and 5-HIAA levels in SERT$^{+/+}$, SERT$^{+/-}$ and SERT$^{-/-}$ rats were analyzed with use of one-way ANOVA. For each genotype, microdialysis measurements were expressed as a percentage of baseline and analyzed by repeated measures ANOVA with time (4 levels: −90 min, −60 min, −30 min and 0 min) as within subject factor and treatment (saline or LPS) as between subject factor to exclude differences between the saline and LPS groups at baseline. Subsequently, post-injection data was compared in a repeated measures ANOVA with time (8 levels: 30 min, 60 min, 90 min, 120 min, 150 min, 180 min, 210 min and 240 min) as within subject factor and treatment (saline or LPS) as between subject factor. In case of a significant time × treatment interaction, effects of LPS on individual time points were analyzed with post hoc *t*-tests with treatment (saline or LPS) as the grouping variable. When the assumption of sphericity was violated, the results were corrected by the Greenhouse-Geisser procedure. Threshold for significance level was set at $p < 0.05$.

5. Conclusions

The present study supports the hypothesis that systemic LPS administration increases 5-HT metabolism by increasing SERT function in the CNS of male rats, as reflected by higher 5-HIAA levels in both the NAc and mPFC, which were reduced or fully absent in partially or completely SERT knockout male rats, respectively.

Author Contributions: Data curation, L.M.J.A. and E.M.v.O.; Formal analysis, G.A.H.K.-B., K.G.C.W. and S.M.K.; Funding acquisition, S.M.K.; Investigation, F.v.H. and K.G.C.W.; Methodology, G.A.H.K.-B., K.G.C.W., L.M.J.A. and E.M.v.O.; Project administration, F.v.H.; Resources, S.M.K.; Supervision, S.M.K.; Validation, F.v.H.; Writing—original draft, G.A.H.K.-B.; Writing—review & editing, O.G. and S.M.K.

Funding: This research received no external funding.

Conflicts of Interest: The authors declare no conflict of interest.

References

1.   Dantzer, R.; O'Connor, J.C.; Freund, G.G.; Johnson, R.W.; Kelley, K.W. From inflammation to sickness and depression: When the immune system subjugates the brain. *Nat. Rev. Neurosci.* **2008**, *9*, 46–56. [CrossRef] [PubMed]

2.   Dantzer, R. Cytokine, sickness behavior, and depression. *Immunol. Allergy Clin. N. Am.* **2009**, *29*, 247–264. [CrossRef] [PubMed]

3.   Konsman, J.P.; Parnet, P.; Dantzer, R. Cytokine-induced sickness behaviour: Mechanisms and implications. *Trends Neurosci.* **2002**, *25*, 154–159. [CrossRef]

4.   Pollak, Y.; Yirmiya, R. Cytokine-induced changes in mood and behaviour: Implications for 'depression due to a general medical condition', immunotherapy and antidepressive treatment. *Int. J. Neuropsychopharmacol.* **2002**, *5*, 389–399. [CrossRef] [PubMed]

5.   Akay, A.; Pekcanlar, A.; Bozdag, K.E.; Altintas, L.; Karaman, A. Assessment of depression in subjects with psoriasis vulgaris and lichen planus. *J. Eur. Acad. Dermatol. Venereol.* **2002**, *16*, 347–352. [CrossRef] [PubMed]

6.   Hauser, W.; Janke, K.H.; Klump, B.; Hinz, A. Anxiety and depression in patients with inflammatory bowel disease: Comparisons with chronic liver disease patients and the general population. *Inflamm. Bowel. Dis.* **2011**, *17*, 621–632. [CrossRef] [PubMed]

7.   Isik, A.; Koca, S.S.; Ozturk, A.; Mermi, O. Anxiety and depression in patients with rheumatoid arthritis. *Clin. Rheumatol.* **2007**, *26*, 872–878. [CrossRef] [PubMed]

8.   Loftus, E.V.; Guérin, A.; Yu, A.P.; Wu, E.Q.; Yang, M.; Chao, J.; Mulani, P.M. Increased risks of developing anxiety and depression in young patients with crohn's disease. *Am. J. Gastroenterol.* **2011**, *106*, 1670–1677. [CrossRef] [PubMed]

9.   Kenny, P.J.; Polis, I.; Koob, G.F.; Markou, A. Low dose cocaine self-administration transiently increases but high dose cocaine persistently decreases brain reward function in rats. *Eur. J. Neurosci.* **2003**, *17*, 191–195. [CrossRef] [PubMed]

10. Borowski, T.; Kokkinidis, L.; Merali, Z.; Anisman, H. Lipopolysaccharide, central in vivo biogenic amine variations, and anhedonia. *Neuroreport* **1998**, *9*, 3797–3802. [CrossRef] [PubMed]

11. Van Heesch, F.; Prins, J.; Konsman, J.P.; Westphal, K.G.; Olivier, B.; Kraneveld, A.D.; Korte, S.M. Lipopolysaccharide-induced anhedonia is abolished in male serotonin transporter knockout rats: An intracranial self-stimulation study. *Brain Behav. Immun.* **2013**, *29*, 98–103. [CrossRef] [PubMed]

12. Smolinska, M.J.; Page, T.H.; Urbaniak, A.M.; Mutch, B.E.; Horwood, N.J. Hck tyrosine kinase regulates TLR4-induced tnf and IL-6 production via AP-1. *J. Immunol.* **2011**, *187*, 6043–6051. [CrossRef] [PubMed]

13. Homberg, J.R.; Olivier, J.D.; Smits, B.M.; Mul, J.D.; Mudde, J.; Verheul, M.; Nieuwenhuizen, O.F.; Cools, A.R.; Ronken, E.; Cremers, T.; et al. Characterization of the serotonin transporter knockout rat: A selective change in the functioning of the serotonergic system. *Neuroscience* **2007**, *146*, 1662–1676. [CrossRef] [PubMed]

14. Siesser, W.B.; Sachs, B.D.; Ramsey, A.J.; Sotnikova, T.D.; Beaulieu, J.M.; Zhang, X.; Caron, M.G.; Gainetdinov, R.R. Chronic SSRI treatment exacerbates serotonin deficiency in humanized TPH2 mutant mice. *ACS Chem. Neurosci.* **2013**, *4*, 84–88. [CrossRef] [PubMed]

15. Mössner, R.; Heils, A.; Stöber, G.; Okladnova, O.; Daniel, S.; Lesch, K.P. Enhancement of serotonin transporter function by tumor necrosis factor alpha but not by interleukin-6. *Neurochem. Int.* **1998**, *33*, 251–254. [CrossRef]

16. Zhu, C.B.; Blakely, R.D.; Hewlett, W.A. The proinflammatory cytokines interleukin-1beta and tumor necrosis factor-alpha activate serotonin transporters. *Neuropsychopharmacology* **2006**, *31*, 2121–2131. [CrossRef] [PubMed]

17. Zhu, C.B.; Lindler, K.M.; Owens, A.W.; Daws, L.C.; Blakely, R.D.; Hewlett, W.A. Interleukin-1 receptor activation by systemic lipopolysaccharide induces behavioral despair linked to MAPK regulation of CNS serotonin transporters. *Neuropsychopharmacology* **2010**, *35*, 2510–2520. [CrossRef] [PubMed]

18. Connor, T.J.; Song, C.; Leonard, B.E.; Anisman, H.; Merali, Z. Stressor-induced alterations in serotonergic activity in an animal model of depression. *Neuroreport* **1999**, *10*, 523–528. [CrossRef] [PubMed]

19. Van Heesch, F.; Prins, J.; Konsman, J.P.; Korte-Bouws, G.A.H.; Westphal, K.G.C.; Rybka, J.; Olivier, B.; Kraneveld, A.D.; Korte, S.M. Lipopolysaccharide increases degradation of central monoamines: An in vivo microdialysis study in the nucleus accumbens and medial prefrontal cortex of mice. *Eur. J. Pharmacol.* **2014**, *725*, 55–63. [CrossRef] [PubMed]

20. Merali, Z.; Lacosta, S.; Anisman, H. Effects of interleukin-1beta and mild stress on alterations of norepinephrine, dopamine and serotonin neurotransmission: A regional microdialysis study. *Brain Res.* **1997**, *761*, 225–235. [CrossRef]

21. Van Heesch, F.; Prins, J.; Korte-Bouws, G.A.; Westphal, K.G.; Lemstra, S.; Olivier, B.; Kraneveld, A.D.; Korte, S.M. Systemic tumor necrosis factor-alpha decreases brain stimulation reward and increases metabolites of serotonin and dopamine in the nucleus accumbens of mice. *Behav. Brain Res.* **2013**, *253*, 191–195. [CrossRef] [PubMed]

22. O'Connor, J.C.; Lawson, M.A.; André, C.; Moreau, M.; Lestage, J.; Castanon, N.; Kelley, K.W.; Dantzer, R. Lipopolysaccharide-induced depressive-like behavior is mediated byindoleamine 2,3 dioxygenase activation in mice. *Mol. Psychiatry* **2009**, *14*, 511–552. [CrossRef] [PubMed]

23. Kim, D.K.; Tolliver, T.J.; Huang, S.J.; Martin, B.J.; Andrews, A.M.; Wichems, C.; Holmes, A.; Lesch, K.P.; Murphy, D.L. Altered serotonin synthesis, turnover and dynamic regulation in multiple brain regions of mice lacking the serotonin transporter. *Neuropharmacology* **2005**, *49*, 798–810. [CrossRef] [PubMed]

24. Schwamborn, R.; Brown, E.; Haase, J. Elevation of cortical serotonin transporter activity upon peripheral immune challenge is regulated independently of p38 mitogen-activated protein kinase activation and transporter phosphorylation. *J. Neurochem.* **2016**, *137*, 423–435. [CrossRef] [PubMed]

25. Molliver, M.E. Serotonergic neuronal systems: What their anatomic organization tells us about function. *J. Clin. Psychopharmacol.* **1987**, *7*, 3S–23S. [CrossRef] [PubMed]

26. Linthorst, A.C.; Flachskamm, C.; Holsboer, F.; Reul, J.M. Activation of serotonergic and noradrenergic neurotransmission in the rat hippocampus after peripheral administration of bacterial endotoxin: involvement of the cyclo-oxygenase pathway. *Neuroscience* **1996**, *72*, 989–997. [CrossRef]

27. Linthorst, A.C.; Flachskamm, C.; Müller-Preuss, P.; Holsboer, F.; Reul, J.M. Effect of bacterial endotoxin and interleukin-1 beta on hippocampal serotonergic neurotransmission, behavioral activity, and free corticosterone levels: an in vivo microdialysis study. *J. Neurosci.* **1995**, *15*, 2920–2934. [CrossRef] [PubMed]

28. Dunn, A.J. Effects of cytokines and infections on brain neurochemistry. *Clin. Neurosci. Res.* **2006**, *6*, 52–68. [CrossRef] [PubMed]

29. Hines, D.J.; Choi, H.B.; Hines, R.M.; Phillips, A.G.; MacVicar, B.A. Prevention of LPS-induced microglia activation, cytokine production and sickness behavior with TLR4 receptor interfering peptides. *PLoS ONE* **2013**, *8*, e60388. [CrossRef] [PubMed]

30. Gorina, R.; Font-Nieves, M.; Márquez-Kisinousky, L.; Santalucia, T.; Planas, A.M. Astrocyte TLR4 activation induces a proinflammatory environment through the interplay between myd88-dependent NFκB signaling, MAPK, and Jak1/Stat1 pathways. *Glia* **2011**, *59*, 242–255. [CrossRef] [PubMed]

31. Zhao, R.; Wang, S.; Huang, Z.; Zhang, L.; Yang, X.; Bai, X.; Zhou, D.; Qin, Z.; Du, G. Lipopolysaccharide-induced serotonin transporter up-regulation involves pkg-i and p38mapk activation partially through a3 adenosine receptor. *Biosci. Trends* **2015**, *9*, 367–376. [CrossRef] [PubMed]

32. Tsao, C.W.; Lin, Y.S.; Cheng, J.T.; Lin, C.F.; Wu, H.T.; Wu, S.R.; Tsai, W.H. Interferon-alpha-induced serotonin uptake in Jurkat T cells via mitogen-activated protein kinase and transcriptional regulation of the serotonin transporter. *J. Psychopharmacol.* **2008**, *22*, 753–760. [CrossRef] [PubMed]

33. Haase, J.; Brown, E. Integrating the monoamine, neurotrophin and cytokine hypotheses of depression—A central role for the serotonin transporter? *Pharmacol. Ther.* **2015**, *147*, 1–11. [CrossRef] [PubMed]

34. Zhu, C.B.; Hewlett, W.A.; Feoktistov, I.; Biaggioni, I.; Blakely, R.D. Adenosine receptor, protein kinase G, and p38 mitogen-activated protein kinase-dependent up-regulation of serotonin transporters involves both transporter trafficking and activation. *Mol. Pharmacol.* **2004**, *65*, 1462–1474. [CrossRef] [PubMed]

35. Zhu, C.B.; Carneiro, A.M.; Dostmann, W.R.; Hewlett, W.A.; Blakely, R.D. P38 MAPK activation elevates serotonin transport activity via a trafficking-independent, protein phosphatase 2a-dependent process. *J. Biol. Chem.* **2005**, *280*, 15649–15658. [CrossRef] [PubMed]

36. Zhu, C.B.; Steiner, J.A.; Munn, J.L.; Daws, L.C.; Hewlett, W.A.; Blakely, R.D. Rapid stimulation of presynaptic serotonin transport by A(3) adenosine receptors. *J. Pharmacol. Exp. Ther.* **2007**, *322*, 332–340. [CrossRef] [PubMed]

37. Morón, J.A.; Zakharova, I.; Ferrer, J.V.; Merrill, G.A.; Hope, B.; Lafer, E.M.; Lin, Z.C.; Wang, J.B.; Javitch, J.A.; Galli, A.; et al. Mitogen-activated protein kinase regulates dopamine transporter surface expression and dopamine transport capacity. *J. Neurosci.* **2003**, *23*, 8480–8488. [CrossRef] [PubMed]

38. Bermingham, D.P.; Blakely, R.D. Kinase-dependent regulation of monoamine neurotransmitter transporters. *Pharmacol. Rev.* **2016**, *68*, 888–953. [CrossRef] [PubMed]

39. Mathews, T.A.; Fedele, D.E.; Coppelli, F.M.; Avila, A.M.; Murphy, D.L.; Andrews, A.M. Gene dose-dependent alterations in extraneuronal serotonin but not dopamine in mice with reduced serotonin transporter expression. *J. Neurosci. Methods* **2004**, *140*, 169–181. [CrossRef] [PubMed]

40. Olivier, J.D.; Van Der Hart, M.G.; Van Swelm, R.P.; Dederen, P.J.; Homberg, J.R.; Cremers, T.; Deen, P.M.; Cuppen, E.; Cools, A.R.; Ellenbroek, B.A. A study in male and female 5-ht transporter knockout rats: An animal model for anxiety and depression disorders. *Neuroscience* **2008**, *152*, 573–584. [CrossRef] [PubMed]

41. Zhou, F.C.; Lesch, K.P.; Murphy, D.L. Serotonin uptake into dopamine neurons via dopamine transporters: A compensatory alternative. *Brain Res.* **2002**, *942*, 109–119. [CrossRef]

42. Olivier, J.D.; Jans, L.A.; Korte-Bouws, G.A.; Korte, S.M.; Deen, P.M.; Cools, A.R.; Ellenbroek, B.A.; Blokland, A. Acute tryptophan depletion dose dependently impairs object memory in serotonin transporter knockout rats. *Psychopharmacology* **2008**, *200*, 243–254. [CrossRef] [PubMed]

43. Bengel, D.; Murphy, D.L.; Andrews, A.M.; Wichems, C.H.; Feltner, D.; Heils, A.; Mössner, R.; Westphal, H.; Lesch, K.P. Altered brain serotonin homeostasis and locomotor insensitivity to 3, 4-methylenedioxymethamphetamine ("Ecstasy") in serotonin transporter-deficient mice. *Mol. Pharmacol.* **1998**, *53*, 649–655. [CrossRef] [PubMed]

44. Hannestad, J.; DellaGioia, N.; Ortiz, N.; Pittman, B.; Bhagwagar, Z. Citalopram reduces endotoxin-induced fatigue. *Brain Behav. Immun.* **2011**, *25*, 256–259. [CrossRef] [PubMed]

45. Galvao-de Almeida, A.; Guindalini, C.; Batista-Neves, S.; de Oliveira, I.R.; Miranda-Scippa, A.; Quarantini, L.C. Can antidepressants prevent interferon-alpha-induced depression? A review of the literature. *Gen. Hosp. Psychiatry* **2010**, *32*, 401–405. [CrossRef] [PubMed]

46. Van Heesch, F.; Prins, J.; Westphal, K.G.C.; Korte-Bouws, G.A.H.; Hoevenaar, W.H.M.; Olivier, B.; Kraneveld, A.D.; Korte, S.M. Pro-inflammatory cytokines affect monoamine (metabolite) levels in the nucleus accumbens and induce anhedonia in mice. In Proceedings of the SfN Neuroscience 42nd Annual Meeting of SFN Neuroscience, New Orleans, LA, USA, 13–17 October 2012.

47. Cunningham, E.T.; Wada, E.; Carter, D.B.; Tracey, D.E.; Battey, J.F.; De Souza, E.B. In situ histochemical localization of type I interleukin-1 receptor messenger rna in the central nervous system, pituitary, and adrenal gland of the mouse. *J. Neurosci.* **1992**, *12*, 1101–1114. [CrossRef] [PubMed]

48. Baganz, N.L.; Lindler, K.M.; Zhu, C.B.; Smith, J.T.; Robson, M.J.; Iwamoto, H.; Deneris, E.S.; Hewlett, W.A.; Blakely, R.D. A requirement of serotonergic p38α mitogen-activated protein kinase for peripheral immune system activation of cns serotonin uptake and serotonin-linked behaviors. *Transl. Psychiatry* **2015**, *5*, e671. [CrossRef] [PubMed]

49. Couch, Y.; Anthony, D.C.; Dolgov, O.; Revischin, A.; Festoff, B.; Santos, A.I.; Steinbusch, H.W.; Strekalova, T. Microglial activation, increased tnf and sert expression in the prefrontal cortex define stress-altered behaviour in mice susceptible to anhedonia. *Brain Behav. Immun.* **2013**, *29*, 136–146. [CrossRef] [PubMed]

50. Smits, B.M.; Mudde, J.B.; van de Belt, J.; Verheul, M.; Olivier, J.; Homberg, J.; Guryev, V.; Cools, A.R.; Ellenbroek, B.A.; Plasterk, R.H.; et al. Generation of gene knockouts and mutant models in the laboratory rat by enu-driven target-selected mutagenesis. *Pharmacogenet. Genom.* **2006**, *16*, 159–169.

51. Paxinos, G.; Franklin, K.B. *The Mouse Brain in Stereotaxic Coordinates*, 2nd ed.; Academic Press: San Diego, CA, USA, 2001.

3

Interactions Between Epilepsy and Plasticity

José J. Jarero-Basulto [1,*], Yadira Gasca-Martínez [1], Martha C. Rivera-Cervantes [1],
Mónica E. Ureña-Guerrero [2], Alfredo I. Feria-Velasco [1,†] and Carlos Beas-Zarate [3,*]

[1] Cellular Neurobiology Laboratory, Cell and Molecular Biology Department, CUCBA,
    University of Guadalajara, 45220 Zapopan, Jalisco, Mexico; gasca.mx@hotmail.com (Y.G.-M.);
    mrivera@academicos.udg.mx (M.C.R.-C.); alfredoferia1340@hotmail.com (A.I.F.-V.)
[2] Neurotransmission Biology Laboratory, Cell and Molecular Biology Department, CUCBA,
    University of Guadalajara, 45220 Zapopan, Jalisco, Mexico; murena@cucba.udg.mx
[3] Development and Neural Regeneration Laboratory, Cell and Molecular Biology Department, CUCBA,
    University of Guadalajara, 45220 Zapopan, Jalisco, Mexico; carlos.beas@academicos.udg.mx
* Correspondence: jose.jarero@academicos.udg.mx (J.J.J.-B.); carlos.beas@academicos.udg.mx (C.B.-Z.)

Abstract: Undoubtedly, one of the most interesting topics in the field of neuroscience is the ability of the central nervous system to respond to different stimuli (normal or pathological) by modifying its structure and function, either transiently or permanently, by generating neural cells and new connections in a process known as neuroplasticity. According to the large amount of evidence reported in the literature, many stimuli, such as environmental pressures, changes in the internal dynamic steady state of the organism and even injuries or illnesses (e.g., epilepsy) may induce neuroplasticity. Epilepsy and neuroplasticity seem to be closely related, as the two processes could positively affect one another. Thus, in this review, we analysed some neuroplastic changes triggered in the hippocampus in response to seizure-induced neuronal damage and how these changes could lead to the establishment of temporal lobe epilepsy, the most common type of focal human epilepsy.

Keywords: seizures; hippocampus; granular cells; plasticity; epilepsy

1. Introduction

The human central nervous system (CNS) is composed of multiple neuronal communication networks, which are closely regulated by their interactions with non-neuronal cells (glial and endothelial cells) [1]. One of the multiple attributes of the CNS is the ability to restructure itself in response to both physiological and pathological stimuli, through a process known as neuroplasticity, which is determined by cell and molecular mechanisms that modify the structure, density, and functionality of synaptic connections. In general, neuroplastic changes include the following: (a) increments in the efficacy of synaptic transmission in pre-existing synapses; (b) induction of new synaptic connections and reordering of pre-existing contacts; and (c) improvement of the ability of neurons to become excited. These changes were considered for a long time as an exclusive event of early developmental postnatal stages that are mainly stimulated as a subjacent process to learning and memory [2], an ability that was supposed to disappear with the ageing [3,4]. However, after several investigations, it was demonstrated that neuroplasticity is as follows: (1) a continuous process of remodelling neuronal circuitries; (2) it can occur at any life stage in response to different stimuli including brain damage; and (3) it comprises short-, medium- and long-time events that could last from minutes to years. In this sense, it must be considered that even the adult brain conserves the ability to generate neuroplastic responses, and they are lesser than those observed in early developmental stages [5]. In addition, in the adulthood, this process usually emerges as an adaptive and compensatory response to cerebral damage, among other processes [6,7]. Therefore, identifying the mechanisms implied in neuroplasticity is critically needed to improve our understanding of several physiological and pathological processes that occur in the CNS.

Additionally, it must be noted that even if neuroplastic changes try to compensate for the damage, in some cases, they can lead to the establishment of chronic neurological disorders or neurodegenerative illnesses [8,9]. For example, abnormal structural modifications to the dendritic spines have been implicated in intellectual disabilities and in childhood epilepsy [10], while insufficient or excessive elimination of synaptic contacts has been described as a basic aetiological mechanism of certain behavioural disorders, such as schizophrenia initiated at adolescence [11,12].

Epilepsy is a chronic disorder of the CNS characterized by the appearance of spontaneous recurrent seizures (SRS) generated by an imbalance of excitatory and inhibitory synaptic transmissions that induce electrical activity that is abnormally synchronized, which initially is focal, but may generalize [13–16]. It is still unknown whether this imbalance is a cause or a consequence of this disease. For some types of epilepsy categorized as idiopathic, the etiology is unknown, but it is thought that they may involve genetic predispositions [17,18]. In other cases, epilepsy is categorized as secondary or acquired because the seizures are the result of another neurological disease or an acute brain injury.

After the detonating neuronal damage, several neuroplastic changes predispose the brain to develop SRS in a process known as epileptogenesis, which leads to the establishment of epilepsy [15,16,19–22]. This process results from progressive cell and molecular changes that lead to neuronal network reorganization; most of these changes occur during a latent period of several years in humans and from weeks to months in experimental models. Because plastic responses of the CNS seem to depend on both the developmental state and the regional susceptibility, not all subjects with brain injuries develop epilepsy [23].

The hippocampus has been clearly identified as an epileptogenic brain region that is highly susceptible to damage, that involves both structural and functional changes, such as neuronal loss, inflammation, blood-brain barrier (BBB) leakage, angiogenesis, neurogenesis, axonal sprouting and synaptogenesis, among others. All these events have been associated with the pathophysiology of the temporal lobe epilepsy (TLE), which remains the most severe and frequent type of pharmacoresistant focally acquired epilepsy [15].

Despite the many physiological implications of neuroplasticity, the aim of this review is to analyse some of the neuroplastic changes triggered in the hippocampus as a response to cell death generated by seizures and how those could lead to the establishment of TLE.

2. Neuroplasticity in the Epileptogenic Hippocampus

The hippocampus is a cortical structure whose anatomy and plasticity have been broadly studied. It is a prominent C-shaped, bulging structure that is localized in the floor of the temporal horn of the lateral ventricle, which is subdivided into three major subfields (CA1–CA3) in rats and into four (CA1–CA4) in humans. Along with the dentate gyrus (DG), the subicular complex, and the entorhinal cortex comprise the hippocampal formation (commonly referred to as the hippocampus) [24,25]. The principal neurons of the hippocampus (pyramidal and granular cells) are excitatory and are surrounded by several types of interneurons (mainly GABAergic) and aminergic axon terminals. However, the major hippocampal circuitry (trisynaptic; Figure 1) is essentially excitatory and is highly sensitive to synaptic remodelling [26,27]. This brain region has a functional relevance in memory and learning processes, motor control and stereotyped behaviours, among others [28]. The highly organized laminar structure of the hippocampus has permitted the clear identification of cellular changes associated with both neuroplastic and epileptogenesis processes [24]. Moreover, as has been mentioned above, the hippocampus is one of the most vulnerable cerebral regions to be damaged, being fundamental in the establishment of the different types of epilepsy [29,30].

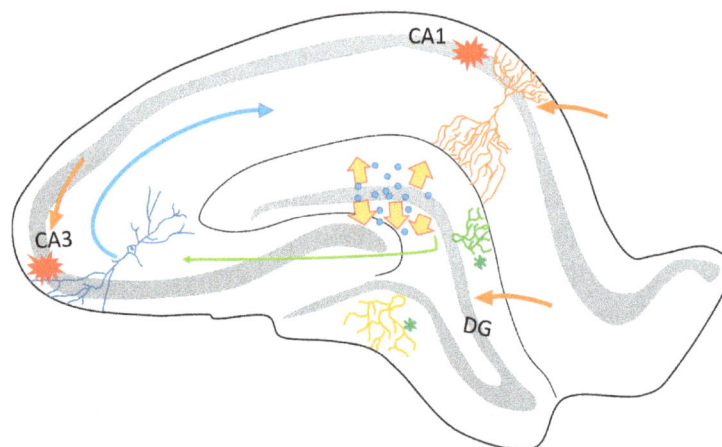

Figure 1. Schematic representation of the structural organization of the rat hippocampus. It is known that the hippocampus is connected to the entorhinal cortex through different anatomical circuitries that have been well described. Particularly, the perforant pathway projects from the DG and the CA3 to the CA1 (green and blue arrows). One of the characteristics of this circuitry is its directionality between the different neuronal layers. The DG, CA3 and the apical layers of CA1 (orange arrows) project mainly via the superficial layers of the entorhinal cortex (II and III). On the other hand, many pieces of evidence have reported that the hippocampus is highly vulnerable to cell loss via seizure activity, particularly in the CA1 and CA3 subfields (red marks). The dispersion of dentate granular cells (yellow arrows) and intense axonal sprouting (asterisks) are common in epileptogenesis process. These structural changes affects the organization and function of hippocampal circuitry and contribute to the establishment of the TLE.

Nearly fifty percent of acquired epilepsies belong to the focal type [31,32], and inside this category, TLE is considered the most frequent type in adults [33–38]. Although the exact cause of TLE is unknown, in most cases, it appears after an initial precipitating injury, such as *status epilepticus* (SE), tumours, vascular malformations, traumatic brain injury, severe infections, inflammation, among others cases [15,16,20–22]. In TLE, the epileptic focus involves limbic structures, such as the hippocampus, entorhinal cortex and amygdala, although less frequent damage is found in the latter two brain regions [39]. Generally, hippocampal sclerosis (HS) or mesial temporal sclerosis can be present [40], which has been found to be related to massive neuronal loss and reactive gliosis in the mid-basal areas that comprise the temporal lobe [41–43]. It is important to consider that, depending on the initial precipitating injury, the HS can be present or absent in the TLE [35,44].

Other changes observed in the hippocampus after epileptic seizures include selective neuronal loss (particularly in the pyramidal layer of CA1 and CA3 subfields, DG and the entorhinal cortex) [41,45,46] and cellular dispersion in the DG [47–52], as well as axonal sprouting in granular cells (Figure 1) [53–56]. These events have been observed in different experimental animal models for the study of epilepsy [46,57,58], as well as in human brain samples obtained from patients with drug-resistant TLE, who have undergone surgery to remove the epileptogenic zone, which is a common strategy that is applied as a treatment in this type of epilepsy [59–61].

It should be mentioned that, even though in some cases the seizures are brief, they may be sufficient to produce alterations in cerebral homeostasis and synaptic functioning and to promote new synaptic connections and aberrant circuitries [62]. Different research groups around the world have proposed that neural networks affected by epileptic episodes suffer neuroplastic modifications that contribute to the adoption of different pathological phenotypes [63,64]. However, this statement requires of more studies to clarify the mechanisms implicated in the structural and functional rearrangement of neural networks in epilepsy [65].

Taking into account several results that were obtained through different methodological strategies, it has been postulated that the neuronal loss produced in the hippocampus by epileptic seizures triggers an intense axonal sprouting in the neighbouring granular cells of the DG [58,61], increasing the number of aberrant synaptic connections that, together with an evident decrement in chandelier hippocampal cells (GABAergic interneurons), which exert a significant inhibitory effect [59], contribute to the establishment of hyperexcitable circuitry that stimulates the excessive release of glutamate (Glu), promoting the epileptic activity and excitotoxic neuronal damage [62].

Although, following the damage generated by seizures, several compensatory changes try to maintain the neuronal homeostasis and to restore the neuronal connections, they are limited by the underlying mechanism of epileptogenesis. In some cases of epilepsy (usually pharmacoresistant type), seizures can become so frequent and intense that repair mechanisms are unable to carry out their function [66]. However, the neuroplastic process remains active without restoring normal function and, on the contrary, tends to facilitate the modifications that promote the epileptogenic process.

3. Axonal Sprouting: Hippocampal Cell Response to Epileptic Seizures

The neuroplastic mechanisms involved in the recovery from lesions or illnesses are not always positive; and in some cases, they are responsible for initiating or enhancing the pathological processes [62]. When a massive loss of neuronal cells occurs, generating deafferentiation of a brain area, axonal sprouting arises as a widespread plastic response in part of the CNS to reorganize itself and try to restore the damage [67]. Nevertheless, the axonal sprouting process has also been described as a sign of different disorders of the CNS in which neuronal death occurs. Particularly in TLE, the prominent neuronal death produced by the seizures in the hippocampus (CA1 and CA3 subfields) and the amygdala, promotes the sprouting of new axons in the surviving dentate granular cells, which attempt to reinnervate the affected brain area, and produces an aberrant synaptic reorganization, which has been implicated in the pathogenesis of this disease [68,69]. In a clinical study, Scheimeiser and collaborators (2017) analysed 319 samples of TLE patients and observed that there was a correlation between the extent of mossy fibre sprouting and neuronal loss [70], but other evidence has suggested that neuronal degeneration is not strictly necessary for the sprouting to begin [71]. On the other hand, the aberrant function of axonal sprouting has also been considered as a consequence of granular cell ageing. Althaus and colleagues (2017) injected retroviruses carrying a synaptophysin-yellow fluorescent protein in a model of TLE in rats (SE induced by pilocarpine administration) and demonstrated that, in both neonatal and adult animals, the newly born granular cells contributed to the aberrant axonal reorganization to a similar extent, at least in this experimental model [72]. These and other results suggest that there is a more complex relationship between granular cells age and their participation in seizure-related plasticity.

The synaptic reorganization of the CNS and neuroanatomical description of the axonal sprouting process involves a very complicated series of events that are difficult to be reproduced in vitro; however, some of them have been characterized in samples of human brains and animal models of TLE [60,73]. Timm's staining method [74,75] has evidenced important structural changes in dentate granular cells with the sprouting of new axonal collaterals [54,76] that establish functional synapses with the dendrites of granular cells inside the inner molecular layer [45,74,77]. The neuronal reorganization of networks may occur in different brain areas generating numerous aberrant connections that promote TLE [46,76].

On the other hand, axonal sprouting is a mechanism regulated by different molecules that play an important role in brain development and in epileptogenesis. In this sense, it is known that the expression of some proteins, such as MAPs (microtubule-associated proteins) [62] and the GAP-43, are essential for this process. In particular, the GAP-43 protein, which is abundant in the neuronal growth cones and is required for growth and restructuration of neuronal axons, it is widely utilized as a specific marker of axonal sprouting [78–83]. Other critical molecules capable of promoting or inhibiting axonal growth are found outside of the cell, such as extracellular matrix molecules and cell adhesion molecules, as well as diffusible molecules such as cytokines produced by glial (reactive) or neuronal cells around the injured region [83]. These molecules also have other important functions, pointing the way that a new axon has to follow to reach to the target regions and cells.

Despite the different approaches that have so far contributed to the understanding of neuroplasticity and epileptogenesis processes, the identification of more participating molecules that are involved and a detailed description of the neuroanatomical profile of axonal sprouting at the level of individual cells are necessary to improve the treatment of this and other neuronal diseases.

4. Transcriptional Changes Related to Seizures and the Neuroplasticity Process

During development or during a pathological event, the neuroplastic process is highly influenced by extrinsic environmental experiences. Through different studies, it has been shown that short- and long-term synaptic plasticity responses may change substantially in the hippocampus and cerebral cortex after epileptic seizures [84–86]. However, the underlying mechanisms of these changes are still generally unclear because of contradictory results that currently exist. Immediate early genes (IEGs) are among the first changes induced in response to different physiological or pathological events. Specifically, changes in the gene expression levels of c-Fos, FosB, c-Jun, Egr1, Egr2, Egr4, FoxP2, Homer-1, Nacc-1, Nurr77, Arc and ApoE among others have been observed; these expression changes have been implicated in both the neuroplastic process and in the establishment of neurological disorders, such as epilepsy [87–98]. Subsequently, it has been proposed that IEGs are activated by the excessive synaptic activation that is generated in hippocampal and neocortical tissues [97,99,100] by high levels of Glu released to the extracellular space [101]. Glu overactivates its specific receptors, promoting excessive neuronal excitation and the overload of cytosolic free-Ca^{2+}, followed by cell death via excitotoxicity [102,103]. Glu-mediated signalling activates kinase cascades, such as the ERK pathway [104,105], that are responsible for phosphorylating several transcription factors that may translocate to the cell nucleus and regulate gene transcription processes [106].

On the other hand, previous studies have documented a complex pattern of long-term changes in plasticity-associated protein expression after seizure activity [107]. Neurotrophins, brain-derived neurotrophic factor (BDNF), insulin-like growth factor (IGF), and vascular endothelial growth factor (VEGF), are just some of the affected proteins [108,109]. In some cases, the low protein expression may be confused with the ageing process, which is known to alter the time course of gene expression, similar to that after seizures activity [110,111]. Additionally, differential changes in the expression of neurotransmitter receptors and modifications to the expression levels of neuropeptides in hippocampal cells, are induced by seizures [112–117], such as neuropeptide Y (NPY) in DG cells (Y1, Y2, and Y5), which has been found to be related to memory, learning and epilepsy.

Although we do not know enough of the specific genes that are involved in the neuroplasticity associated with epilepsy, it has been considered that each stimulus may initiate its own molecular pathway activation in the brain depending on the damage intensity generated to the neural networks [118]. The results of studies regarding changes in the expression of genes and the modifications of proteins in a temporal profile to determine its variability could have important implications for the development of new treatments for seizures disorders.

5. Changes in the Neurotransmission Systems by Seizures Related to Neuroplasticity

Neurotransmission systems are implied in neuroplasticity as both inducers and as targets of the process. In this sense, although more than fifty transmitter substances have been described, two of them appear to be particularly relevant in all neurological processes, including neuroplasticity and epileptogenesis, namely, Glu and γ-aminobutyric acid (GABA). Both are highly concentrated amino acids that converge biochemically and functionally in most of the regions of the vertebrate CNS; they exerting opposite effects, at least in the adulthood, wherein Glu normally depolarizes and excites neurons, while GABA hyperpolarizes and inhibits them [119–121]. In general, it is accepted that principal cortical and hippocampal projection neurons (pyramidal and granular cells) release Glu as a primary neurotransmitter, and most of the surrounding interneurons release GABA, among other neurotransmitters [119,122,123]. Glu-mediated excitation is essential for the neural activation implied in basically all nervous functions [120,121], while GABA-mediated inhibition is involved in excitation threshold maintenance and in the control of neuronal firing frequency and occurrence [14,122,124]. Subsequently, in general, the cross-talk between glutamatergic and GABAergic synapses builds, defines and remodels the neuronal circuitries [14,125] influenced by other neurotransmitters (such as acetylcholine, serotonin and dopamine, among others) and also, by the astrocytes activity because they do not only reuptake and metabolize these neurotransmitters, but they respond specifically to GABA and release Glu [126].

It has been broadly demonstrated that extracellular Glu levels are significantly increased in precipitant conditions of neuronal damage and during the seizures [122,127,128] that Glu-mediated excessive neuronal excitation leads to neuronal damage through a process known as excitotoxicity, which has been widely resembled in the hippocampus with several Glu analogues (Figure 2) [61,62,122,127,129–131]. Subsequently, neuronal damage and seizures may self-promote and regulate reciprocally in a positive feedback mechanism, wherein Glu is the neurotransmitter clearly implied. In addition, both GABAergic and glutamatergic cells may die, but interneurons seem to be more susceptible [61,129,130]. The effects of Glu depend on activation of several types of specific plasma membrane receptors (GluR), three of which are of the ionotropic (iGluR) type and are named by the selective agonists they are receptors for, namely, NMDA, AMPA (α-amino-3-hydroxy-5 methyl-4-isoxazole propionate) and kainate, which act as ligand-gated sodium/calcium channels; and eight of which are of the metabotropic type (mGluR), which are dependent on G proteins [119,120]. The iGluR antagonists block or reduce both neuronal death by Glu-mediated excitotoxicity and acute seizures generation but have poor efficacy in TLE epilepsy treatment [122]. Instead, GABA interacts with two general types of receptors, namely, one ionotropic known as GABA-A that acts as a ligand-gated chloride channel and the other as GABA-B, which is metabotropic and dependent on G proteins; [119] in this case, GABA-A receptor activation seems to be a common mechanism involved in the antiepileptic action of several drugs [122]. In addition, neuroplastic changes affect the neuronal signalling mediated by these neurotransmitters, as well as their transport, synthesis or degradation, such that neuronal inhibition is decreased and excitation is improved, resulting in the brain being more susceptible to seizures and to epileptogenesis [14,61,62,65,121,127,132,133].

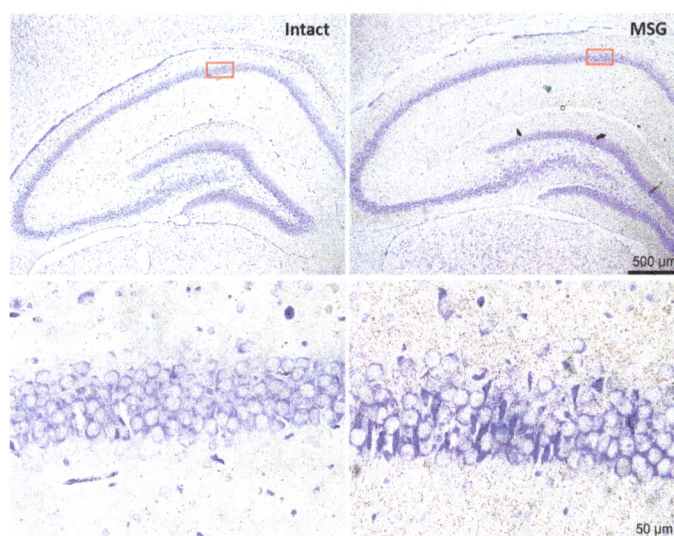

Figure 2. Representative images of neuronal excitotoxic damage in rat hippocampus after subcutaneous monosodium glutamate neonatally administered. Photomicrographs were taken at the level of the dorsal hippocampus, with a focus on the CA1 area (square red). Nissl stain. Scale bars correspond to 500 and 50 μm in upper and lower panels, respectively (for methodological details see: Rivera-Cervantes [131]).

During early development, both Glu and GABA exert neurotrophic effects, activating neuronal migration and axonal growth; moreover, GABA also controls these processes and promotes neurites outgrowth in the definition of dendritic arbors [125]. In later stages, long-lasting neuroplastic changes may be induced in the hippocampus by long-term potentiation (LTP) or long-term depression (LTD), which increase or decrease synaptic efficacy, respectively. Similar stimulation protocols or neural activity patterns can induce LTP in glutamatergic synapses and LTD in GABAergic, a condition that has been proposed as being determinant in both learning and epileptogenesis [14,61,62,122,127]. Establishment of LTP requires both pre- and post-synaptic depolarization, and GluRs activation, particularly of the NMDA receptors [14,61,62], whose composition, density and distribution are significantly modified in resected tissues of TLE patients and in samples obtained from several TLE experimental models [61,62].

Another plastic change that seems to be implicated in epileptogenesis involves to GABAergic neurotransmission, and it is related to the mechanisms that lead to GABA-mediated excitation through GABA-A receptor activation, which include changes in expression, viability or activity and cell distribution of two cation-chloride cotransporters (CCCs), namely, NKCC1 (chloride importer) and KCC2 (chloride exporter). When functional expression of KCC2 is higher than that of NKCC1, then GABA-A receptor activation promotes chloride entry and neuronal hyperpolarization, but when that relationship between these two CCCs is inverted, then GABA-A receptor activation depolarizes the neuron, and this condition has been related to seizures susceptibility and epileptogenesis in early development and in TLE [14,134,135].

Two important aspects should be noted. First, all statements mentioned above are based on the analysis of experimental acute and chronic epilepsy models, and of surgically TLE samples; second, not only have Glu and GABA been implicated in the plastic changes that mediate epileptogenesis, but also synaptic strength is highly susceptible to growth factors, other neurotransmitters, neuromodulators and hormones, which cannot be fully detailed in this review.

6. Neuronal and Glial Responses in the Hippocampus after Epileptic Seizures

Because neurons are not alone into the brain, one of the difficulties in the study of neuroplasticity and epilepsy, as in other neurological processes, was identifying all changes that occur in different cells in the orchestration of whatever process is being studied. However, in this section, we focused on the cells most closely related to synapses efficacy: neurons, astrocytes, and microglial cells. In addition to the modifications mentioned above, neurons that survive the degenerative process triggered by seizures modify the expression pattern and secretion of different neuropeptides and the density and distribution of their receptors, which may reduce the damage but also may reduce neuronal activation of GABA neurons or may increase Glu neurons activation [136], such as NPY and its receptors Y1 and Y2, whose expression is increased in both mossy fibres and GABAergic interneurons of the rat hippocampus in response to recurrent seizures. Similarly, the expression of those receptors also appears to be increased in surgically resected TLE samples, apparently reducing Glu release and neuronal excitation [113,137]. It should be mentioned that, even though interneurons are more vulnerable to the damage caused by seizures in comparison to dentate granular cells, dentate mossy cells are more sensitive than interneurons, and they respond to seizures extremely quickly and it is very complicated to identify the early changes produced in them [138]. Although some neuropeptides may reduce excitability, the progressive interneuron loss associated with seizures may promote a hyperexcitable state that complicates the control of them [139,140].

On the other hand, glial cells also respond to seizures and neuronal damage through a process known as "glial reactivity", which comprises both morphological and biochemical changes. The morphological changes include cell proliferation and ramification of the cell processes of both astrocytes and microglial cells [141]; additionally, reactive astrocytes have shown a reduced capacity to maintain extracellular homeostasis at the level of ions, nutrients, and neurotransmitters, improving the hyperexcitable state [142], and even releasing Glu [126]. In addition, the BBB can be dramatically damaged, not only by changes in the functional expression of transport proteins expressed by the astrocyte but also because the astroglial feet retract and lose contact with endothelial cells [141]. Consequently, glial reactivity has a strong influence on neuronal functioning, particularly in the plastic changes related to epileptogenesis [143–146]. Furthermore, reactive glial cells increase the synthesis and secretion of chemokines and cytokines [147,148], which may improve astrocytes and microglial cells activation in a positive feedback signalling process. For example, pro-inflammatory cytokines, such as NF-κB and interleukin (IL)-1β, as well as its signalling receptor IL-1R1, are highly expressed by neurons and glial cells in TLE [149,150]. Recent studies carried out in different experimental models of epileptogenesis showed that epileptic seizures may induce glial reactivity [151–154] and increase pro-inflammatory cytokine levels, particularly in cerebral regions involved in the processes of both epileptogenesis and neuroplasticity [155–157]. These and other data allow the suggestion that seizures induce a strong inflammatory response that significantly modifies the functional interactions among microglial cells, astrocytes and neurons, which could be an important link between the two boarded processes here.

7. Neurogenic and Synaptogenic Responses to Epileptic Seizures

The integration of newborn neurons into the pre-existing circuitries of the adult hippocampus seems to have an important role in learning and memory in physiological conditions, but in pathological states this may induce aberrant synaptic reorganization neuroplasticity, contributing to the alterations [158,159]. Hippocampal neurogenesis has been considered an important factor in the pathophysiology of TLE over the last two decades [160–166]. Most of the neurogenesis occurs during early development, although certain brains regions maintain this neurogenic capacity throughout the lifespan, such as the DG wherein new cells appear to arise from the subgranular zone.

The neurogenic process that occurs after seizures has been demonstrated using experimental models and during other pathological events [167–169]. Weeks after the initial stimulus is presented, some neurons mature and are able to integrate into nearby neural circuitries [170,171], while many others may lose their way migrating towards the hilus and the CA3 area, where they constitute part of the pathophysiological changes. Electrophysiological studies have shown that the new cells have membrane properties similar to the mature cells located in the granular layer [171]. However, small differences have been observed, such as the presence of dendrites on both sides of the soma and the tendency to show epileptiform discharges spontaneously, with a frequency of 0.5 to 0.05 Hz.

In addition, the seizure type determines the neurogenic response, the amount of neuron newly produced, and aberrant migration; in particular, both excitotoxicity damage and neuronal denervation promote neuritogenesis [26]. As described above, in order for these modifications to be carried out, the expression of IEGs is necessary because they are responsible for the initiation of structural and functional changes through the regulation of secondary or late gene expression [172]. Both in the human hippocampus and in different experimental models, an intense re-innervation of the granular cells of the DG by mossy fibres has been observed, which contributes to the amplification of excitatory glutamatergic components, thus facilitating the unleashing of epileptiform seizures [160,173]. This cellular re-innervation could constitute a mechanism for the development and maintenance of epilepsy.

Another alteration in the hippocampus is the GABAergic cells loss and, consequently, the alteration in the mechanisms that regulate neuronal excitability, which are dependent on GABA as a predominant inhibitory neurotransmitter in adulthood. The disconnection of GABAergic interneurons from the hilus generates a disinhibition of the DG and the CA3 region, which also facilitates the discharge in the glutamatergic cells [40,174].

As was described earlier in this review, a large variety of plastic changes are generated in response to neuronal damage, especially after prolonged or repetitive seizures. Although, differential effects of the neurogenic role in epilepsy establishment are present and dependent on multiple factors, generally it is accepted that the outcome depends on synaptogenesis of the new neurons.

8. Conclusions

The neuroplastic process has been considered both a cause and consequence of epilepsy, which represents more complexity than only the CNS restructuring. After seizure activity in the hippocampus not only does neuronal death occurs but also cell and molecular events that restructure and modify neuronal networks and synaptic communication occur; these modifications can reestablish normal functions or contribute to the development of neuronal illnesses, such as TLE. Growing evidence obtained through both experimental models and human brain samples has tried to explain some of the mechanisms involved in this type of illness, although many of them are contradictory. Specifically, in animal models, different factors must be considered, such as the mechanisms of damage induction, the animal species used, ages, genders, among others. Nevertheless, many groups of investigators continue to research the mechanisms implicated in neuroplasticity associated with epilepsy at different levels, especially in brain areas such as the hippocampus, which has a very important role in these processes (Figure 3).

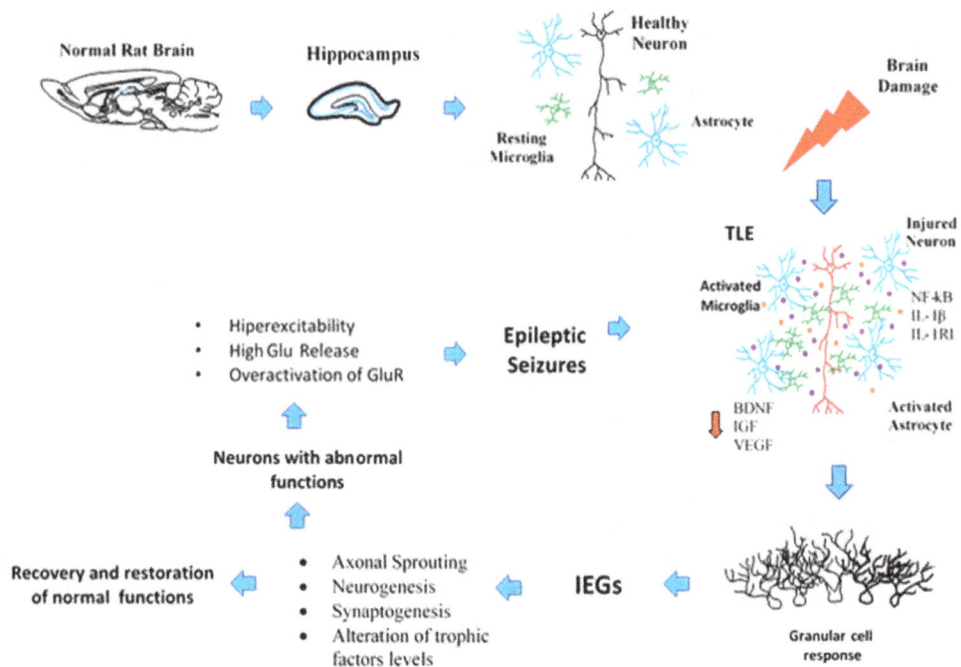

Figure 3. Schematic representation of the progressive events that lead to neuroplasticity and epileptogenic processes. First, the upper images refer to the undamaged hippocampus (blue colour) in a rat brain with most of the diverse cell populations (layers) represented (neuron: black colour; astrocytes: blue colour; and microglial cells: green colour). After non-lethal damage to the brain (red ray), reactive glial cells release pro-inflammatory chemokines and cytokines and modify neuronal activity (neuron: red colour; astrocytes: blue colour, and microglial cells: green colour; released pro-inflammatory molecules: purple colour; trophic factors levels are altered: red arrow). Then, through IEGs transcription, dentate granular cells respond to the damage through plastic changes that try to restore normal function but can also contribute to epileptogenesis, in a global process where in the mechanisms could affect on another.

Finally, one of the most important goals is to accomplish a clearly identification and understanding of the mechanisms and signalling pathways involved in neuronal death, plasticity, and epilepsy to identify new targets that may be used to develop therapeutic strategies to prevent or decrease the damages that lead to the establishment of neurological illnesses such as epilepsy.

Acknowledgments: This work was supported by the Guadalajara University (Lab_130 Research Strengthening Project); and CONACYT grant #177594. México. Additionally the authors express gratitude for language editing to Macias-Veles R.J.

Author Contributions: J.J.J.-B. and Y.G.-M. responsible for conception and design of this review. M.C.R.-C. and M.E.U.-G. integration and interpretation of information. A.I.F.-V. and C.B.-Z. editing and revising critically this work and contributing with important intellectual content. All authors contributed to and approved the final version of the manuscript.

Conflicts of Interest: The authors declare no conflict of interest.

References

1. Nieto-Sampedro, M.; Nieto-Diaz, M. Neural plasticity: Changes with age. *J. Neural Transm.* **2005**, *112*, 3–27. [CrossRef] [PubMed]

2. Hebb, D.O. Spontaneous neurosis in chimpanzees; theoretical relations with clinical and experimental phenomena. *Psychosom. Med.* **1947**, *9*, 3–19. [CrossRef] [PubMed]

3. Agnati, L.F.; Benfenati, F.; Solfrini, V.; Biagini, G.; Fuxe, K.; Guidolin, D.; Carani, C.; Zini, I. Brain aging and neuronal plasticity. *Ann. N. Y. Acad. Sci.* **1992**, *673*, 180–186. [CrossRef] [PubMed]

4. Agnati, L.F.; Zoli, M.; Biagini, G.; Fuxe, K. Neuronal plasticity and ageing processes in the frame of the 'red queen theory'. *Acta Physiol. Scand.* **1992**, *145*, 301–309. [CrossRef] [PubMed]

5. Bach-y-Rita, P. Brain plasticity as a basis for recovery of function in humans. *Neuropsychologia* **1990**, *28*, 547–554. [CrossRef]

6. Kaas, J.H.; Merzenich, M.M.; Killackey, H.P. The reorganization of somatosensory cortex following peripheral nerve damage in adult and developing mammals. *Annu. Rev. Neurosci.* **1983**, *6*, 325–356. [CrossRef] [PubMed]

7. Wall, P.D.; Egger, M.D. Formation of new connexions in adult rat brains after partial deafferentation. *Nature* **1971**, *232*, 542–545. [CrossRef] [PubMed]

8. Malinow, R.; Malenka, R.C. Ampa receptor trafficking and synaptic plasticity. *Annu. Rev. Neurosci.* **2002**, *25*, 103–126. [CrossRef] [PubMed]

9. Ismail, F.Y.; Fatemi, A.; Johnston, M.V. Cerebral plasticity: Windows of opportunity in the developing brain. *Eur. J. Paediatr. Neurol.* **2017**, *21*, 23–48. [CrossRef] [PubMed]

10. Phillips, M.; Pozzo-Miller, L. Dendritic spine dysgenesis in autism related disorders. *Neurosci. Lett.* **2015**, *601*, 30–40. [CrossRef] [PubMed]

11. Glausier, J.R.; Lewis, D.A. Dendritic spine pathology in schizophrenia. *Neuroscience* **2013**, *251*, 90–107. [CrossRef] [PubMed]

12. Sekar, A.; Bialas, A.R.; de Rivera, H.; Davis, A.; Hammond, T.R.; Kamitaki, N.; Tooley, K.; Presumey, J.; Baum, M.; Van Doren, V.; et al. Schizophrenia risk from complex variation of complement component 4. *Nature* **2016**, *530*, 177–183. [CrossRef] [PubMed]

13. Hirtz, D.; Thurman, D.J.; Gwinn-Hardy, K.; Mohamed, M.; Chaudhuri, A.R.; Zalutsky, R. How common are the "common" neurologic disorders? *Neurology* **2007**, *68*, 326–337. [CrossRef] [PubMed]

14. Bonansco, C.; Fuenzalida, M. Plasticity of hippocampal excitatory-inhibitory balance: Missing the synaptic control in the epileptic brain. *Neural Plast.* **2016**, *2016*, 8607038. [CrossRef] [PubMed]

15. Pitkanen, A.; Sutula, T.P. Is epilepsy a progressive disorder? Prospects for new therapeutic approaches in temporal-lobe epilepsy. *Lancet Neurol.* **2002**, *1*, 173–181. [CrossRef]

16. Lewis, D.V. Losing neurons: Selective vulnerability and mesial temporal sclerosis. *Epilepsia* **2005**, *46* (Suppl. 7), 39–44. [CrossRef] [PubMed]

17. Hirose, S.; Okada, M.; Kaneko, S.; Mitsudome, A. Are some idiopathic epilepsies disorders of ion channels?: A working hypothesis. *Epilepsy Res.* **2000**, *41*, 191–204. [CrossRef]

18. Berkovic, S.F.; Scheffer, I.E. Genetics of the epilepsies. *Epilepsia* **2001**, *42* (Suppl. 5), 16–23. [CrossRef] [PubMed]

19. Borkum, J.M. Migraine triggers and oxidative stress: A narrative review and synthesis. *Headache* **2016**, *56*, 12–35. [CrossRef] [PubMed]

20. Mathern, G.W.; Pretorius, J.K.; Babb, T.L. Influence of the type of initial precipitating injury and at what age it occurs on course and outcome in patients with temporal lobe seizures. *J. Neurosurg.* **1995**, *82*, 220–227. [CrossRef] [PubMed]

21. Mathern, G.W.; Babb, T.L.; Leite, J.P.; Pretorius, K.; Yeoman, K.M.; Kuhlman, P.A. The pathogenic and progressive features of chronic human hippocampal epilepsy. *Epilepsy Res.* **1996**, *26*, 151–161. [CrossRef]

22. French, J.A.; Williamson, P.D.; Thadani, V.M.; Darcey, T.M.; Mattson, R.H.; Spencer, S.S.; Spencer, D.D. Characteristics of medial temporal lobe epilepsy: I. Results of history and physical examination. *Ann. Neurol.* **1993**, *34*, 774–780. [CrossRef] [PubMed]

23. Engel, J., Jr. Ilae classification of epilepsy syndromes. *Epilepsy Res.* **2006**, *70* (Suppl. 1), S5–S10. [CrossRef] [PubMed]

24. Amaral, D.G.; Witter, M.P. The three-dimensional organization of the hippocampal formation: A review of anatomical data. *Neuroscience* **1989**, *31*, 571–591. [CrossRef]

25. Hennerici, M.G.; Szabo, K. Preface. Hippocampus from a neurologist's point of view. *Front. Neurol. Neurosci.* **2014**, *34*, IX. [CrossRef] [PubMed]

26. Marrone, D.F.; Petit, T.L. The role of synaptic morphology in neural plasticity: Structural interactions underlying synaptic power. *Brain Res. Brain Res. Rev.* **2002**, *38*, 291–308. [CrossRef]

27. Drapeau, E.; Mayo, W.; Aurousseau, C.; Le Moal, M.; Piazza, P.V.; Abrous, D.N. Spatial memory performances of aged rats in the water maze predict levels of hippocampal neurogenesis. *Proc. Natl. Acad. Sci. USA* **2003**, *100*, 14385–14390. [CrossRef] [PubMed]

28. Shah, P.; Bassett, D.S.; Wisse, L.E.M.; Detre, J.A.; Stein, J.M.; Yushkevich, P.A.; Shinohara, R.T.; Pluta, J.B.; Valenciano, E.; Daffner, M.; et al. Mapping the structural and functional network architecture of the medial temporal lobe using 7t mri. *Hum. Brain Mapp.* **2017**. [CrossRef] [PubMed]

29. Mathern, G.W.; Adelson, P.D.; Cahan, L.D.; Leite, J.P. Hippocampal neuron damage in human epilepsy: Meyer's hypothesis revisited. *Prog. Brain Res.* **2002**, *135*, 237–251. [PubMed]

30. Mathern, G.W.; Leiphart, J.L.; De Vera, A.; Adelson, P.D.; Seki, T.; Neder, L.; Leite, J.P. Seizures decrease postnatal neurogenesis and granule cell development in the human fascia dentata. *Epilepsia* **2002**, *43* (Suppl. 5), 68–73. [CrossRef] [PubMed]

31. Engel, J., Jr. Intractable epilepsy: Definition and neurobiology. *Epilepsia* **2001**, *42* (Suppl. 6), 3. [CrossRef]

32. Thom, M.; Eriksson, S.; Martinian, L.; Caboclo, L.O.; McEvoy, A.W.; Duncan, J.S.; Sisodiya, S.M. Temporal lobe sclerosis associated with hippocampal sclerosis in temporal lobe epilepsy: Neuropathological features. *J. Neuropathol. Exp. Neurol.* **2009**, *68*, 928–938. [CrossRef] [PubMed]

33. Panayiotopoulos, C.P. Evidence-based epileptology, randomized controlled trials, and sanad: A critical clinical view. *Epilepsia* **2007**, *48*, 1268–1274. [CrossRef] [PubMed]

34. McHugh, J.C.; Delanty, N. Epidemiology and classification of epilepsy: Gender comparisons. *Int. Rev. Neurobiol.* **2008**, *83*, 11–26. [PubMed]

35. Tellez-Zenteno, J.F.; Ladino, L.D. [Temporal epilepsy: Clinical, diagnostic and therapeutic aspects]. *Rev. Neurol.* **2013**, *56*, 229–242. [PubMed]

36. Kobayashi, E.; Santos, N.F.; Torres, F.R.; Secolin, R.; Sardinha, L.A.; Lopez-Cendes, I.; Cendes, F. Magnetic resonance imaging abnormalities in familial temporal lobe epilepsy with auditory auras. *Arch. Neurol.* **2003**, *60*, 1546–1551. [CrossRef] [PubMed]

37. Theodore, W.H.; Epstein, L.; Gaillard, W.D.; Shinnar, S.; Wainwright, M.S.; Jacobson, S. Human herpes virus 6b: A possible role in epilepsy? *Epilepsia* **2008**, *49*, 1828–1837. [CrossRef] [PubMed]

38. Cendes, F.; Kobayashi, E.; Lopes-Cendes, I. Familial temporal lobe epilepsy with auditory features. *Epilepsia* **2005**, *46* (Suppl. 10), 59–60. [CrossRef] [PubMed]

39. Yilmazer-Hanke, D.M.; Wolf, H.K.; Schramm, J.; Elger, C.E.; Wiestler, O.D.; Blumcke, I. Subregional pathology of the amygdala complex and entorhinal region in surgical specimens from patients with pharmacoresistant temporal lobe epilepsy. *J. Neuropathol. Exp. Neurol.* **2000**, *59*, 907–920. [CrossRef] [PubMed]

40. Sloviter, R.S. Hippocampal epileptogenesis in animal models of mesial temporal lobe epilepsy with hippocampal sclerosis: The importance of the "latent period" and other concepts. *Epilepsia* **2008**, *49* (Suppl. 9), 85–92. [CrossRef] [PubMed]

41. Benbadis, S.; Helmers, S.; Hirsch, L.; Sirven, J.; Vale, F.L.; Wheless, J. Yes, neurostimulation has a role in the management of epilepsy. *Neurology* **2014**, *83*, 845–847. [CrossRef] [PubMed]

42. Schwartzkroin, P.A. Hippocampal slices in experimental and human epilepsy. *Adv. Neurol.* **1986**, *44*, 991–1010. [PubMed]

43. Bercovici, E.; Kumar, B.S.; Mirsattari, S.M. Neocortical temporal lobe epilepsy. *Epilepsy Res Treat* **2012**, *2012*, 103160. [CrossRef] [PubMed]

44. Blumcke, I.; Thom, M.; Aronica, E.; Armstrong, D.D.; Bartolomei, F.; Bernasconi, A.; Bernasconi, N.; Bien, C.G.; Cendes, F.; Coras, R.; et al. International consensus classification of hippocampal sclerosis in temporal lobe epilepsy: A task force report from the ilae commission on diagnostic methods. *Epilepsia* **2013**, *54*, 1315–1329. [CrossRef] [PubMed]

45. Ben-Ari, Y.; Cossart, R. Kainate, a double agent that generates seizures: Two decades of progress. *Trends Neurosci.* **2000**, *23*, 580–587. [CrossRef]

46. Cross, D.J.; Cavazos, J.E. Synaptic reorganization in subiculum and ca3 after early-life status epilepticus in the kainic acid rat model. *Epilepsy Res.* **2007**, *73*, 156–165. [CrossRef] [PubMed]

47. Spencer, D.D.; Spencer, S.S. Hippocampal resections and the use of human tissue in defining temporal lobe epilepsy syndromes. *Hippocampus* **1994**, *4*, 243–249. [CrossRef] [PubMed]

48. Spencer, S.S. Substrates of localization-related epilepsies: Biologic implications of localizing findings in humans. *Epilepsia* **1998**, *39*, 114–123. [CrossRef] [PubMed]

49. Spencer, S.S.; Spencer, D.D. Entorhinal-hippocampal interactions in medial temporal lobe epilepsy. *Epilepsia* **1994**, *35*, 721–727. [CrossRef] [PubMed]

50. Toyoda, I.; Bower, M.R.; Leyva, F.; Buckmaster, P.S. Early activation of ventral hippocampus and subiculum during spontaneous seizures in a rat model of temporal lobe epilepsy. *J. Neurosci.* **2013**, *33*, 11100–11115. [CrossRef] [PubMed]

51. Berkovic, S.F.; Andermann, F.; Olivier, A.; Ethier, R.; Melanson, D.; Robitaille, Y.; Kuzniecky, R.; Peters, T.; Feindel, W. Hippocampal sclerosis in temporal lobe epilepsy demonstrated by magnetic resonance imaging. *Ann. Neurol.* **1991**, *29*, 175–182. [CrossRef] [PubMed]

52. Uemori, T.; Toda, K.; Seki, T. Seizure severity-dependent selective vulnerability of the granule cell layer and aberrant neurogenesis in the rat hippocampus. *Hippocampus* **2017**, *27*, 1054–1068. [CrossRef] [PubMed]

53. Cavazos, J.E.; Zhang, P.; Qazi, R.; Sutula, T.P. Ultrastructural features of sprouted mossy fiber synapses in kindled and kainic acid-treated rats. *J Comp. Neurol.* **2003**, *458*, 272–292. [CrossRef] [PubMed]

54. Buckmaster, P.S. Mossy fiber sprouting in the dentate gyrus. In *Jasper's Basic Mechanisms of the Epilepsies*, 4th ed.; Noebels, J.L., Avoli, M., Rogawski, M.A., Olsen, R.W., Delgado-Escueta, A.V., Eds.; National Center for Biotechnology Information: Bethesda, MD, USA, 2012.

55. Ribak, C.E.; Shapiro, L.A.; Yan, X.X.; Dashtipour, K.; Nadler, J.V.; Obenaus, A.; Spigelman, I.; Buckmaster, P.S. Seizure-induced formation of basal dendrites on granule cells of the rodent dentate gyrus. In *Jasper's Basic Mechanisms of the Epilepsies*, 4th ed.; Noebels, J.L., Avoli, M., Rogawski, M.A., Olsen, R.W., Delgado-Escueta, A.V., Eds.; National Center for Biotechnology Information: Bethesda, MD, USA, 2012.

56. Parent, J.M.; Kron, M.M. Neurogenesis and epilepsy. In *Jasper's Basic Mechanisms of the Epilepsies*, 4th ed.; Noebels, J.L., Avoli, M., Rogawski, M.A., Olsen, R.W., Delgado-Escueta, A.V., Eds.; National Center for Biotechnology Information: Bethesda, MD, USA, 2012.

57. Cornejo, B.J.; Mesches, M.H.; Coultrap, S.; Browning, M.D.; Benke, T.A. A single episode of neonatal seizures permanently alters glutamatergic synapses. *Ann. Neurol.* **2007**, *61*, 411–426. [CrossRef] [PubMed]

58. Morimoto, K.; Fahnestock, M.; Racine, R.J. Kindling and status epilepticus models of epilepsy: Rewiring the brain. *Prog. Neurobiol.* **2004**, *73*, 1–60. [CrossRef] [PubMed]

59. Arellano, J.I.; Munoz, A.; Ballesteros-Yanez, I.; Sola, R.G.; DeFelipe, J. Histopathology and reorganization of chandelier cells in the human epileptic sclerotic hippocampus. *Brain* **2004**, *127*, 45–64. [CrossRef] [PubMed]

60. Proper, E.A.; Oestreicher, A.B.; Jansen, G.H.; Veelen, C.W.; van Rijen, P.C.; Gispen, W.H.; de Graan, P.N. Immunohistochemical characterization of mossy fibre sprouting in the hippocampus of patients with pharmaco-resistant temporal lobe epilepsy. *Brain J. Neurol.* **2000**, *123 Pt 1*, 19–30. [CrossRef]

61. McNamara, J.O.; Huang, Y.Z.; Leonard, A.S. Molecular signaling mechanisms underlying epileptogenesis. *Sci. STKE* **2006**, *2006*, re12. [CrossRef] [PubMed]

62. Ben-Ari, Y. Cell death and synaptic reorganizations produced by seizures. *Epilepsia* **2001**, *42* (Suppl. 3), 5–7. [CrossRef] [PubMed]

63. Tuunanen, J.; Lukasiuk, K.; Halonen, T.; Pitkanen, A. Status epilepticus-induced neuronal damage in the rat amygdaloid complex: Distribution, time-course and mechanisms. *Neuroscience* **1999**, *94*, 473–495. [CrossRef]

64. Riba-Bosch, A.; Perez-Clausell, J. Response to kainic acid injections: Changes in staining for zinc, fos, cell death and glial response in the rat forebrain. *Neuroscience* **2004**, *125*, 803–818. [CrossRef] [PubMed]

65. Scharfman, H.E. The neurobiology of epilepsy. *Curr. Neurol. Neurosci. Rep.* **2007**, *7*, 348–354. [CrossRef] [PubMed]

66. Mathern, G.W.; Babb, T.L.; Vickrey, B.G.; Melendez, M.; Pretorius, J.K. The clinical-pathogenic mechanisms of hippocampal neuron loss and surgical outcomes in temporal lobe epilepsy. *Brain J. Neurol.* **1995**, *118 Pt 1*, 105–118. [CrossRef]

67. Steward, O. Cholinergic sprouting is blocked by repeated induction of electroconvulsive seizures, a manipulation that induces a persistent reactive state in astrocytes. *Exp. Neurol.* **1994**, *129*, 103–111. [CrossRef] [PubMed]

68. Larner, A.J. Axonal sprouting and synaptogenesis in temporal lobe epilepsy: Possible pathogenetic and therapeutic roles of neurite growth inhibitory factors. *Seizure* **1995**, *4*, 249–258. [CrossRef]

69. Sloviter, R.S. The functional organization of the hippocampal dentate gyrus and its relevance to the pathogenesis of temporal lobe epilepsy. *Ann. Neurol.* **1994**, *35*, 640–654. [CrossRef] [PubMed]

70. Schmeiser, B.; Zentner, J.; Prinz, M.; Brandt, A.; Freiman, T.M. Extent of mossy fiber sprouting in patients with mesiotemporal lobe epilepsy correlates with neuronal cell loss and granule cell dispersion. *Epilepsy Res.* **2017**, *129*, 51–58. [CrossRef] [PubMed]

71. Stringer, J.L.; Agarwal, K.S.; Dure, L.S. Is cell death necessary for hippocampal mossy fiber sprouting? *Epilepsy Res.* **1997**, *27*, 67–76. [CrossRef]

72. Althaus, A.L.; Zhang, H.; Parent, J.M. Axonal plasticity of age-defined dentate granule cells in a rat model of mesial temporal lobe epilepsy. *Neurobiol. Dis.* **2016**, *86*, 187–196. [CrossRef] [PubMed]

73. Sutula, T.P.; Dudek, F.E. Unmasking recurrent excitation generated by mossy fiber sprouting in the epileptic dentate gyrus: An emergent property of a complex system. *Prog. Brain Res.* **2007**, *163*, 541–563. [PubMed]

74. Sutula, T.; Cascino, G.; Cavazos, J.; Parada, I.; Ramirez, L. Mossy fiber synaptic reorganization in the epileptic human temporal lobe. *Ann. Neurol.* **1989**, *26*, 321–330. [CrossRef] [PubMed]

75. Sloviter, R.S. A simplified timm stain procedure compatible with formaldehyde fixation and routine paraffin embedding of rat brain. *Brain Res. Bull.* **1982**, *8*, 771–774. [CrossRef]

76. Buckmaster, P.S.; Zhang, G.F.; Yamawaki, R. Axon sprouting in a model of temporal lobe epilepsy creates a predominantly excitatory feedback circuit. *J. Neurosci.* **2002**, *22*, 6650–6658. [PubMed]

77. Babb, T.L. Bilateral pathological damage in temporal lobe epilepsy. *Can. J. Neurol. Sci.* **1991**, *18*, 645–648. [CrossRef] [PubMed]

78. Bendotti, C.; Pende, M.; Samanin, R. Expression of gap-43 in the granule cells of rat hippocampus after seizure-induced sprouting of mossy fibres: In situ hybridization and immunocytochemical studies. *Eur. J. Neurosci.* **1994**, *6*, 509–515. [CrossRef] [PubMed]

79. Represa, A.; Pollard, H.; Moreau, J.; Ghilini, G.; Khrestchatisky, M.; Ben-Ari, Y. Mossy fiber sprouting in epileptic rats is associated with a transient increased expression of alpha-tubulin. *Neurosci. Lett.* **1993**, *156*, 149–152. [CrossRef]

80. Shen, E.Y.; Lai, Y.J. In vivo microdialysis study of excitatory and inhibitory amino acid levels in the hippocampus following penicillin-induced seizures in mature rats. *Acta Paediatr. Taiwan* **2002**, *43*, 313–318. [PubMed]

81. Tessier-Lavigne, M.; Goodman, C.S. The molecular biology of axon guidance. *Science* **1996**, *274*, 1123–1133. [CrossRef] [PubMed]

82. Oestreicher, A.B.; De Graan, P.N.; Gispen, W.H.; Verhaagen, J.; Schrama, L.H. B-50, the growth associated protein-43: Modulation of cell morphology and communication in the nervous system. *Prog. Neurobiol.* **1997**, *53*, 627–686. [CrossRef]

83. Naffah-Mazzacoratti, M.G.; Funke, M.G.; Sanabria, E.R.; Cavalheiro, E.A. Growth-associated phosphoprotein expression is increased in the supragranular regions of the dentate gyrus following pilocarpine-induced seizures in rats. *Neuroscience* **1999**, *91*, 485–492. [CrossRef]

84. Abegg, M.H.; Savic, N.; Ehrengruber, M.U.; McKinney, R.A.; Gahwiler, B.H. Epileptiform activity in rat hippocampus strengthens excitatory synapses. *J. Physiol.* **2004**, *554*, 439–448. [CrossRef] [PubMed]

85. Muller, L.; Tokay, T.; Porath, K.; Kohling, R.; Kirschstein, T. Enhanced nmda receptor-dependent ltp in the epileptic ca1 area via upregulation of nr2b. *Neurobiol. Dis.* **2013**, *54*, 183–193. [CrossRef] [PubMed]

86. Zhou, J.L.; Shatskikh, T.N.; Liu, X.; Holmes, G.L. Impaired single cell firing and long-term potentiation parallels memory impairment following recurrent seizures. *Eur. J. Neurosci.* **2007**, *25*, 3667–3677. [CrossRef] [PubMed]

87. Davis, S.; Bozon, B.; Laroche, S. How necessary is the activation of the immediate early gene zif268 in synaptic plasticity and learning? *Behav. Brain Res.* **2003**, *142*, 17–30. [CrossRef]

88. Rakhade, S.N.; Jensen, F.E. Epileptogenesis in the immature brain: Emerging mechanisms. *Nat. Rev. Neurol.* **2009**, *5*, 380–391. [CrossRef] [PubMed]

89. Plath, N.; Ohana, O.; Dammermann, B.; Errington, M.L.; Schmitz, D.; Gross, C.; Mao, X.; Engelsberg, A.; Mahlke, C.; Welzl, H.; et al. Arc/arg3.1 is essential for the consolidation of synaptic plasticity and memories. *Neuron* **2006**, *52*, 437–444. [CrossRef] [PubMed]

90. Gass, P.; Katsura, K.; Zuschratter, W.; Siesjo, B.; Kiessling, M. Hypoglycemia-elicited immediate early gene expression in neurons and glia of the hippocampus: Novel patterns of fos, jun, and krox expression following excitotoxic injury. *J. Cereb. Blood Flow Metab.* **1995**, *15*, 989–1001. [CrossRef] [PubMed]

91. Hughes, P.E.; Alexi, T.; Walton, M.; Williams, C.E.; Dragunow, M.; Clark, R.G.; Gluckman, P.D. Activity and injury-dependent expression of inducible transcription factors, growth factors and apoptosis-related genes within the central nervous system. *Prog. Neurobiol.* **1999**, *57*, 421–450. [CrossRef]

92. Knapska, E.; Kaczmarek, L. A gene for neuronal plasticity in the mammalian brain: Zif268/egr-1/ngfi-a/krox-24/tis8/zenk? *Prog. Neurobiol.* **2004**, *74*, 183–211. [CrossRef] [PubMed]

93. Yutsudo, N.; Kamada, T.; Kajitani, K.; Nomaru, H.; Katogi, A.; Ohnishi, Y.H.; Ohnishi, Y.N.; Takase, K.; Sakumi, K.; Shigeto, H.; et al. Fosb-null mice display impaired adult hippocampal neurogenesis and spontaneous epilepsy with depressive behavior. *Neuropsychopharmacology* **2013**, *38*, 895–906. [CrossRef] [PubMed]

94. Sia, G.M.; Clem, R.L.; Huganir, R.L. The human language-associated gene srpx2 regulates synapse formation and vocalization in mice. *Science* **2013**, *342*, 987–991. [CrossRef] [PubMed]

95. Meyer, D.; Bonhoeffer, T.; Scheuss, V. Balance and stability of synaptic structures during synaptic plasticity. *Neuron* **2014**, *82*, 430–443. [CrossRef] [PubMed]

96. Yang, C.P.; Gilley, J.A.; Zhang, G.; Kernie, S.G. Apoe is required for maintenance of the dentate gyrus neural progenitor pool. *Development* **2011**, *138*, 4351–4362. [CrossRef] [PubMed]

97. Herdegen, T.; Leah, J.D. Inducible and constitutive transcription factors in the mammalian nervous system: Control of gene expression by jun, fos and krox, and creb/atf proteins. *Brain Res. Brain Res. Rev.* **1998**, *28*, 370–490. [CrossRef]

98. Retchkiman, I.; Fischer, B.; Platt, D.; Wagner, A.P. Seizure induced c-fos mrna in the rat brain: Comparison between young and aging animals. *Neurobiol. Aging* **1996**, *17*, 41–44. [CrossRef]

99. Rakhade, S.N.; Shah, A.K.; Agarwal, R.; Yao, B.; Asano, E.; Loeb, J.A. Activity-dependent gene expression correlates with interictal spiking in human neocortical epilepsy. *Epilepsia* **2007**, *48* (Suppl. 5), 86–95. [CrossRef] [PubMed]

100. Rakhade, S.N.; Yao, B.; Ahmed, S.; Asano, E.; Beaumont, T.L.; Shah, A.K.; Draghici, S.; Krauss, R.; Chugani, H.T.; Sood, S.; et al. A common pattern of persistent gene activation in human neocortical epileptic foci. *Ann. Neurol.* **2005**, *58*, 736–747. [CrossRef] [PubMed]

101. Luo, P.; Fei, F.; Zhang, L.; Qu, Y.; Fei, Z. The role of glutamate receptors in traumatic brain injury: Implications for postsynaptic density in pathophysiology. *Brain Res. Bull.* **2011**, *85*, 313–320. [CrossRef] [PubMed]

102. Lai, T.W.; Zhang, S.; Wang, Y.T. Excitotoxicity and stroke: Identifying novel targets for neuroprotection. *Prog. Neurobiol.* **2014**, *115*, 157–188. [CrossRef] [PubMed]

103. Algattas, H.; Huang, J.H. Traumatic brain injury pathophysiology and treatments: Early, intermediate, and late phases post-injury. *Int. J. Mol. Sci.* **2013**, *15*, 309–341. [CrossRef] [PubMed]

104. Curia, G.; Gualtieri, F.; Bartolomeo, R.; Vezzali, R.; Biagini, G. Resilience to audiogenic seizures is associated with p-erk1/2 dephosphorylation in the subiculum of fmr1 knockout mice. *Front. Cell. Neurosci.* **2013**, *7*, 46. [CrossRef] [PubMed]

105. Giordano, C.; Costa, A.M.; Lucchi, C.; Leo, G.; Brunel, L.; Fehrentz, J.A.; Martinez, J.; Torsello, A.; Biagini, G. Progressive seizure aggravation in the repeated 6-hz corneal stimulation model is accompanied by marked increase in hippocampal p-erk1/2 immunoreactivity in neurons. *Front. Cell. Neurosci.* **2016**, *10*, 281. [CrossRef] [PubMed]

106. Greer, P.L.; Greenberg, M.E. From synapse to nucleus: Calcium-dependent gene transcription in the control of synapse development and function. *Neuron* **2008**, *59*, 846–860. [CrossRef] [PubMed]

107. Popa-Wagner, A.; Fischer, B.; Schmoll, H.; Platt, D.; Kessler, C. Increased expression of microtubule-associated protein 1b in the hippocampus, subiculum, and perforant path of rats treated with a high dose of pentylenetetrazole. *Exp. Neurol.* **1997**, *148*, 73–82. [CrossRef] [PubMed]

108. Martinez-Levy, G.A.; Rocha, L.; Lubin, F.D.; Alonso-Vanegas, M.A.; Nani, A.; Buentello-Garcia, R.M.; Perez-Molina, R.; Briones-Velasco, M.; Recillas-Targa, F.; Perez-Molina, A.; et al. Increased expression of bdnf transcript with exon vi in hippocampi of patients with pharmaco-resistant temporal lobe epilepsy. *Neuroscience* **2016**, *314*, 12–21. [CrossRef] [PubMed]

109. Forster, E.; Naumann, T.; Deller, T.; Straube, A.; Nitsch, R.; Frotscher, M. Cholinergic sprouting in the rat fascia dentata after entorhinal lesion is not linked to early changes in neurotrophin messenger rna expression. *Neuroscience* **1997**, *80*, 731–739. [CrossRef]

110. Popa-Wagner, A.; Schroder, E.; Schmoll, H.; Walker, L.C.; Kessler, C. Upregulation of map1b and map2 in the rat brain after middle cerebral artery occlusion: Effect of age. *J. Cereb. Blood Flow Metab.* **1999**, *19*, 425–434. [CrossRef] [PubMed]

111. Schmoll, H.; Badan, I.; Grecksch, G.; Walker, L.; Kessler, C.; Popa-Wagner, A. Kindling status in sprague-dawley rats induced by pentylenetetrazole: Involvement of a critical development period. *Am. J. Pathol.* **2003**, *162*, 1027–1034. [CrossRef]

112. Kofler, N.; Kirchmair, E.; Schwarzer, C.; Sperk, G. Altered expression of npy-y1 receptors in kainic acid induced epilepsy in rats. *Neurosci. Lett.* **1997**, *230*, 129–132. [CrossRef]

113. Schwarzer, C.; Kofler, N.; Sperk, G. Up-regulation of neuropeptide y-y2 receptors in an animal model of temporal lobe epilepsy. *Mol. Pharmacol.* **1998**, *53*, 6–13. [CrossRef] [PubMed]

114. Schwarzer, C.; Williamson, J.M.; Lothman, E.W.; Vezzani, A.; Sperk, G. Somatostatin, neuropeptide y, neurokinin b and cholecystokinin immunoreactivity in two chronic models of temporal lobe epilepsy. *Neuroscience* **1995**, *69*, 831–845. [CrossRef]

115. Madsen, T.M.; Greisen, M.H.; Nielsen, S.M.; Bolwig, T.G.; Mikkelsen, J.D. Electroconvulsive stimuli enhance both neuropeptide y receptor y1 and y2 messenger rna expression and levels of binding in the rat hippocampus. *Neuroscience* **2000**, *98*, 33–39. [CrossRef]

116. Vezzani, A.; Moneta, D.; Mule, F.; Ravizza, T.; Gobbi, M.; French-Mullen, J. Plastic changes in neuropeptide y receptor subtypes in experimental models of limbic seizures. *Epilepsia* **2000**, *41* (Suppl. 6), S115–S121. [CrossRef] [PubMed]

117. Vezzani, A.; Sperk, G.; Colmers, W.F. Neuropeptide y: Emerging evidence for a functional role in seizure modulation. *Trends Neurosci.* **1999**, *22*, 25–30. [CrossRef]

118. Murphy, T.H.; Corbett, D. Plasticity during stroke recovery: From synapse to behaviour. *Nat. Rev. Neurosci.* **2009**, *10*, 861–872. [CrossRef] [PubMed]

119. Petroff, O.A. Gaba and glutamate in the human brain. *Neuroscientist* **2002**, *8*, 562–573. [CrossRef] [PubMed]

120. Martinez-Lozada, Z.; Ortega, A. Glutamatergic transmission: A matter of three. *Neural Plast.* **2015**, *2015*, 787396. [CrossRef] [PubMed]

121. Platt, S.R. The role of glutamate in central nervous system health and disease—A review. *Vet. J.* **2007**, *173*, 278–286. [CrossRef] [PubMed]

122. Foster, A.C.; Kemp, J.A. Glutamate- and gaba-based cns therapeutics. *Curr. Opin. Pharmacol.* **2006**, *6*, 7–17. [CrossRef] [PubMed]

123. Kann, O. The interneuron energy hypothesis: Implications for brain disease. *Neurobiol. Dis.* **2016**, *90*, 75–85. [CrossRef] [PubMed]

124. Stafstrom, C.E. Epilepsy comorbidities: How can animal models help? *Adv. Exp. Med. Biol.* **2014**, *813*, 273–281. [PubMed]

125. Ruediger, T.; Bolz, J. Neurotransmitters and the development of neuronal circuits. *Adv. Exp. Med. Biol.* **2007**, *621*, 104–115. [PubMed]

126. Perea, G.; Gomez, R.; Mederos, S.; Covelo, A.; Ballesteros, J.J.; Schlosser, L.; Hernandez-Vivanco, A.; Martin-Fernandez, M.; Quintana, R.; Rayan, A.; et al. Activity-dependent switch of gabaergic inhibition into glutamatergic excitation in astrocyte-neuron networks. *eLife* **2016**, *5*. [CrossRef] [PubMed]

127. Guerriero, R.M.; Giza, C.C.; Rotenberg, A. Glutamate and gaba imbalance following traumatic brain injury. *Curr. Neurol. Neurosci. Rep.* **2015**, *15*, 27. [CrossRef] [PubMed]

128. Lopez-Perez, S.J.; Urena-Guerrero, M.E.; Morales-Villagran, A. Monosodium glutamate neonatal treatment as a seizure and excitotoxic model. *Brain Res.* **2010**, *1317*, 246–256. [CrossRef] [PubMed]

129. Struzynska, L. A glutamatergic component of lead toxicity in adult brain: The role of astrocytic glutamate transporters. *Neurochem. Int.* **2009**, *55*, 151–156. [CrossRef] [PubMed]

130. Gareri, P.; Condorelli, D.; Belluardo, N.; Russo, E.; Loiacono, A.; Barresi, V.; Trovato-Salinaro, A.; Mirone, M.B.; Ferreri Ibbadu, G.; De Sarro, G. Anticonvulsant effects of carbenoxolone in genetically epilepsy prone rats (geprs). *Neuropharmacology* **2004**, *47*, 1205–1216. [CrossRef] [PubMed]

131. Rivera-Carvantes, M.C.; Jarero-Basulto, J.J.; Feria-Velasco, A.I.; Beas-Zarate, C.; Navarro-Meza, M.; Gonzalez-Lopez, M.B.; Gudino-Cabrera, G.; Garcia-Rodriguez, J.C. Changes in the expression level of mapk pathway components induced by monosodium glutamate-administration produce neuronal death in the hippocampus from neonatal rats. *Neuroscience* **2017**, *365*, 57–69. [CrossRef] [PubMed]

132. Barker-Haliski, M.; White, H.S. Glutamatergic mechanisms associated with seizures and epilepsy. *Cold Spring Harb. Perspect. Med.* **2015**, *5*, a022863. [CrossRef] [PubMed]

133. Meldrum, B.S. The role of glutamate in epilepsy and other cns disorders. *Neurology* **1994**, *44*, S14–S23. [PubMed]

134. Murguia-Castillo, J.; Beas-Zarate, C.; Rivera-Cervantes, M.C.; Feria-Velasco, A.I.; Urena-Guerrero, M.E. Nkcc1 and kcc2 protein expression is sexually dimorphic in the hippocampus and entorhinal cortex of neonatal rats. *Neurosci. Lett.* **2013**, *552*, 52–57. [CrossRef] [PubMed]

135. Kaila, K.; Ruusuvuori, E.; Seja, P.; Voipio, J.; Puskarjov, M. Gaba actions and ionic plasticity in epilepsy. *Curr. Opin. Neurobiol.* **2014**, *26*, 34–41. [CrossRef] [PubMed]

136. Dobolyi, A.; Kekesi, K.A.; Juhasz, G.; Szekely, A.D.; Lovas, G.; Kovacs, Z. Receptors of peptides as therapeutic targets in epilepsy research. *Curr. Med. Chem.* **2014**, *21*, 764–787. [CrossRef] [PubMed]

137. Vezzani, A.; Sperk, G. Overexpression of npy and y2 receptors in epileptic brain tissue: An endogenous neuroprotective mechanism in temporal lobe epilepsy? *Neuropeptides* **2004**, *38*, 245–252. [CrossRef] [PubMed]

138. Scharfman, H.E. The enigmatic mossy cell of the dentate gyrus. *Nat. Rev. Neurosci.* **2016**, *17*, 562–575. [CrossRef] [PubMed]

139. Scharfman, H.E.; Smith, K.L.; Goodman, J.H.; Sollas, A.L. Survival of dentate hilar mossy cells after pilocarpine-induced seizures and their synchronized burst discharges with area ca3 pyramidal cells. *Neuroscience* **2001**, *104*, 741–759. [CrossRef]

140. Blumcke, I.; Zuschratter, W.; Schewe, J.C.; Suter, B.; Lie, A.A.; Riederer, B.M.; Meyer, B.; Schramm, J.; Elger, C.E.; Wiestler, O.D. Cellular pathology of hilar neurons in ammon's horn sclerosis. *J. Comp. Neurol.* **1999**, *414*, 437–453. [CrossRef]

141. Curia, G.; Lucchi, C.; Vinet, J.; Gualtieri, F.; Marinelli, C.; Torsello, A.; Costantino, L.; Biagini, G. Pathophysiogenesis of mesial temporal lobe epilepsy: Is prevention of damage antiepileptogenic? *Curr. Med. Chem.* **2014**, *21*, 663–688. [CrossRef] [PubMed]

142. D'Ambrosio, R. The role of glial membrane ion channels in seizures and epileptogenesis. *Pharmacol. Ther.* **2004**, *103*, 95–108. [CrossRef] [PubMed]

143. Hinterkeuser, S.; Schroder, W.; Hager, G.; Seifert, G.; Blumcke, I.; Elger, C.E.; Schramm, J.; Steinhauser, C. Astrocytes in the hippocampus of patients with temporal lobe epilepsy display changes in potassium conductances. *Eur. J. Neurosci.* **2000**, *12*, 2087–2096. [CrossRef] [PubMed]

144. Bordey, A.; Spencer, D.D. Distinct electrophysiological alterations in dentate gyrus versus ca1 glial cells from epileptic humans with temporal lobe sclerosis. *Epilepsy Res.* **2004**, *59*, 107–122. [CrossRef] [PubMed]

145. Bowser, D.N.; Khakh, B.S. Atp excites interneurons and astrocytes to increase synaptic inhibition in neuronal networks. *J. Neurosci.* **2004**, *24*, 8606–8620. [CrossRef] [PubMed]

146. Bonansco, C.; Couve, A.; Perea, G.; Ferradas, C.A.; Roncagliolo, M.; Fuenzalida, M. Glutamate released spontaneously from astrocytes sets the threshold for synaptic plasticity. *Eur. J. Neurosci.* **2011**, *33*, 1483–1492. [CrossRef] [PubMed]

147. Du, F.; Williamson, J.; Bertram, E.; Lothman, E.; Okuno, E.; Schwarcz, R. Kynurenine pathway enzymes in a rat model of chronic epilepsy: Immunohistochemical study of activated glial cells. *Neuroscience* **1993**, *55*, 975–989. [CrossRef]

148. Vezzani, A.; Ravizza, T.; Moneta, D.; Conti, M.; Borroni, A.; Rizzi, M.; Samanin, R.; Maj, R. Brain-derived neurotrophic factor immunoreactivity in the limbic system of rats after acute seizures and during spontaneous convulsions: Temporal evolution of changes as compared to neuropeptide y. *Neuroscience* **1999**, *90*, 1445–1461. [CrossRef]

149. Ravizza, T.; Gagliardi, B.; Noe, F.; Boer, K.; Aronica, E.; Vezzani, A. Innate and adaptive immunity during epileptogenesis and spontaneous seizures: Evidence from experimental models and human temporal lobe epilepsy. *Neurobiol. Dis.* **2008**, *29*, 142–160. [CrossRef] [PubMed]

150. Crespel, A.; Coubes, P.; Rousset, M.C.; Brana, C.; Rougier, A.; Rondouin, G.; Bockaert, J.; Baldy-Moulinier, M.; Lerner-Natoli, M. Inflammatory reactions in human medial temporal lobe epilepsy with hippocampal sclerosis. *Brain Res.* **2002**, *952*, 159–169. [CrossRef]

151. Koepp, M.J.; Arstad, E.; Bankstahl, J.P.; Dedeurwaerdere, S.; Friedman, A.; Potschka, H.; Ravizza, T.; Theodore, W.H.; Baram, T.Z. Neuroinflammation imaging markers for epileptogenesis. *Epilepsia* **2017**, *58* (Suppl. 3), 11–19. [CrossRef] [PubMed]

152. Pivonkova, H.; Anderova, M. Altered homeostatic functions in reactive astrocytes and their potential as a therapeutic target after brain ischemic injury. *Curr. Pharm. Des.* **2017**, *23*, 5056–5074. [CrossRef] [PubMed]

153. Shapiro, L.A.; Wang, L.; Ribak, C.E. Rapid astrocyte and microglial activation following pilocarpine-induced seizures in rats. *Epilepsia* **2008**, *49* (Suppl. 2), 33–41. [CrossRef] [PubMed]

154. Turrin, N.P.; Rivest, S. Innate immune reaction in response to seizures: Implications for the neuropathology associated with epilepsy. *Neurobiol. Dis.* **2004**, *16*, 321–334. [CrossRef] [PubMed]

155. De Simoni, M.G.; Perego, C.; Ravizza, T.; Moneta, D.; Conti, M.; Marchesi, F.; De Luigi, A.; Garattini, S.; Vezzani, A. Inflammatory cytokines and related genes are induced in the rat hippocampus by limbic status epilepticus. *Eur. J. Neurosci.* **2000**, *12*, 2623–2633. [CrossRef] [PubMed]

156. Plata-Salaman, C.R.; Ilyin, S.E.; Turrin, N.P.; Gayle, D.; Flynn, M.C.; Romanovitch, A.E.; Kelly, M.E.; Bureau, Y.; Anisman, H.; McIntyre, D.C. Kindling modulates the il-1beta system, tnf-alpha, tgf-beta1, and neuropeptide mrnas in specific brain regions. *Brain Res. Mol. Brain Res.* **2000**, *75*, 248–258. [CrossRef]

157. Ravizza, T.; Vezzani, A. Status epilepticus induces time-dependent neuronal and astrocytic expression of interleukin-1 receptor type i in the rat limbic system. *Neuroscience* **2006**, *137*, 301–308. [CrossRef] [PubMed]

158. Arisi, G.M.; Garcia-Cairasco, N. Doublecortin-positive newly born granule cells of hippocampus have abnormal apical dendritic morphology in the pilocarpine model of temporal lobe epilepsy. *Brain Res.* **2007**, *1165*, 126–134. [CrossRef] [PubMed]

159. Overstreet-Wadiche, L.S.; Bromberg, D.A.; Bensen, A.L.; Westbrook, G.L. Seizures accelerate functional integration of adult-generated granule cells. *J. Neurosci.* **2006**, *26*, 4095–4103. [CrossRef] [PubMed]

160. Kuruba, R.; Hattiangady, B.; Shetty, A.K. Hippocampal neurogenesis and neural stem cells in temporal lobe epilepsy. *Epilepsy Behav.* **2009**, *14* (Suppl. 1), 65–73. [CrossRef] [PubMed]

161. Parent, J.M.; Yu, T.W.; Leibowitz, R.T.; Geschwind, D.H.; Sloviter, R.S.; Lowenstein, D.H. Dentate granule cell neurogenesis is increased by seizures and contributes to aberrant network reorganization in the adult rat hippocampus. *J. Neurosci.* **1997**, *17*, 3727–3738. [PubMed]

162. Scharfman, H.E.; Goodman, J.H.; Sollas, A.L. Granule-like neurons at the hilar/ca3 border after status epilepticus and their synchrony with area ca3 pyramidal cells: Functional implications of seizure-induced neurogenesis. *J. Neurosci.* **2000**, *20*, 6144–6158. [PubMed]

163. Scharfman, H.E.; Sollas, A.L.; Smith, K.L.; Jackson, M.B.; Goodman, J.H. Structural and functional asymmetry in the normal and epileptic rat dentate gyrus. *J. Comp. Neurol.* **2002**, *454*, 424–439. [CrossRef] [PubMed]

164. Scharfman, H.E.; Sollas, A.E.; Berger, R.E.; Goodman, J.H.; Pierce, J.P. Perforant path activation of ectopic granule cells that are born after pilocarpine-induced seizures. *Neuroscience* **2003**, *121*, 1017–1029. [CrossRef]

165. Hattiangady, B.; Rao, M.S.; Shetty, A.K. Chronic temporal lobe epilepsy is associated with severely declined dentate neurogenesis in the adult hippocampus. *Neurobiol. Dis.* **2004**, *17*, 473–490. [CrossRef] [PubMed]

166. Pirttila, T.J.; Lukasiuk, K.; Hakansson, K.; Grubb, A.; Abrahamson, M.; Pitkanen, A. Cystatin c modulates neurodegeneration and neurogenesis following status epilepticus in mouse. *Neurobiol. Dis.* **2005**, *20*, 241–253. [CrossRef] [PubMed]

167. Scott, B.W.; Wang, S.; Burnham, W.M.; De Boni, U.; Wojtowicz, J.M. Kindling-induced neurogenesis in the dentate gyrus of the rat. *Neurosci. Lett.* **1998**, *248*, 73–76. [CrossRef]

168. Scott, B.W.; Wojtowicz, J.M.; Burnham, W.M. Neurogenesis in the dentate gyrus of the rat following electroconvulsive shock seizures. *Exp. Neurol.* **2000**, *165*, 231–236. [CrossRef] [PubMed]

169. Gray, W.P.; Sundstrom, L.E. Kainic acid increases the proliferation of granule cell progenitors in the dentate gyrus of the adult rat. *Brain Res.* **1998**, *790*, 52–59. [CrossRef]

170. Markakis, E.A.; Gage, F.H. Adult-generated neurons in the dentate gyrus send axonal projections to field ca3 and are surrounded by synaptic vesicles. *J. Comp. Neurol.* **1999**, *406*, 449–460. [CrossRef]

171. Scharfman, H.E. Epileptogenesis in the parahippocampal region. Parallels with the dentate gyrus. *Ann. N. Y. Acad. Sci.* **2000**, *911*, 305–327. [CrossRef] [PubMed]

172. Kovacs, K.J. C-fos as a transcription factor: A stressful (re)view from a functional map. *Neurochem. Int.* **1998**, *33*, 287–297. [CrossRef]

173. Leite, J.P.; Neder, L.; Arisi, G.M.; Carlotti, C.G., Jr.; Assirati, J.A.; Moreira, J.E. Plasticity, synaptic strength, and epilepsy: What can we learn from ultrastructural data? *Epilepsia* **2005**, *46* (Suppl. 5), 134–141. [CrossRef] [PubMed]

174. Sloviter, R.S. Permanently altered hippocampal structure, excitability, and inhibition after experimental status epilepticus in the rat: The "dormant basket cell" hypothesis and its possible relevance to temporal lobe epilepsy. *Hippocampus* **1991**, *1*, 41–66. [CrossRef] [PubMed]

4

2017 FDA Peptide Harvest

Othman Al Musaimi [1,2,†] **⬤**, **Danah Al Shaer** [1,2,†] **⬤**, **Beatriz G. de la Torre** [3,*] **⬤** and **Fernando Albericio** [2,4,5,*] **⬤**

[1]   College of Health Sciences, University of KwaZulu-Natal, Durban 4000, South Africa;
      musamiau@gmail.com (O.A.M.); danah.shaer@gmail.com (D.A.S.)
[2]   School of Chemistry, University of KwaZulu-Natal, Durban 4001, South Africa
[3]   KRISP, College of Health Sciences, University of KwaZulu-Natal, Durban 4001, South Africa
[4]   CIBER-BBN, Networking Centre on Bioengineering, Biomaterials and Nanomedicine,
      University of Barcelona, 08028 Barcelona, Spain
[5]   Department of Organic Chemistry, University of Barcelona, 08028 Barcelona, Spain
*   Correspondence: garciadelatorreb@ukzn.ac.za (B.G.d.l.T.); albericio@ukzn.ac.za (F.A.)

†   These authors contributed equally to this work.

Abstract: 2017 was an excellent year in terms of new drugs (chemical entities and biologics) approved by the FDA, with a total of 46. In turn, one of the highlights was the number of peptides (six) included in this list. Here, the six peptides are analyzed in terms of chemical structure, synthetic strategy used for their production, source, therapeutic use, and mode of action.

Keywords: pharmaceutical market; drugs; drug discovery; solid-phase peptide synthesis

1. Introduction

The financial investment associated with the pharmaceutical industry is one of the largest in the industrial sector—surpassed only by the telecommunications sector. However, the number of new products (drugs) entering the market each year is relatively low. In this context, 2017 was an exceptional year, in that 46 new drugs were approved by the US Food and Drug Administration (FDA) [1]—the highest figure in the last twenty-five years. Drugs can be broadly divided into two main groups. The first encompasses biologics (12 approved in 2017, accounting for 25% of the total number of drugs approved), which are prepared by means of biotechnological techniques. The second group comprises chemical entities (34 approved in 2017), which are prepared using chemical synthesis [2]. In turn, chemical entities can be grouped into two categories, the so-called small molecules, which also include some natural products, and TIDES (peptides and oligonucleotides). Figure 1 shows the drugs approved by the FDA in 2017 and classified on the basis of their chemical structure. Thus, in a clockwise direction, biologics (antibodies, enzymes, and antibodies drug conjugates) appear first, followed by peptides, modified amino acids, and more traditional small molecules.

Along a similar line, 2017 was an excellent year for peptides, with the FDA approving five peptides and one peptidomimetic, which together accounted for 13% of the drugs accepted that year.

However, the 2017 figures should be interpreted with care. They cannot be taken as a trend since the arrival of a drug onto the market involves many unpredictable variables.

From a structural point of view, the six peptides in the 2017 harvest show almost the full range of diversity, probably lacking only a homodetic cyclic peptide and/or a cyclodepsipeptide. In this regard, in addition to a peptidomimetic macimorelin (MacrilenTM), the 2017 harvest included two linear peptides angiotensin II (GiaprezaTM) and abaloparatide (TymlosTM) with 8 and 34 amino acids, respectively, and a peptide plecanatide (TrulanceTM) containing two disulphide bridges. It also included the following two unique branched peptides: semaglutide (OzempicTM) with a chain pending at a Lys residue, which contains two mini-PEG amino acids, a Glu residue linked to the chain through the ω-carboxylic group, and a C18 diacid; and etelcalcetide (ParsabivTM), which is formed by a linear chain of seven D-amino acids with a disulphide bridge between a D-Cys with a single L-Cys. Interestingly, three of these peptides (macimorelin, abaloparatide, and semaglutide) contain a residue of the non-proteinogenic aminoisobutyric (Aib) acid, with the purpose of conferring stability against peptidases.

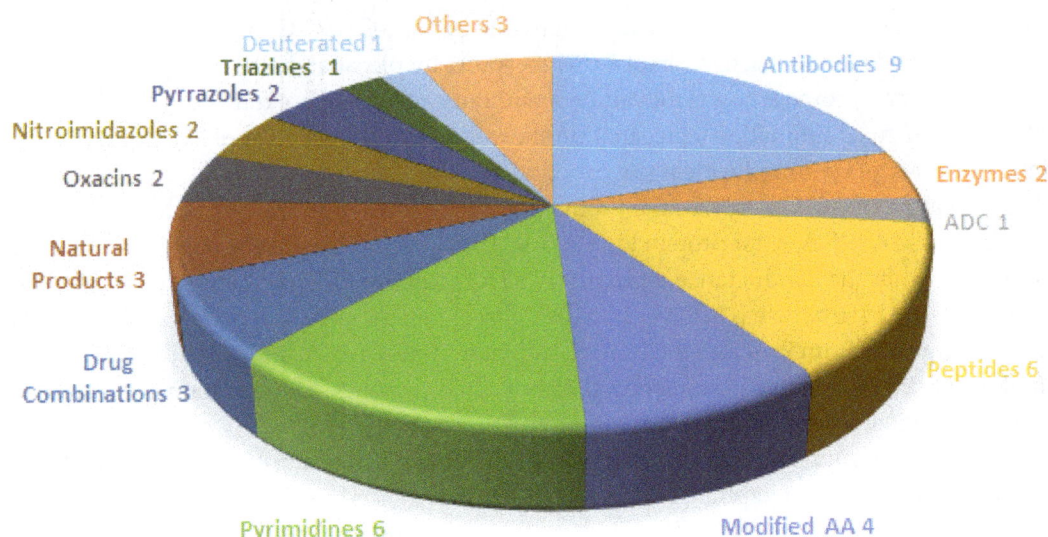

Figure 1. New drugs approved by the FDA in 2017 and classified on the basis of chemical structure.

Only one of these peptides have been developed by two so-called big pharmas (semaglutide by Novo Nordisk A/S) and the rest by biotech companies. Macimorelin had its roots in Fehrentz and Martinez's group at the University of Montpellier (France). The five peptides other than macimorelin were produced using the solid-phase technique.

2. Plecanatide (Trulance)

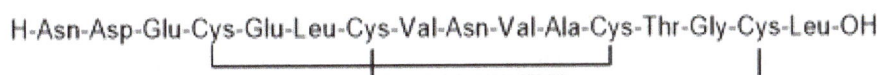

This peptide has a linear sequence of 16 amino acids with two disulphide bridges pairing Cys 4 with Cys12 and Cys7 with Cys15. Its C-terminal residue is in acid form (molecular weight of 1681.9 Da) (Figure 2a). It is manufactured using solid-phase technique.

Figure 2. Structure of (**a**) plecanatide and (**b**) the related linaclotide.

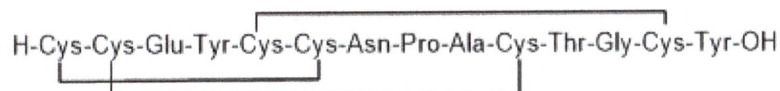

Plecanatide differs from uroguanylin (the endogenous counterpart of plecanatide) only in the replacement of Asp3 by Glu3 [3].

It was developed by Synergy Pharmaceuticals (New York City, NY, USA) and was approved by the FDA on 7 January 2017 for the treatment of chronic idiopathic constipation (CIC) and irritable bowel syndrome with constipation (IBS-C) [4]. Plecanatide is an agonist of guanylate cyclase-C, it increases intestinal transit and fluid through a build-up of guanosine $3',5'$-cyclic monophosphate (cGMP) [5] and has a similar mode of action as linaclotide (Constella-Linzess) (Figure 2b), which is a 14-amino acid peptide containing three disulphide bridges which are located between Cys1 and Cys6, between Cys2 and Cys10, and between Cys5 and Cys13. Linaclotide was approved by the FDA in 2012 [6].

Plecanatide draws water into the gastrointestinal (GI) tract, thereby softening stool and encouraging its natural passage. It activates guanylate cyclase-C (GC-C) on endothelial cells within the GI [7]. The pH-dependent activation of GC-C receptors by plecanatide (as it has the acidic residues Asp2 and Glu3) may promote bowel movements without causing severe diarrhea [3,7]. Furthermore, in molecular dynamics simulations, plecanatide showed optimal activity at pH 5, indicating that the proximal intestine (pH 5–6) is the ideal site of action [8].

The activation of GC-C catalyzes the production of the second messenger cGMP, which leads to the protein kinase A (PKA)- and protein kinase G II (PKGII)-mediated phosphorylation of the cystic fibrosis transmembrane conductance regulator (CFTR) protein [9]. Upon activation, CFTR secretes chloride ($Cl-$) and bicarbonate ($HCO3-$) into the GI tract lumen, followed by the passive secretion of positively charged sodium ions into the lumen, and water follows by osmosis [10].

In the GI tract, plecanatide is metabolized by intestinal enzymes. The excretion of plecanatide has not been studied in humans [3].

Plecanatide is administered orally as is linaclotide. These two examples showcase the feasibility of the oral administration of peptides.

3. Etelcalcetide (Parsabiv)

This is an octapeptide formed by a linear chain of seven D-amino acids containing a D-Cys, which is linked through a disulphide bridge to an L-Cys. The C-terminal residue is in amide form (molecular weight of 1048.3 Da), and it is manufactured using a solid-phase technique (Figure 3). The presence of amino acids in D configuration confers the peptide chain resistance to proteolytic degradation. The presence of disulphide bonds facilitates the biotransformation process, especially with endogenous thiols in blood, and this is considered a main metabolic pathway of etelcalcetide [11–13].

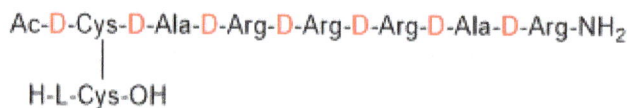

$$\text{Ac-D-Cys-D-Ala-D-Arg-D-Arg-D-Arg-D-Ala-D-Arg-NH}_2$$
$$|$$
$$\text{H-L-Cys-OH}$$

Figure 3. Structure of etelcalcetide. Amino acids of D configuration are shown in red.

Etelcalcetide was developed by KAI Pharmaceuticals Inc. (South of San Francisco, CA, USA), a wholly subsidiary of Amgen Inc. (Thousand Oaks, CA, USA) and approved by the FDA on 7 February 2017 [14]. It is used for the treatment of secondary hyperparathyroidism (SHPT) in chronic kidney disease (CKD) in adult patients on hemodialysis [11,12,15–18]. Cardiovascular calcination is common in CKD patients, and it occurs as a result of impaired mineral homeostasis and secondary hyperparathyroidism [16]. As a calcimimetic agent, etelcalcetide binds to the calcium-sensing receptor (CaSR) through a disulphide bridge between the D-Cys of the etelcalcetide molecule and L-Cys of the CaSRs, thereby enhancing activation of the receptor by means of extracellular calcium. Accordingly, activation of CaSRs on parathyroid chief cells decreases the secretion of parathyroid hormone (PTH), as well as fibroblast growth factor-23 (FGF23), which is stimulated by PTH [12,13,15–21]. Furthermore, etelcalcetide decreases phosphorus in the blood. Interestingly, high blood phosphorus occurs in vascular calcification [16].

A serious side effect of etelcalcetide is that it reduces serum calcium levels, which might lead to hypocalcemia. Therefore, monitoring serum calcium (after etelcalcetide dosing is initiated), as well as PTH, is deemed necessary [13,15,21]. Etelcalcetide can cause vomiting and nausea [11,13,20,21].

4. Abaloparatide (Tymlos)

This is a linear C-terminal amide peptide that contains 34 amino acids. The C-terminal residue is in amide form (molecular weight of 3960.7 Da) (Figure 4a). It is manufactured by a hybrid solution–solid phase approach.

Abaloparatide can be considered a second generation teriparatide (Forteo) (Figure 4b), which is a recombinant form of PTH (84 amino acids), formed by the N-terminal fragment (34 amino acids) of PTH. Abaloparatide contains exactly the same number of amino acids as teriparatide but has multiple substitutions. It has 41% homology with teriparatide [22]. Interestingly, abaloparatide has an Aib residue at position 29.

(a) Abaloparatide

H-Ala-Val-Ser-Glu-His-Gln-Leu-Leu-His-Asp-Lys-Gly-Lys-Ser-Ile-Gln-Asp-
Leu-Arg-Arg-Arg-Glu-Leu-Leu-Glu-Lys-Leu-Leu-**Aib**-Lys-Leu-His-Thr-Ala-NH$_2$

(b) Teriparatide

H-Ser-Val-Ser-Glu-Ile-Gln-Leu-Met-His-Asn-Leu-Gly-Lys-His-Leu-Asn-Ser-
Met-Glu-Arg-Val-Glu-Trp-Leu-Arg-Lys-Lys-Leu-Gln-Asp-Val-His-Asn-Phe-OH

Figure 4. Structure of (**a**) abaloparatide and (**b**) teriparatide. The residues modified are shown in red. The non-proteinogenic amino acid Aib is shown in bold.

Abaloparatide was developed by the biotech company Radius Health, Inc. (Waltham, MA, USA) and approved by the FDA on 28 April 2017 [23].

Abaloparatide works as an anabolic (bone-growing) agent through the selective activation of the parathyroid hormone 1 receptor (PTH1R), a G protein-coupled receptor (GPCR) expressed in osteoblasts and osteocytes [22]. This receptor can be present in two distinct conformation states (R0 and RG), which differ in their signaling response. Ligands that bind selectively to the RG state result in a shorter signaling response, whereas those that bind selectively to the R0 state lead to a prolonged response [24]. Abaloparatide preferentially binds to the RG state of PTH1R, which in turn elicits a transient downstream cyclic AMP signaling response towards a more anabolic signaling pathway [22,24].

Abaloparatide outperforms teriparatide as an anabolic agent, as shown by the increased messenger ribonucleic acid (RNA) expression level for the receptor activator of nuclear factor kappa-B ligand (RANKL) and macrophage colony-stimulating factor in a human osteoblastic cell line. Although the molecular mechanisms underlying the differences between abaloparatide and teriparatide are not well understood, they may be related to conformational differences that determine the affinities of the drugs for PTHR1 [22].

5. Semaglutide (Ozempic)

Semaglutide contains a linear sequence of 31 amino acids, with a moiety pending from the ε-amino function of Lys20 (the numeration of the amino acids in semaglutide is done by taking as reference the numeration in the parent peptide GLP-1), which contains a Glu residue linked to the ε-amino group of Lys side-chain through the γ-carboxylic group, two mini-PEG amino acids [8-amino-3,6-dioxaoctanoic acid (ADO)] and a C18 diacid (Figure 5a). The C-terminal is in the form of a carboxylic acid (molecular weight of 4113.6 Da). It is manufactured using a solid-phase approach.

Semaglutide is a member of the glucagon like peptide-1 (GLP-1) family, derived from the GLP-1 (sequence 7-37), and can be considered the second generation of liraglutide (Figure 5b), which was accepted by the FDA in 2010 [25]. Liraglutide differs from GLP-1 (7-37) (Figure 5b) in the presence of Arg in position 34 instead of Lys and of a moiety at Lys20, which is a reduced version of the one in semaglutide. When comparing the structures of semaglutide and liraglutide, in addition to the pending moiety, semaglutide has Aib instead of Ala in position 8, thereby reducing the susceptibility of semaglutide to degradation by dipeptidyl peptidase-4 [26–28]. Both semaglutide and liraglutide were developed by Novo Nordisk A/S (Måløv, Denmark). Semaglutide was approved by the FDA on 21 December 2017 [29].

(a) Semaglutide

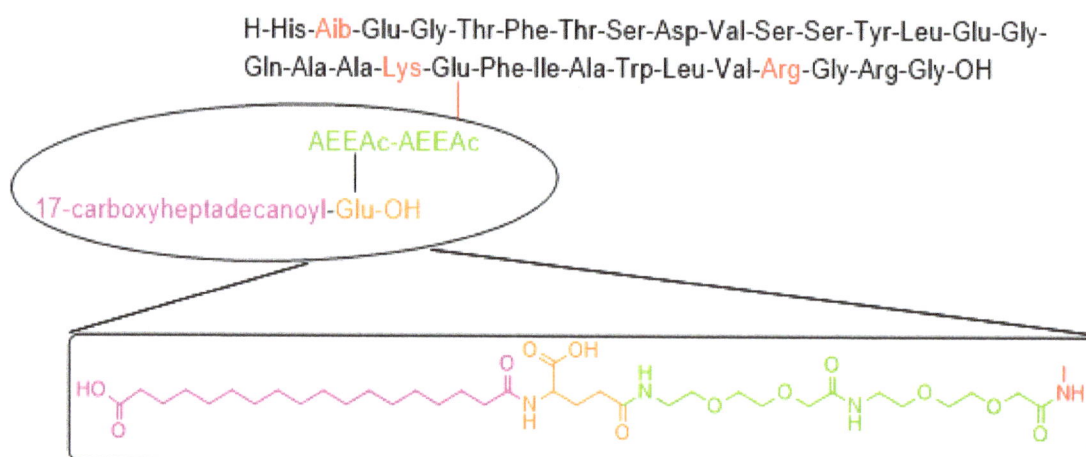

(b) Liraglutide

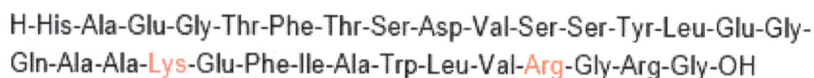

Figure 5. Structure of (**a**) semaglutide and (**b**) its related liraglutide. Changes in structure with respect to GLP-1 (7-37) are shown in color.

The GLP-1 family stimulates insulin and decreases glucagon secretion. However, GLP-1 has a short half-life (1–2 min) as a result of proteolytic degradation, thus hindering its use as a potential treatment for type 2 diabetes [27]. Liraglutide is the first once-daily glucagon-like peptide-1 analogue designed to resist enzymatic degradation and thus have a longer half-life [26,27,30]. The presence of the 17-carboxyheptadecanoyl fatty acid moiety results in its binding to human albumin, which is responsible for the longer-acting activity of liraglutide in comparison with other members of the same family. The rationale behind the design of semaglutide, which allows once-weekly administration, is to increase the affinity of the pending fatty acid moiety for albumin. Moreover, semaglutide has no serious adverse effects, only some mild gastrointestinal disorders [27].

6. Macimorelin (Macrilen)

Macimorelin is a small pseudopeptide formed by three residues: Aib as N-terminus, D-Trp at the central position, and a mimetic of D-Trp—a gem diamino moiety—which is formylated at its N-terminus (Figure 6) (molecular weight of 474.6 Da). It is prepared by solution synthesis.

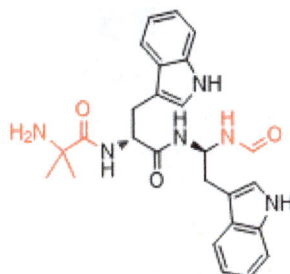

Figure 6. Structure of macimorlein. Modifications with respect to a tripeptide are shown in red.

Macimorelin was discovered by Fehrentz and Martinez's group at the University of Montpellier [31] and developed by the biotech company Aeterna Zentaris GmbH (Frankfurt, Germany). It was approved by the FDA on 20 December 2017 [32]. Administered orally, it is used for the diagnosis of adult growth hormone deficiency (AGHD).

Macimorelin acts as a growth hormone secretagogue (GHS) mimicking ghrelin, which is a 28-amino acid peptide produced by the stomach and is the endogenous ligand for this GHS receptor [31,33–36]. In addition to being orally bioavailable, macimorelin is selective, tolerable, and also safe, with only mild adverse effects—such as an unpleasant taste—being reported [34,35,37].

By acting in an almost identical manner to ghrelin [37], macimorelin outperforms other GHS such as the expensive recombinant human GH.

7. Angiotensin II (Giapreza)

Angiotensin II is a simple linear octapeptide formed by natural amino acids of the L series and its structure is identical to the human hormone of the same name. The C-terminal is in the form of carboxylic acid (molecular weight of 1046.2 Da) (Figure 7). It is manufactured using the solid-phase approach.

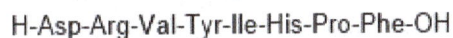

H-Asp-Arg-Val-Tyr-Ile-His-Pro-Phe-OH

Figure 7. Structure of angiotensin II.

Angiotensin II was developed by a biotech company, La Jolla Pharmaceutical Company (San Diego, CA, USA), and approved by the FDA on 21 December 2017 [38]. It is recommended as a vasoconstrictor to increase blood pressure in adults with septic or other distributive shock. It is administered intravenously because its half-life is approximately 30 s.

Angiotensin II is related to the renin–angiotensin System (RAS). From a drug discovery perspective, it can be considered unique among the drugs approved by the FDA in recent years. Its roots can be found in the last part of the XIX century, when Tigerstedt and Bergman discovered the effect of renal extracts on arterial pressure [39]. In the 1930s, two independent groups, one in Argentina with Leloir, Houssay, Fernandez Braun, among others, and that of Page in the US, discovered that RAS is the hormone system that regulates blood pressure and fluid balance [40]. In 1957, again two groups—one in the US (Schwarz and colleagues) [41] and the second in Switzerland (GIBA Geigy) [42]—described the first synthesis of angiotensin II. Seventy years after its first synthesis, this octapeptide reached the market.

Angiotensin II is formed after the removal of two C-terminal residues of angiotensin I by the angiotensin-converting enzyme (ACE). In turn, angiotensin I is the N-terminal part of angiotensinogen, an α-2-globulin produced constitutively and released into the circulation mainly by the liver.

As a summary, Table 1 shows the six peptides approved by the FDA in 2017 highlighting several parameters (chemical modification, source, therapeutic use, mode of action, and administration) that have been key to their development.

Table 1. Summary of the peptides approved by the FDA in 2017.

Generic Name (Trade Name)	Company	Mode of Action	Therapeutic Use	Administration
Plecanatide (Trulance)	Synergy Pharmaceuticals, Inc.	Activation of guanylate cyclase-C	Gastrointestinal laxative	Oral
Etelcalcetide (Parsabiv)	KAI Pharmaceuticals, Inc. *	Activation of CaSR on parathyroid chief cells	Secondary hyperpara-thyroidism in adult patients with chronic kidney disease on hemodialysis	IV
Abaloparatide (Tymlos)	Radius Health, Inc.	Selective activation of the parathyroid hormone 1 receptor	Osteoporosis	SC
Semaglutide (Ozempic)	Novo Nordisk, Inc.	Acts as a Glucagon-like Peptide-1 agonist	Treatment of type 2 diabetes mellitus	SC
Macimorelin (Macrilen)	Aeterna Zentaris, Inc.	Mimic the endogenous ligand for the secretagogue (Ghrelin)	For the diagnosis of adult growth hormone deficiency	Oral
Angiotensin II (Giapreza)	La Jolla Pharm Co.	Acts on the CNS to increase ADH production	Control of blood pressure in adults with sepsis or other critical conditions	IV

* Wholly owned subsidiary of Amgen, Inc.; IV: intra venous; SC: subcutaneous.

Finally, it is important to recall the trend of the peptide market. This market was worth US\$5.3 billion in 2003, rising to US\$8 billion in 2005 and US\$14.1 billion in 2011, and it is expected to reach a value of US\$25.4 billion and US\$46.6 billion by the end of 2018 and 2024, respectively [43–45]. Furthermore, there are currently hundreds of peptides in preclinical testing stages and around 150 peptides in clinical development. Many of these molecules are showing a promising therapeutic impact [36,43,46–48].

It is to be hoped that the coming years will bring about the approval of a similar number of peptides to those accepted by the FDA in 2017 and that the trends of the market in terms of peptide development continue, thus making these molecules one of the best options to treat many diseases.

Author Contributions: All authors have participated in searching for information, in writing the manuscript, and have approved the final version.

Acknowledgments: The work in the laboratory of the authors was funded in part by the following: National Research Foundation (NRF) (CSUR # 105892 and Blue Sky's Research Program # 110960) and the University of KwaZulu-Natal (South Africa); the Spanish Ministry of Economy, Industry and Competitiveness (MINECO) (CTQ2015-67870-P); and the Generalitat de Catalunya (2014 SGR 137) (Spain).

Conflicts of Interest: The authors declare no conflict of interest.

References

1. De la Torre, B.G.; Albericio, F. The pharmaceutical industry in 2017. An analysis of fda drug approvals from the perspective of molecules. *Molecules* **2018**, *23*, 533. [CrossRef] [PubMed]
2. Mullard, A. 2017 fda drug approvals. *Nat. Rev. Drug Discov.* **2018**, *17*, 81–85. [CrossRef] [PubMed]
3. Al-Salama, Z.T.; Syed, Y.Y. Plecanatide: First global approval. *Drugs* **2017**, *77*, 593–598. [CrossRef] [PubMed]
4. FDA. Plecanatide (Trulance) Approval Letter. 2017. Available online: https://www.accessdata.fda.gov/drugsatfda_docs/appletter/2017/208745orig1s000ltr.pdf (accessed on 3 May 2018).

5. Thomas, R.H.; Luthin, D.R. Current and emerging treatments for irritable bowel syndrome with constipation and chronic idiopathic constipation: Focus on prosecretory agents. *Pharmacotherapy* **2015**, *35*, 613–630. [CrossRef] [PubMed]

6. Góngora-Benítez, M.; Tulla-Puche, J.; Albericio, F. Constella™(eu)-linzess™(USA): The last milestone in the long journey of the peptide linaclotide and its implications for the future of peptide drugs. *Future Med. Chem.* **2013**, *5*, 291–300. [CrossRef] [PubMed]

7. Shailubhai, K.; Comiskey, S.; Foss, J.A.; Feng, R.; Barrow, L.; Comer, G.M.; Jacob, G.S. Plecanatide, an oral guanylate cyclase c agonist acting locally in the gastrointestinal tract, is safe and well-tolerated in single doses. *Dig. Dis. Sci.* **2013**, *58*, 2580–2586. [CrossRef] [PubMed]

8. Brancale, A.; Shailubhai, K.; Ferla, S.; Ricci, A.; Bassetto, M.; Jacob, G.S. Mo1316 structural and dynamic features of plecanatide: Insights from molecular dynamics simulations. *Gastroenterology* **2016**, *150*, S695. [CrossRef]

9. Hamra, F.K.; Forte, L.R.; Eber, S.L.; Pidhorodeckyj, N.V.; Krause, W.J.; Freeman, R.H.; Chinii, D.T.; Tompkinsii, J.A.; Fok, K.F.; Smith, C.E.; et al. Uroguanylin: Structure and activity of a second endogenous peptide that stimulatesintestinal guanylate cyclase. *Proc. Natl. Acad. Sci. USA* **1993**, *90*, 10464–10468. [CrossRef] [PubMed]

10. Gadsby, D.C.; Vergani, P.; Csanady, L. The abc protein turned chloride channel whose failure causes cystic fibrosis. *Nature* **2006**, *440*, 477–483. [CrossRef] [PubMed]

11. Subramanian, R.; Zhu, X.; Kerr, S.J.; Esmay, J.D.; Louie, S.W.; Edson, K.Z.; Walter, S.; Fitzsimmons, M.; Wagner, M.; Soto, M.; et al. Nonclinical pharmacokinetics, disposition, and drug-drug interaction potential of a novel d-amino acid peptide agonist of the calcium-sensing receptor amg 416 (etelcalcetide). *Drug Metab. Dispos.* **2016**, *44*, 1319–1331. [CrossRef] [PubMed]

12. Edson, K.Z.; Wu, B.M.; Iyer, A.; Goodman, W.; Skiles, G.L.; Subramanian, R. Determination of etelcalcetide biotransformation and hemodialysis kinetics to guide the timing of its dosing. *Kidney Int. Rep.* **2016**, *1*, 24–33. [CrossRef] [PubMed]

13. Cozzolino, M.; Galassi, A.; Conte, F.; Mangano, M.; Di Lullo, L.; Bellasi, A. Treatment of secondary hyperparathyroidism: The clinical utility of etelcalcetide. *Ther. Clin. Risk Manag.* **2017**, *13*, 679–689. [CrossRef] [PubMed]

14. FDA. Etelcalcetide (Parsabiv) Approval Letter. 2017. Available online: https://www.accessdata.fda.gov/drugsatfda_docs/nda/2017/208325Orig1s000Approv.pdf (accessed on 3 May 2018).

15. Baker, D.E. Formulary drug review: Etelcalcetide. *Hosp. Pharm.* **2017**, *52*, 669–674. [CrossRef] [PubMed]

16. Yu, L.; Tomlinson, J.E.; Alexander, S.T.; Hensley, K.; Han, C.Y.; Dwyer, D.; Stolina, M.; Dean, C., Jr.; Goodman, W.G.; Richards, W.G.; et al. Etelcalcetide, a novel calcimimetic, prevents vascular calcification in a rat model of renal insufficiency with secondary hyperparathyroidism. *Calcif. Tissue Int.* **2017**, *101*, 641–653. [CrossRef] [PubMed]

17. Li, X.; Yu, L.; Asuncion, F.; Grisanti, M.; Alexander, S.; Hensley, K.; Han, C.Y.; Niu, Q.T.; Dwyer, D.; Villasenor, K.; et al. Etelcalcetide (amg 416), a peptide agonist of the calcium-sensing receptor, preserved cortical bone structure and bone strength in subtotal nephrectomized rats with established secondary hyperparathyroidism. *Bone* **2017**, *105*, 163–172. [CrossRef] [PubMed]

18. Martin, K.J.; Bell, G.; Pickthorn, K.; Huang, S.; Vick, A.; Hodsman, P.; Peacock, M. Velcalcetide (amg 416), a novel peptide agonist of the calcium-sensing receptor, reduces serum parathyroid hormone and fgf23 levels in healthy male subjects. *Nephrol. Dial. Transplant.* **2014**, *29*, 385–392. [CrossRef] [PubMed]

19. Lavi-Moshayoff, V.; Wasserman, G.; Meir, T.; Silver, J.; Naveh-Many, T. PTH increases fgf23 gene expression and mediates the high-fgf23 levels of experimental kidney failure: A bone parathyroid feedback loop. *Am. J. Physiol. Renal Physiol.* **2010**, *299*, F882–F889. [CrossRef] [PubMed]

20. Block, G.A.; Bushinsky, D.A.; Cheng, S.; Cunningham, J.; Dehmel, B.; Drueke, T.B.; Ketteler, M.; Kewalramani, R.; Martin, K.J.; Moe, S.M.; et al. Effect of etelcalcetide vs cinacalcet on serum parathyroid hormone in patients receiving hemodialysis with secondary hyperparathyroidism: A randomized clinical trial. *JAMA* **2017**, *317*, 156–164. [CrossRef] [PubMed]

21. Eidman, K.E.; Wetmore, J.B. Managing hyperparathyroidism in hemodialysis: Role of etelcalcetide. *Int. J. Nephrol. Renovasc. Dis.* **2018**, *11*, 69–80. [CrossRef] [PubMed]

22. Tella, S.H.; Kommalapati, A.; Correa, R. Profile of abaloparatide and its potential in the treatment of postmenopausal osteoporosis. *Cureus* **2017**, *9*, e1300. [CrossRef] [PubMed]

23. FDA. Abaloparatide (Tymlos) Approval Letter. 2017. Available online: https://www.accessdata.fda.gov/drugsatfda_docs/nda/2017/208743Orig1s000Approv.pdf (accessed on 3 May 2018).

24. Yang, L.; Morriello, G.; Pan, Y.; Nargund, R.P.; Barakat, K.; Prendergast, K.; Cheng, K.; Chan, W.W.-S.; Smith, R.G.; Patchett, A.A. Tripeptide growth hormone secretagogues. *Bioorg. Med. Chem. Lett.* **1998**, *8*, 759–764. [CrossRef]

25. FDA. Liraglutide Approval Letter. 2010. Available online: https://www.accessdata.fda.gov/drugsatfda_docs/label/2017/022341s027lbl.pdf (accessed on 3 May 2018).

26. Lau, J.; Bloch, P.; Schaffer, L.; Pettersson, I.; Spetzler, J.; Kofoed, J.; Madsen, K.; Knudsen, L.B.; McGuire, J.; Steensgaard, D.B.; et al. Discovery of the once-weekly glucagon-like peptide-1 (glp-1) analogue semaglutide. *J. Med. Chem.* **2015**, *58*, 7370–7380. [CrossRef] [PubMed]

27. Jensen, L.; Helleberg, H.; Roffel, A.; van Lier, J.J.; Bjornsdottir, I.; Pedersen, P.J.; Rowe, E.; Derving Karsbol, J.; Pedersen, M.L. Absorption, metabolism and excretion of the glp-1 analogue semaglutide in humans and nonclinical species. *Eur. J. Pharm. Sci.* **2017**, *104*, 31–41. [CrossRef] [PubMed]

28. Pratley, R.E.; Aroda, V.R.; Lingvay, I.; Lüdemann, J.; Andreassen, C.; Navarria, A.; Viljoen, A. Semaglutide versus dulaglutide once weekly in patients with type 2 diabetes (sustain 7): A randomised, open-label, phase 3b trial. *Lancet Diabetes Endocrinol.* **2018**, 1–12. [CrossRef]

29. FDA. Semaglutide (Ozempic) Approval Letter. 2017. Available online: https://www.accessdata.fda.gov/drugsatfda_docs/appletter/2017/209637s000ltr.pdf (accessed on 3 May 2018).

30. Jacobsen, L.V.; Flint, A.; Olsen, A.K.; Ingwersen, S.H. Liraglutide in type 2 diabetes mellitus: Clinical pharmacokinetics and pharmacodynamics. *Clin. Pharmacokinet.* **2016**, *55*, 657–672. [CrossRef] [PubMed]

31. Guerlavais, V.; Boeglin, D.; Mousseaux, D.; Oiry, C.; Heitz, A.; Deghenghi, R.; Locatelli, V.; Torsello, A.; Ghé, C.; Catapano, F.; et al. New Active Series of Growth Hormone Secretagogues. *J. Med. Chem.* **2003**, *46*, 1196–1203. [CrossRef] [PubMed]

32. FDA. Macimorelin (Macimorelin) Approval Letter. 2017. Available online: https://www.accessdata.fda.gov/drugsatfda_docs/nda/2017/205598Orig1s000Approv.pdf (accessed on 3 May 2018).

33. Garcia, J.M.; Swerdloff, R.; Wang, C.; Kyle, M.; Kipnes, M.; Biller, B.M.; Cook, D.; Yuen, K.C.; Bonert, V.; Dobs, A.; et al. Macimorelin (aezs-130)-stimulated growth hormone (gh) test: Validation of a novel oral stimulation test for the diagnosis of adult gh deficiency. *J. Clin. Endocrinol. Metab.* **2013**, *98*, 2422–2429. [CrossRef] [PubMed]

34. Broglio, F.; Boutignon, F.; Benso, A.; Gottero, C.; Prodam, F.; Arvat, E.; Ghè, C.; Catapano, F.; Torsello, A.; Locatelli, V.; et al. Ep1572: A novel peptido-mimetic gh secretagogue with potent and selective gh-releasing activity in man. *J. Endocrinol. Investig.* **2002**, *25*, RC26–RC28. [CrossRef] [PubMed]

35. Kojima, M.; Hosoda, H.; Matsuo, H.; Kangawa, K. Ghrelin: Discovery of the natural endogenous ligand for the growth hormone secretagogue receptor. *Trends Endocrinol. Metab.* **2001**, *12*, 118–126. [CrossRef]

36. Varamini, P.; Toth, I. Recent advances in oral delivery of peptide hormones. *Expert Opin. Drug Deliv.* **2016**, *13*, 507–522. [CrossRef] [PubMed]

37. Piccoli, F.; Degen, L.; MacLean, C.; Peter, S.; Baselgia, L.; Larsen, F.; Beglinger, C.; Drewe, J. Pharmacokinetics and pharmacodynamic effects of an oral ghrelin agonist in healthy subjects. *J. Clin. Endocrinol. Metab.* **2007**, *92*, 1814–1820. [CrossRef] [PubMed]

38. FDA. Angiotensin II (Giapreza) Aproval Letter. 2017. Available online: https://www.accessdata.fda.gov/drugsatfda_docs/nda/2017/209360Orig1s000Approv.pdf (accessed on 3 May 2018).

39. Tigerstedt, R.; Bergman, P.G. Niere und kreislauf. *Arch. Physiol.* **1898**, *8*, 223–271. [CrossRef]

40. Basso, N.; Terragno, N.A. History about the discovery of the renin-angiotensin system. *Hypertension* **2001**, *38*, 1246–1249. [CrossRef] [PubMed]

41. Schwarz, H.; Bumpus, F.M.; Page, I.H. Synthesis of a biologically active octapeptide similar to natural isoleucine angiotonin octapeptide. *J. Am. Chem. Soc.* **1957**, *79*, 5697–5703. [CrossRef]

42. Rittel, W.; Iselin, B.; Kappeler, H.; Riniker, B.; Schwyzer, R. Synthese eines hochwirksamen Hypertensin II-amids (L-Asparaginyl-L-arginyl-L-valyl-L-tyrosyl-L-isoleucyl-L-histidyl-L-prolyl-L-phenylalanin). *Helvetica Chim. Acta* **1957**, *40*, 614–624. [CrossRef]

43. Fosgerau, K.; Hoffmann, T. Peptide therapeutics: Current status and future directions. *Drug Discov. Today* **2015**, *20*, 122–128. [CrossRef] [PubMed]

44. Kaur, K.; Singh, I.; Kaur, P.; Kaur, R. Food and drug administration (fda) approved peptide drugs. *Asian J. Res. Biol. Pharm. Sci.* **2015**, *3*, 75–88.

45. Ghosh, S. Peptide therapeutics market: Forecast and analysis 2015–2025. *Oligos Pept. Chim. Oggi Chem. Today* **2016**, *34*, 5–7.

46. Albericio, F.; Kruger, H.G. Therapeutic peptides. *Future Med. Chem.* **2012**, *4*, 1527–1531. [CrossRef] [PubMed]

47. Lau, J.L.; Dunn, M.K. Therapeutic peptides: Historical perspectives, current development trends, and future directions. *Bioorg. Med. Chem.* **2017**. [CrossRef] [PubMed]

48. Henninot, A.; Collins, J.C.; Nuss, J.M. The current state of peptide drug discovery: Back to the future? *J. Med. Chem.* **2018**, *61*, 1382–1414. [CrossRef] [PubMed]

5

Controlled-Deactivation CB1 Receptor Ligands as a Novel Strategy to Lower Intraocular Pressure

Sally Miller [1], Shashank Kulkarni [2,†], Alex Ciesielski [1], Spyros P. Nikas [2] ⓘ, Ken Mackie [1], Alexandros Makriyannis [2] and Alex Straiker [1,*]

[1] The Gill Center for Biomolecular Science, The Department of Psychological and Brain Sciences, Indiana University, Bloomington, IN 47405, USA; sallmill@indiana.edu (S.M.); agciesie@umail.iu.edu (A.C.); kmackie@indiana.edu (K.M.)

[2] Center for Drug Discovery, Departments of Chemistry & Chemical Biology and Pharmaceutical Sciences, Northeastern University, Boston, MA 02115, USA; kulkarni.sha@northeastern.edu (S.K.); s.nikas@northeastern.edu (S.P.N.); a.makriyannis@northeastern.edu (A.M.)

* Correspondence: straiker@indiana.edu

† Present affiliation: EMD Serono R&D Institute, Billerica, MA 01821, USA.

Abstract: Nearly half a century has passed since the demonstration that cannabis and its chief psychoactive component Δ^9-THC lowers intraocular pressure (IOP). Elevated IOP remains the chief hallmark and therapeutic target for glaucoma, a condition that places millions at risk of blindness. It is likely that Δ^9-THC exerts much of its IOP-lowering effects via the activation of CB1 cannabinoid receptors. However, the initial promise of CB1 as a target for treating glaucoma has not thus far translated into a credible therapeutic strategy. We have recently shown that blocking monoacylglycerol lipase (MAGL), an enzyme that breaks the endocannabinoid 2-arachidonoyl glycerol (2-AG), substantially lowers IOP. Another strategy is to develop cannabinoid CB1 receptor agonists that are optimized for topical application to the eye. Recently we have reported on a controlled-deactivation approach where the "soft" drug concept of enzymatic deactivation was combined with a "depot effect" that is commonly observed with Δ^9-THC and other lipophilic cannabinoids. This approach allowed us to develop novel cannabinoids with a predictable duration of action and is particularly attractive for the design of CB1 activators for ophthalmic use with limited or no psychoactive effects. We have tested a novel class of compounds using a combination of electrophysiology in autaptic hippocampal neurons, a well-characterized model of endogenous cannabinoid signaling, and measurements of IOP in a mouse model. We now report that AM7410 is a reasonably potent and efficacious agonist at CB1 in neurons and that it substantially (30%) lowers IOP for as long as 5 h after a single topical treatment. This effect is absent in CB1 knockout mice. Our results indicate that the direct targeting of CB1 receptors with controlled-deactivation ligands is a viable approach to lower IOP in a murine model and merits further study in other model systems.

Keywords: cannabinoid; glaucoma; ocular pressure; CB1

1. Introduction

Nearly half a century has passed since the demonstration that cannabis and its chief psychoactive component Δ^9-THC lowers intraocular pressure (IOP) [1]. Elevated IOP remains the chief hallmark and therapeutic target for glaucoma, a condition that places millions at risk of blindness. It is likely that Δ^9-THC exerts much of its IOP-lowering effects via the activation of the cannabinoid signaling system (reviewed in [2]), particularly CB1 cannabinoid receptors since it is an agonist at CB1 [3] and CB1 activation lowers ocular pressure [4]. However, the initial promise of CB1 as a target for treating glaucoma has not thus far translated into a credible therapeutic strategy. We have recently shown that blocking monoacylglycerol lipase (MAGL), an enzyme that breaks the endocannabinoid 2-arachidonoyl glycerol (2-AG), substantially lowers IOP for 8 h [5]. Another strategy is to develop cannabinoid CB1 receptor agonists that are optimized for topical application to the eye. THC and related synthetic cannabinoids are reported to only modestly and briefly reduce IOP and risk ocular irritation and toxicity, as well as having the potential for unwanted CNS side effects [6–8]. Furthermore, the design of drugs for topical ocular application requires improvements in the bioactivity of the compound with a balance of physicochemical properties for enhanced corneal permeability and ocular bioavailability [7,9]. In this regard, the major problem with the currently known classical cannabinoids is their high lipophilicity (e.g., cLogP > 9 for (-)-Δ^8-THC-DMH, **1**, Figure 1), and this needs to be improved while maintaining or enhancing in vivo efficacy. Recently, we reported on a controlled-deactivation approach where the "soft" drug concept of enzymatic deactivation was combined with a "depot effect" which is related to the compound's lipophilicity as well as its tissue distribution and retention [10–13]. Specifically, we have shown that the incorporation of a metabolically labile carboxy ester group (soft spot) at strategic positions within the THC structure leads to potent and efficacious CB1 agonists (**2**, Figure 1) that are bioconverted to inactive metabolites (**3**) by plasma esterases. Importantly, the rate of hydrolytic cleavage can be accordingly modulated using stereochemical features adjacent to the ester group (enzymatic effect) [10,11]. The depot effect is dependent on the compound's polar characteristics and can be regulated by varying its log P and polar surface area (PSA) values [10,11,13]. This controlled-deactivation approach allowed us to develop novel cannabinoids with a predictable duration of action and an improved druggability, and it is particularly attractive for the design of CB1 activators for ophthalmic use with limited or no psychoactive effects. These potent CB1 agonists are expected to exhibit greater ocular tissue exposure because of their enhanced polarity, and after achieving their therapeutic effect in the eye, they will be deactivated in the blood circulation by esterases.

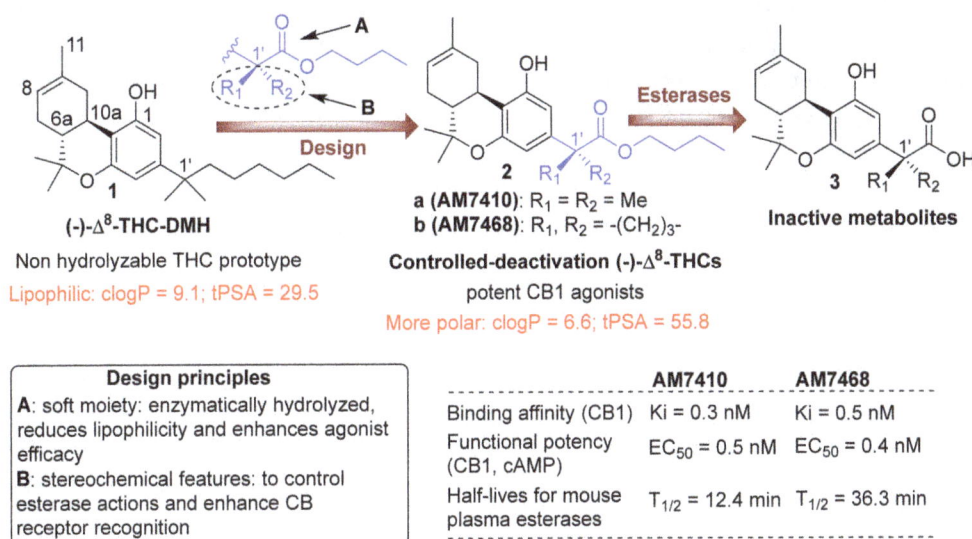

Figure 1. Top panel: design of first-generation side chain carboxylated cannabinoid analogs, with controllable deactivation and increasing polarity, and structures of the prototype (-)-Δ^8-THC-DMH and inactive metabolites. Lower panel: design principles and biological activity data for representative analogs.

We have tested this novel class of compounds using a combination of electrophysiology in autaptic hippocampal neurons, a well-characterized model of endogenous cannabinoid signaling, and measurements of IOP in a normotensive mouse model.

2. Methods

2.1. Animals

Experiments were conducted at the Indiana University campus. All mice used for IOP experiments were handled according to the guidelines of the Indiana University animal care committee (ethics committee name: BIACUC, protocol number: 16-007). Mice (age 3–8 months) were kept on a 12 h (06:00–18:00) light–dark cycle and fed *ad libitum*. Only male mice were used for these experiments and were obtained from Envigo (Indianapolis, IN, USA) or were kindly provided by Dr. Ken Mackie (Indiana University, Bloomington, IN, USA). The mice were C57BL/6J (C57) strain except CB1$^{-/-}$ mice that were on a CD1 strain background. We have previously shown that mice on a CD1 background see a drop in ocular pressure upon topical treatment with CB1 cannabinoid agonists WIN55212 and CP55940 that are absent in CB1 knockouts [4]. Mice were allowed to acclimatize to the animal care facility for at least a week prior to their use in experiments. CB1$^{-/-}$ mice were kindly provided by Dr. Ken Mackie. The knockouts are global knockouts. CB1$^{-/-}$ animals were originally received from Dr. Catherine Ledent (Catholic University, Leuven, Belgium) as heterozygotes [14].

2.2. Intraocular Pressure Measurements

The IOP was measured in mice by rebound tonometry using a Tonolab (Icare Finland Oy, Helsinki, Finland). This instrument uses a light plastic-tipped probe to briefly make contact with the cornea; after the probe encounters the eye the instrument measures the speed at which the probe rebounds in order to calculate IOP.

To obtain reproducible IOP measurements, mice were anesthetized with isoflurane (3% induction). The anesthetized mouse was then placed on a platform in a prone position, where anesthesia was maintained with 2% isoflurane. Baseline IOP measurements were taken in both eyes. A 'measurement' consisted of the average value of six readings. One eye was then treated with the drug dissolved in Tocrisolve (Tocris Biosciences, Bristol, UK), a soya-based solvent [15], 5 μL final volume applied topically) while the other eye was treated with the vehicle. The animal was then allowed to recover. After an hour, the animal was again anesthetized as above. The IOP was then measured in the drug-treated and the vehicle-treated contralateral eye.

The IOP measurements following drug administration were analyzed by paired t-tests comparing drug-treated eyes to the contralateral vehicle-treated eyes. In animals that were injected with the drug, the ocular pressures of animals were compared with those of vehicle-injected animals and compared using an unpaired t-test.

2.3. Hippocampal Culture Preparation

Mouse hippocampal neurons isolated from the CA1–CA3 region were cultured on microislands as described previously [16,17]. Neurons were obtained from animals (age postnatal day 0–2) and plated onto a feeder layer of hippocampal astrocytes that had been laid down previously [18]. Cultures were grown in high-glucose (20 mM) Dulbecco's Modified Eagle's Medium (DMEM) that contained 10% horse serum, had no mitotic inhibitors, and was used for recordings after eight days in culture and for no more than three hours after removal from the culture medium.

2.4. Electrophysiology

When a single neuron is grown on a small island of permissive substrate, it forms synapses—or "autapses"—onto itself. All experiments were performed on isolated autaptic neurons. Whole cell voltage-clamp recordings from autaptic neurons were carried out at room temperature using an Axopatch 200A amplifier (Molecular Devices, Sunnyvale, CA, USA). The extracellular solution contained (in mM) 119 NaCl, 5 KCl, 2.5 CaCl$_2$, 1.5 MgCl$_2$, 30 glucose, and 20 HEPES. A continuous flow of solution through the bath chamber (~2 mL/min) ensured rapid drug application and clearance.

Drugs were typically prepared as stocks, and then they were diluted into an extracellular solution at their final concentration and used on the same day.

Recording pipettes of 1.8–3 MΩ were filled with (in mM) 121.5 KGluconate, 17.5 KCl, 9 NaCl, 1 MgCl$_2$, 10 HEPES, 0.2 EGTA, 2 MgATP, and 0.5 LiGTP. The access resistance and the holding current were monitored and only cells with both a stable access resistance and a holding current were included for data analysis. The conventional stimulus protocol was as follows: the membrane potential was held at −70 mV, and the excitatory postsynaptic currents (EPSCs) were evoked every 20 s by triggering an unclamped action current with a 1.0 ms depolarizing step. The resultant evoked waveform consisted of a brief stimulus artifact and a large downward spike representing inward sodium currents, followed by the slower EPSC. The size of the recorded EPSCs was calculated by integrating the evoked current to yield a charge value (in pC). Calculating the charge value in this manner yields an indirect measure of the amount of neurotransmitter released while minimizing the effects of cable distortion on currents generated far from the site of the recording electrode (the soma). Data were acquired at a sampling rate of 5 kHz.

The depolarisation suppression of excitation (DSE) stimuli was as follows: After establishing a 10–20 s 0.5 Hz baseline, the DSE was evoked by depolarizing to 0 mV for 50 ms, 100 ms, 300 ms, 500 ms, 1 s, 3 s, and 10 s, followed in each case by the resumption of a 0.5 Hz stimulus protocol for 20–80+ s, allowing EPSCs to recover to baseline values. This approach allowed us to determine the sensitivity of the synapses to DSE induction. To allow for a comparison, baseline values (prior to the DSE stimulus) were normalized to one. DSE inhibition values were presented as fractions of 1, i.e., a 50% inhibition from the baseline response was $0.50 \pm$ standard error of the mean. The x-axis of DSE depolarization–response curves are log-scale seconds of the duration of the depolarization used to elicit the DSE. Depolarization–response curves were obtained to determine the pharmacological properties of endogenous 2-AG signaling by depolarizing neurons for progressively longer durations (50 ms, 100 ms, 300 ms, 500 ms, 1 s, 3 s, and 10 s). The data were fitted with a nonlinear regression, allowing for a calculation of an ED50, the effective dose or duration of depolarization at which a 50% inhibition is achieved. Statistical significance in these curves was taken as non-overlapping 95% confidence intervals.

3. Results

3.1. AM7410 as a Controlled-Deactivation CB1 Ligand

Through the controlled-deactivation ligand development project we have identified the 1′-gem-dimethyl analog AM7410, which exhibits remarkably high affinities for both CB1 and CB2 receptors (Figure 1). The ligand is susceptible to enzymatic hydrolysis by plasma esterases while its metabolite (AM7408) is inactive at the CB receptors. In further in vitro and in vivo experiments, AM7410 was shown to be a potent CB1 receptor agonist and exhibited CB1-mediated hypothermic and analgesic effects.

3.2. AM7410 Is a Potent and Efficacious Ligand at CB1 Receptors

We tested the activity of AM7410 in an endogenous neuronal model of cannabinoid signaling. Autaptic hippocampal neurons are a simple, well-characterized preparation that comprises a full circuit of cannabinoid signaling since these neurons produce 2-AG post-synaptically [19], which then acts on presynaptic CB1 receptors, which in turn suppress neurotransmitter release [20]. This retrograde synaptic plasticity is induced by a brief depolarization of the neuron (see Methods) and is termed depolarization induced suppression of excitation or inhibition (DSE/DSI) depending on the neurotransmitter in question [21]. The suppression of neurotransmitter release by a study drug can thus be compared to the suppression elicited by endogenously released 2-AG. As shown in Figure 2, we tested AM7410 at 1 nM, 10 nM, 100 nM, and 1 uM ($n = 6$ at each concentration), which yielded an EC50 of 6.2 nM, which is comparable to our results for WIN55212 [20]. The maximal inhibition due to treatment with AM7410 was similar to that for the maximal inhibition of neurotransmission seen with DSE (relative EPSC charge after AM7410: 0.52 ± 0.07, $n = 6$; after DSE: 0.48 ± 0.07, $n = 6$). Thus, AM7410 is both a potent and efficacious activator of CB1 cannabinoid receptors in this neuronal system.

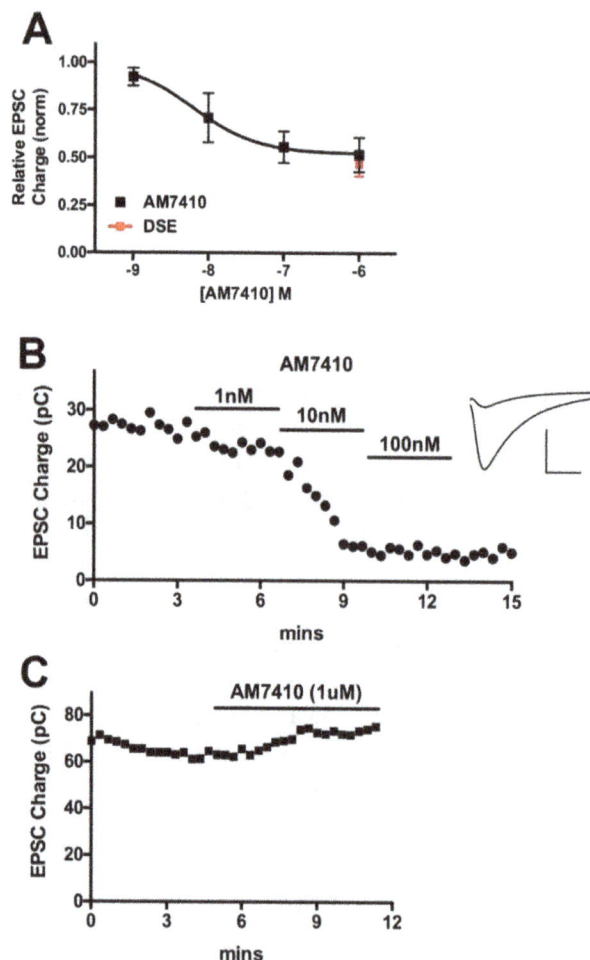

Figure 2. AM7410 is a potent and efficacious CB1 receptor agonist. (**A**) AM7410 inhibits excitatory neurotransmission in autaptic hippocampal neurons in a concentration-dependent manner. Maximal inhibition is similar to maximal inhibition from DSE in the same neurons; (**B**) Time course shows time course of inhibition of EPSCs after treatment with various concentrations of AM7410. Inset shows sample EPSCs before treatment and after treatment with 100 nM AM7410; (**C**) Sample time course shows absence of AM7410 effect in CB1$^{-/-}$ neuron.

3.3. AM7410 Lowers Ocular Pressure in a Normotensive Mouse Model

We tested whether the topical application of AM7410 would lower intraocular pressure using rebound tonometry in a normotensive mouse model. The mouse is an established model system for the study of IOP [22,23], offering access to assorted genetic mutants such as CB1 knockout mice, among other things. We have made use of this system in several studies of the regulation of ocular pressure by endocannabinoids [5,24].

We found that AM7410 applied topically at 3 mM in mice did not lower IOP at 1 h but reduced IOP by 30% at 5 h relative to vehicle-treated contralateral eyes (Figure 3A,B, $n = 7, 7$). This effect was absent in CB1 knockout mice (Figure 3C,D, $n = 8, 8$). We also tested the inactive metabolite of AM7410, AM7408, at 5 h and found it to have no effect (Figure 3E, $n = 8$). 3 mM was chosen because the cornea represents a formidable barrier to drug penetration, necessitating high topical concentrations to assure that a sufficient amount of a given drug penetrates to the intraocular target. Therapeutic topical concentrations of approved glaucoma drugs range as high as 2% (e.g., dorzolamide [25]).

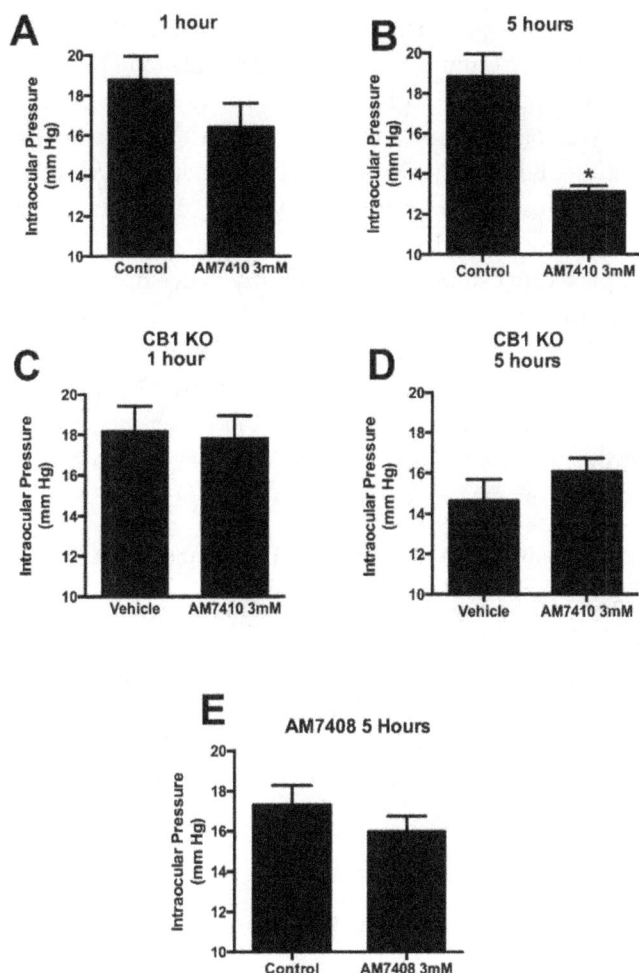

Figure 3. AM7410 lowers intraocular pressure in a normotensive model. (**A,B**) AM7410 applied topically at 3 mM lowers ocular pressure at 5 h post-treatment; (**C,D**) The effect of AM7410 on ocular pressure is absent in CB1 knockout (KO) mice; (**E**) The inactive metabolite AM7408 does not lower ocular pressure at 5 h. *, $p < 0.05$ by paired t-test.

4. Discussion

Our chief findings are that the controlled-deactivation CB1 ligand AM7410 is a potent and efficacious agonist at CB1 in a neuronal model of endogenous cannabinoid signaling and that this compound, when applied topically in a normotensive mouse model, substantially reduces intraocular pressure (IOP) by 30% 5 h after treatment, while its metabolite has no effect.

There are currently six classes of drugs available for the treatment of glaucoma through the lowering of ocular pressure. Not all patients respond to a given drug, and each drug has its own side effect profile (including itching, burning, redness, and altered eye color) that proves to be intolerable in some patients. In addition, because glaucoma is a lifelong disease requiring one or more treatments with eye drops each day, patients develop tolerance to some treatments. There is therefore a continued need for the development of new treatments to effectively lower ocular pressure, but it is generally held that the bar for entry of a new compound is high, with the expectation that a new entrant substantially lowers IOP. AM7410 represents an example of a cannabinoid-based compound that fulfills this expectation, with a 30% drop in IOP in a normotensive model.

The eye is an ideal setting for the use of a controlled-deactivation ligand. Designed to be rapidly metabolized in the bloodstream, this compound can be applied topically and is allowed to cross the cornea into the ocular chamber where it acts. Once it enters the capillary beds of various ocular tissues, the compound exerts its pharmacological action and is converted to AM7408, a compound that did not lower IOP when applied topically (Figure 2). It may be possible to regulate the duration of the effect of a controlled-deactivation ligand by a rational molecular design of the ligand, thus "tuning" the duration of action. This is supported, for example, by in vitro data comparing the half-lives for plasma esterases of the 1′-gem-dimethyl analog AM7410 and its bulkier 1′-cyclobutyl counterpart AM7468 (Figure 1), as well as by in vivo work we published earlier [10,11]. An additional advantage of the controlled-deactivation CB1 agonists is that they allow structural modifications to produce very polar cannabinoids that are expected to exhibit higher solubility in eye drop preparations as well as in the tears, which results in an increased ocular absorption and ocular drug bioavailability [9,10,13].

In summary, we find that the controlled-deactivation CB1 ligand AM7410 is a potent and efficacious agonist at CB1 in neurons and that it substantially (30%) lowers IOP at least 5 h after a single topical treatment. Our results indicate that the direct targeting of CB1 receptors with controlled-deactivation ligands is a viable approach to lower IOP in a murine model and merits further study in other model systems.

Author Contributions: Conceptualization, A.S., A.M., and S.P.N.; Methodology, A.S.; Formal Analysis, S.M., A.S.; Investigation, A.S., A.C., S.M.; Resources, S.K., A.M., K.M., and S.P.N.; Data Curation, A.S.; Writing-Original Draft Preparation, A.S.; Writing-Review & Editing, S.P.N., A.M. and K.M.; Project Administration, A.S., A.M. and S.P.N.; Funding Acquisition, A.S., A.M. and K.M.

Acknowledgments: This work was supported by grants from the National Institute on Drug Abuse, DA009158 (AM), DA007215 (AM), DA09064 (AM), DA021696 (KM), and the NEI, EY24625 (AS).

Conflicts of Interest: The authors declare no conflict of interest. The funding sponsors had no role in the design of the study; in the collection, analyses, or interpretation of data; in the writing of the manuscript, and in the decision to publish the results

References

1. Hepler, R.S.; Frank, I.R. Marihuana smoking and intraocular pressure. *JAMA* **1971**, *217*, 1392. [CrossRef] [PubMed]

2. Piomelli, D. The molecular logic of endocannabinoid signalling. *Nat. Rev. Neurosci.* **2003**, *4*, 873–884. [CrossRef] [PubMed]

3. Matsuda, L.A.; Lolait, S.J.; Brownstein, M.J.; Young, A.C.; Bonner, T.I. Structure of a cannabinoid receptor and functional expression of the cloned cDNA. *Nature* **1990**, *346*, 561–564. [CrossRef] [PubMed]

4. Hudson, B.D.; Beazley, M.; Szczesniak, A.M.; Straiker, A.; Kelly, M.E. Indirect sympatholytic actions at beta-adrenoceptors account for the ocular hypotensive actions of cannabinoid receptor agonists. *J. Pharmacol. Exp. Ther.* **2011**, *339*, 757–767. [CrossRef] [PubMed]

5. Miller, S.; Leishman, E.; Hu, S.S.; Elghouche, A.; Daily, L.; Murataeva, N.; Bradshaw, H.; Straiker, A. Harnessing the Endocannabinoid 2-Arachidonoylglycerol to Lower Intraocular Pressure in a Murine Model. *Investig. Ophthalmol. Vis. Sci.* **2016**, *57*, 3287–3296. [CrossRef] [PubMed]

6. Cairns, E.A.; Toguri, J.T.; Porter, R.F.; Szczesniak, A.M.; Kelly, M.E. Seeing over the horizon—Targeting the endocannabinoid system for the treatment of ocular disease. *J. Basic Clin. Physiol. Pharmacol.* **2016**, *27*, 253–265. [CrossRef] [PubMed]

7. Jarvinen, T.; Pate, D.W.; Laine, K. Cannabinoids in the treatment of glaucoma. *Pharmacol. Ther.* **2002**, *95*, 203–220. [CrossRef]

8. Panahi, Y.; Manayi, A.; Nikan, M.; Vazirian, M. The arguments for and against cannabinoids application in glaucomatous retinopathy. *Biomed. Pharmacother.* **2017**, *86*, 620–627. [CrossRef] [PubMed]

9. Shirasaki, Y. Molecular design for enhancement of ocular penetration. *J. Pharm. Sci.* **2008**, *97*, 2462–2496. [CrossRef] [PubMed]

10. Nikas, S.P.; Sharma, R.; Paronis, C.A.; Kulkarni, S.; Thakur, G.A.; Hurst, D.; Wood, J.T.; Gifford, R.S.; Rajarshi, G.; Liu, Y.; et al.   Probing the carboxyester side chain in controlled deactivation (−)-delta(8)-tetrahydrocannabinols. *J. Med. Chem.* **2015**, *58*, 665–681. [CrossRef] [PubMed]

11. Sharma, R.; Nikas, S.P.; Paronis, C.A.; Wood, J.T.; Halikhedkar, A.; Guo, J.J.; Thakur, G.A.; Kulkarni, S.; Benchama, O.; Raghav, J.G.; et al. Controlled-deactivation cannabinergic ligands. *J. Med. Chem.* **2013**, *56*, 10142–10157. [CrossRef] [PubMed]

12. Sharma, R.; Nikas, S.P.; Guo, J.J.; Mallipeddi, S.; Wood, J.T.; Makriyannis, A. C-ring cannabinoid lactones: A novel cannabinergic chemotype. *ACS Med. Chem. Lett.* **2014**, *5*, 400–404. [CrossRef] [PubMed]

13. Kulkarni, S.; Nikas, S.P.; Sharma, R.; Jiang, S.; Paronis, C.A.; Leonard, M.Z.; Zhang, B.; Honrao, C.; Mallipeddi, S.; Raghav, J.G.; et al. Novel C-Ring-Hydroxy-Substituted Controlled Deactivation Cannabinergic Analogues. *J. Med. Chem.* **2016**, *59*, 6903–6919. [CrossRef] [PubMed]

14. Ledent, C.; Valverde, O.; Cossu, G.; Petitet, F.; Aubert, J.F.; Beslot, F.; Böhme, G.A.; Imperato, A.; Pedrazzini, T.; Roques, B.P.; et al. Unresponsiveness to cannabinoids and reduced addictive effects of opiates in CB1 receptor knockout mice. *Science* **1999**, *283*, 401–404. [CrossRef] [PubMed]

15. Oltmanns, M.H.; Samudre, S.S.; Castillo, I.G.; Hosseini, A.; Lichtman, A.H.; Allen, R.C.; Lattanzio, F.A.; Williams, P.B. Topical WIN55212-2 alleviates intraocular hypertension in rats through a CB1 receptor mediated mechanism of action. *J. Ocul. Pharmacol. Ther.* **2008**, *24*, 104–115. [CrossRef] [PubMed]

16. Bekkers, J.M.; Stevens, C.F. Excitatory and inhibitory autaptic currents in isolated hippocampal neurons maintained in cell culture. *Proc. Natl. Acad. Sci. USA* **1991**, *88*, 7834–7838. [CrossRef] [PubMed]

17. Furshpan, E.J.; MacLeish, P.R.; O'Lague, P.H.; Potter, D.D. Chemical transmission between rat sympathetic neurons and cardiac myocytes developing in microcultures: Evidence for cholinergic, adrenergic, and dual-function neurons. *Proc. Natl. Acad. Sci. USA* **1976**, *73*, 4225–4229. [CrossRef] [PubMed]

18. Levison, S.W.; McCarthy, K.D. Characterization and partial purification of AIM: A plasma protein that induces rat cerebral type 2 astroglia from bipotential glial progenitors. *J. Neurochem.* **1991**, *57*, 782–794. [CrossRef] [PubMed]

19. Jain, T.; Wager-Miller, J.; Mackie, K.; Straiker, A. Diacylglycerol lipasealpha (DAGLalpha) and DAGLbeta cooperatively regulate the production of 2-arachidonoyl glycerol in autaptic hippocampal neurons. *Mol. Pharmacol.* **2013**, *84*, 296–302. [CrossRef] [PubMed]

20. Straiker, A.; Mackie, K. Depolarization-induced suppression of excitation in murine autaptic hippocampal neurones. *J. Physiol.* **2005**, *569 Pt 2*, 501–517. [CrossRef] [PubMed]

21. Wilson, R.I.; Nicoll, R.A. Endogenous cannabinoids mediate retrograde signalling at hippocampal synapses. *Nature* **2001**, *410*, 588–592. [CrossRef] [PubMed]

22. McKinnon, S.J.; Schlamp, C.L.; Nickells, R.W. Mouse models of retinal ganglion cell death and glaucoma. *Exp. Eye Res.* **2009**, *88*, 816–824. [CrossRef] [PubMed]

23. Akaishi, T.; Odani-Kawabata, N.; Ishida, N.; Nakamura, M. Ocular hypotensive effects of anti-glaucoma agents in mice. *J. Ocul. Pharmacol. Ther.* **2009**, *25*, 401–408. [CrossRef] [PubMed]

24. Caldwell, M.; Hu, S.S.; Viswanathan, S.; Bradshaw, H.; Kelly, M.E.; Straiker, A. A GPR18-based signaling system regulates IOP in murine eye. *Br. J. Pharmacol.* **2013**, *169*, 834–843. [CrossRef] [PubMed]

25. Bell, N.P.; Ramos, J.L.; Feldman, R.M. Safety, tolerability, and efficacy of fixed combination therapy with dorzolamide hydrochloride 2% and timolol maleate 0.5% in glaucoma and ocular hypertension. *Clin. Ophthalmol.* **2010**, *4*, 1331–1346. [CrossRef] [PubMed]

6

The Implication of the Brain Insulin Receptor in Late Onset Alzheimer's Disease Dementia

Jaume Folch [1,2], Miren Ettcheto [1,2,3,4], Oriol Busquets [1,2,3,4], Elena Sánchez-López [2,5,6], Rubén D. Castro-Torres [2,3,4,7,8], Ester Verdaguer [2,4,7], Patricia R. Manzine [3,9], Saghar Rabiei Poor [3], María Luisa García [5,6], Jordi Olloquequi [10], Carlos Beas-Zarate [8], Carme Auladell [2,4,7] and Antoni Camins [2,3,4,*]

[1] Departament de Bioquímica i Biotecnologia, Facultat de Medicina i Ciències de la Salut, Universitat Rovira i Virgili, 43201 Reus, Spain; jaume.folch@urv.cat (J.F.); emiren@gmail.com (M.E.); oriolbusquets@gmail.com (O.B.)

[2] Biomedical Research Networking Centre in Neurodegenerative Diseases (CIBERNED), 28031 Madrid, Spain; esanchezlopez@ub.edu (E.S.-L.); rubendario@gmail.com (R.D.C.-T.); everdaguer@ub.edu (E.V.); cauladell@ub.edu (C.A.)

[3] Departament de Farmacologia, Toxicologia i Química Terapèutica, Facultat de Farmàcia i Ciències de l'Alimentació, Universitat de Barcelona, Av. Joan XXIII 27/31, E-08028 Barcelona, Spain; patricia_manzine@yahoo.com.br (P.R.M.); shagar.rabii@gmail.com (S.R.P.)

[4] Institut de Neurociències, Universitat de Barcelona, E-08028 Barcelona, Spain

[5] Unitat de Farmàcia, Tecnologia Farmacèutica i Fisico-química, Facultat de Farmàcia i Ciències de l'Alimentació, Universitat de Barcelona, E-08028 Barcelona, Spain; rdcm@ub.edu

[6] Institute of Nanoscience and Nanotechnology (IN2UB), University of Barcelona, Barcelona E-08028, Spain

[7] Departament de Biologia Cel·lular, Fisiologia i Immunologia, Facultat de Biologia, Universitat de Barcelona, E-08028 Barcelona, Spain

[8] Laboratorio de Regeneración y Desarrollo Neural, Instituto de Neurobiología, Departamento de Biología Celular y Molecular, Centro Universitario de Ciencias Biológicas y Agropecuarias, Universidad de Guadalajara, Zapopan 44600, Mexico; carlosbeas55@gmail.com

[9] Department of Gerontology, Federal University of São Carlos (UFSCar), São Carlos 13565-905, Brazil

[10] Instituto de Ciencias Biomédicas, Facultad de Ciencias de la Salud, Universidad Autónoma de Chile, Talca 3460000, Chile; jolloquequi@gmail.com

* Correspondence: camins@ub.edu

Abstract: Alzheimer's disease (AD) is progressive neurodegenerative disorder characterized by brain accumulation of the amyloid β peptide (Aβ), which form senile plaques, neurofibrillary tangles (NFT) and, eventually, neurodegeneration and cognitive impairment. Interestingly, epidemiological studies have described a relationship between type 2 diabetes mellitus (T2DM) and this pathology, being one of the risk factors for the development of AD pathogenesis. Information as it is, it would point out that, impairment in insulin signalling and glucose metabolism, in central as well as peripheral systems, would be one of the reasons for the cognitive decline. Brain insulin resistance, also known as Type 3 diabetes, leads to the increase of Aβ production and TAU phosphorylation, mitochondrial dysfunction, oxidative stress, protein misfolding, and cognitive impairment, which are all hallmarks of AD. Moreover, given the complexity of interlocking mechanisms found in late onset AD (LOAD) pathogenesis, more data is being obtained. Recent evidence showed that Aβ42 generated in the brain would impact negatively on the hypothalamus, accelerating the "peripheral" symptomatology of AD. In this situation, Aβ42 production would induce hypothalamic dysfunction that would favour peripheral hyperglycaemia due to down regulation of the liver insulin receptor. The objective of this review is to discuss the existing evidence supporting the concept that brain insulin resistance and altered glucose metabolism play an important role in pathogenesis of LOAD. Furthermore, we discuss AD treatment approaches targeting insulin signalling using anti-diabetic drugs and mTOR inhibitors.

Keywords: Alzheimer's; insulin resistance; amyloid; TAU; cognition; insulin receptor; type 2 diabetes

1. Introduction

Prevention is a key factor when trying to reduce the impact of age-related diseases like cardiovascular alterations, cancer and dementias. These pathologies do not only create substantial personal and family burdens but, unsustainable increases in the public health economic costs in developed populations. The most common form of dementia is Alzheimer's disease (AD) [1–7]. The number of patients diagnosed with AD is rapidly increasing worldwide and becoming a common cause of death in aging populations [4–7]. Moreover, no effective treatments have been established yet to prevent or delay the progression of AD [8,9].

AD has been classified into two groups, depending on its onset: the first classification is familial AD, related to genetic alterations of the amyloid beta precursor protein (AβPP) and preselinins (PS1) [1–5]. This subgroup represents approximately about 3% of the diseased patients [1,4]. The other classification group is the late onset form (LOAD), also known as sporadic. It accounts for the remaining 97% of diagnoses [1,4]. Historically, the neuropathological characteristics of AD were described through the amyloidogenic hypothesis by Selkoe (1992) [9,10]. They were: cognitive loss, abnormal accumulations of Aβ and hyperphosphorylation of TAU protein in areas of the cerebral cortex and hippocampus [6–10]. Initially, the Aβ peptide is generated from the catabolism of AβPP, a plasmatic membrane protein with a single domain found in different cellular types, including neurons, astrocytes and oligodendrocytes [10,11]. This protein is cleaved by α-, β-, and γ-secretase enzymes, as well as, a complex of proteins containing presenilin 1 (PS1) [4,10,11]. In neuropathological situations, AβPP is metabolized predominantly by the amyloidogenic pathway in which the Aβ cleaving enzyme 1 (BACE 1; β-secretase) breaks AβPP by the N-terminal end while γ-secretases cleave the C-terminal end, obtaining Aβ40 and Aβ42 fragments that remain in the extracellular space [4,10].

Since the presence of amyloid plaques has been repeatedly demonstrated not to be strictly correlated with AD symptoms, considerable research has focused on understanding its actual role. Now, one of the working hypotheses is that Aβ42 accumulates in the form of several soluble species, oligomers and protofibres, which contain potentially high toxic properties [11]. As the concentration of these molecules increases, they continue to aggregate into insoluble fibres that are the main constituents of Aβ plaques. Nevertheless, some authors suggest that the cognitive impairment correlates best with alterations on the TAU protein than the Aβ plaques, suggesting a predominant role for TAU in the pathogenesis of AD [4,9–11]. Therefore, in the field of AD research, there are multiple approaches to consider when trying to understand the origin of this disease.

Another hallmark that has been associated as a risk factor for LOAD is the ε4 allele of the apolipoprotein E (APOE) gene [12–16]. This information was demonstrated when studying how the response to intranasal insulin differed between carriers of different apolipoprotein ε4 alleles [14]. APOE genotype influences peripheral glucose and insulin metabolism. Also, as it occurs in other diseases, gender has an influence in the affection and incidence of pathology. APOE positive carrier women have higher risk than men to develop LOAD and, respond less favourably to insulin related therapies [13–16]. Importantly, the molecular basis of this association has remained elusive for decades. Yet, recent findings determined that APOE4 interacts with insulin receptors (IR), impairing its trafficking between endosomes and the plasmatic membranes, by trapping them and favouring the development of impaired insulin signalling [16]. Furthermore, the association between T2DM and LOAD amyloid pathology is specific among carriers of the apolipoprotein E (APOE) ε4 gene allele, compared to the common ε3 allele and the protective ε2 allele [16]. All these new data reinforce the metabolic hypothesis that T2DM appears as a key factor involved in LOAD [17–20].

Currently, only symptomatic therapies are available and their effects are modest (acetylcholinesterase inhibitors and NMDA antagonists) [8]. Memantine (MEM), a low-affinity voltage-dependent uncompetitive antagonist of NMDA receptors (NMDAR), is currently being prescribed for the treatment of AD, jointly with acetylcholinesterase inhibitors such as galantamine, donepezil, and rivastigmine [20–22]. Since it is a low-affinity antagonist, it blocks the NMDAR but it is rapidly displaced from it, avoiding prolonged receptor blockade and the associated negative side effects on learning and memory that have been observed in high affinity NMDAR antagonists. Unfortunately, and despite its high prevalence and mortality, there are no effective disease-modifying therapies at present.

For the last 25 years, the main focus of research has been on senile plaques, considering them the main source of the symptoms of AD. Consequently, therapeutic approaches have focused on this biomarker. Recent studies at preclinical level and in LOAD patients show that an antibody (aducanumab) penetrates in the brain and reduces soluble and insoluble Aβ42 in a dose-dependent manner [23]. In patients with mild LOAD, a year of treatment by administering monthly intravenous infusions of aducanumab, reduces cerebral Aβ and patients show cognitive improvements. These results suggest that the amyloidogenic hypothesis may contribute to the development of LOAD exacerbating its consequences, possibly along with other factors such as metabolic alterations, glia activation, mitochondrial alteration and oxidative stress, among others [23]. Thus, the classical definition of AD that attributes the main role to plaques and tangles as the main responsible source of the neuropathophysiology should be modified.

Accordingly, the main objective of this review is to summarize the information regarding metabolic alterations and the appearance of LOAD, especially associated with type II diabetes mellitus (T2DM). Finally, the pathways associated with the IR signalling and its inhibition will be presented. Our aim is to evaluate the possible application of drugs involved in the regulation/modulation of brain IR in LOAD treatment, in order to improve cognitive performance and deter the development of AD.

2. The Hippocampal Insulin Receptor Is a Key Target in Physiological Cognitive Processes and Neurodegeneration

In 1985, previous to the establishment of the amyloidogenic hypothesis as the paradigm for the study of AD, Hoyer, proposed the concept of central insulin resistance and dysfunctional insulin signalling in LOAD (Table 1) [24–28]. Insulin resistance is defined as a situation in the human organism in which it does not respond sufficiently to the physiological levels of insulin [29–39]. It is involved in the onset of the metabolic syndrome. Yet, even though this idea had already been theorized, these conclusions did not begin to be established until the publication of the Rotterdam study, a clinical report that described the connection between T2DM and LOAD, revealing that those patients that had been diagnosed with diabetes had higher risk of dementia [33,34]. Subsequent clinical and epidemiological studies have confirmed this potential association demonstrating that the alteration of metabolic parameters, such as hyperglycaemia and hyperinsulinemia, correlates positively with the development of pathology related to LOAD, mainly with the cognitive loss [35–41].

Table 1. Examples of IR signalling pathway alterations in the brain in late onset Alzheimer's disease.

Reference	Physiological Alterations	Pathological Effects
Biessels and Reagan, 2015 [36]	Down regulation in neurogenesis were associated with reductions in dendritic spine density in CA1 pyramidal neurons.	Learning and memory loss.
Hoyer, S., 2004 [26]	Decline in ATP levels (mitochondrial alteration). PKB activity inhibition GSK3 activity increase.	Amount in TAU phosphorylation. Oxidative stress increases
De Felice, F.G., 2014 [29]	Neuroinflammation and TNFα increase associated with neuronal ER stress and JNK activation	Brain IR down regulation and synaptic alteration.
Grillo, C.A., 2015 [42]	Hippocampal-specific insulin resistance using a lentiviral vector expressing an IR antisense sequence	Down regulation of GluN2B and GluA1 phosphorylation at synapses. Memory failure independent of peripheral metabolic alterations.
Hoyer, S., 1994 [28]	Insulin modulates levels of acetylcholine and norepinephrine neurotransmitters,	Cognition loss

Table 1. *Cont.*

Reference	Physiological Alterations	Pathological Effects
Frolich, L.D., 1999 [25]	Formation and deposition of advanced glycation end products (AGEs)	Up-regulate APP via oxidative stress and Aβ production enhancement
De Felice and Ferreira, 2014 [30]	mTOR dysregulation	Learning and memory deficits, cell cycle reentry
Craft, S. 2012 [6]	Insulin resistance increases vascular dysfunction	Vascular dementia
Craft, S. 2005 [43]	Insulin resistance inhibits IDE activity	Aβ levels Increase

Under physiological conditions when insulin binds to the IR, a cascade regulates key downstream serine/threonine kinases such as, protein kinases B (AKT/PKB), mechanistic target of rapamycin (mTOR), and extracellular signal-regulated kinases (ERK), that eventually phosphorylate serine/threonine residues of the insulin receptor substrates (IRS), inhibiting insulin signalling in a negative feedback regulation (Figure 1) [35–41,44–46]. In neurons, the phosphoinositide 3-kinase (PI3K), AKT, glycogen synthase kinase 3β (GSK3β), BCL-2 agonist of cell death (BAD), fork-head box (FOX), mTOR and the mitogen activated protein kinase (MAPK) pathways are critical for cell survival signalling and are regulated by the activity of the IR [43,47,48]. Therefore, alteration of the physiological activity on these pathways might be the source of alteration in normal neuronal performance, supporting the hypothesis that brain insulin resistance could promote LOAD, precisely by inhibition of these pathways [39,41,45].

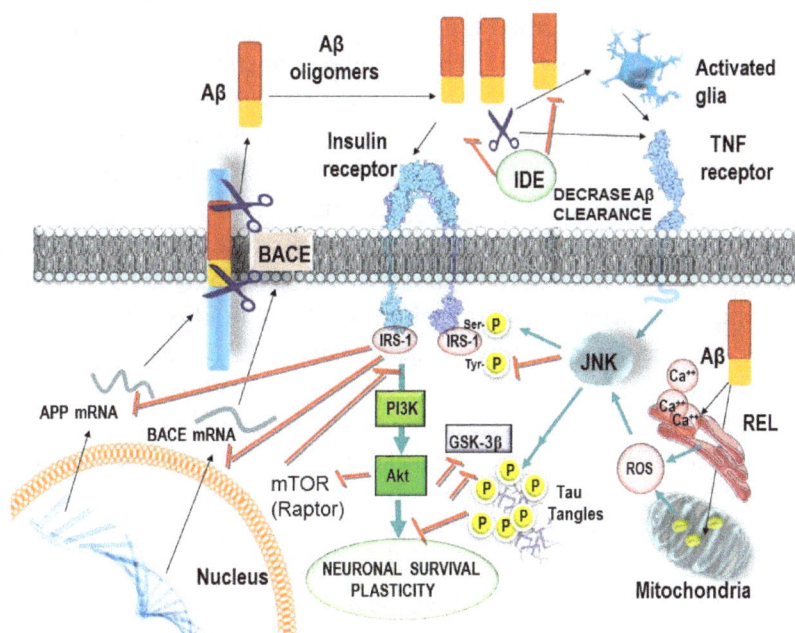

Figure 1. Consequences of insulin and Aβ interactions on reduced neuronal IR signalling. In type 2 diabetes, there can be decreased or increased levels of insulin in brain, along with IR desensitization. Soluble Aβ oligomers block IR. Increased Aβ levels will compete for insulin degrading enzyme (IDE) against cerebral insulin. Reduced IR signalling results in downstream negative effects on PI3K activity and proteins like PKB/AKT. Consequences of this include: reduced glucose metabolism and increased oxidative stress which modulate APP and JNK activity. Moreover, reduced GSK3β phosphorylation leads to up-regulation in TAU phosphorylation and Aβ formation. Likewise, Aβ promotes the activation of microglia increasing the levels of cytokines, mainly TNFα that activates JNK that subsequently inhibits the brain IR. On the other hand, Aβ can alter the endoplasmic reticulum and the mitochondria, generating free oxygen radicals that modulate APP and JNK.

The metabolic hypothesis associated with the appearance of LOAD is based on the fact that cerebral IRs are widely distributed in the brain, existing in higher densities in the olfactory bulb, hypothalamus, cerebral cortex and hippocampus [28,49]. Frölich and colleagues reported a significant reduced level of CNS IRs in LOAD patients [24–28]. Research from the group led by de la Monte, demonstrated significant decreases in insulin and insulin growth factor (IGF-I) receptor levels in LOAD frontal cortex, hippocampus, and hypothalamus of AD patients [45,50]. In addition, the same research group correlated the decrease in gene expression and protein levels of insulin, IGF1 receptors and other downstream molecules, with impaired acetylcholine production and cognitive performance in LOAD brains. Another recent study strengthened this hypothesis by demonstrating significant alterations in mRNA expression profiles of genes related to insulin signalling in the cortex and hippocampus [51]. Intriguingly, the highest differences in mRNA expression were detected in the hippocampal region of the brain, the main area associated with the cognitive process [51].

A recently published work by the group of Butterfield, reported new information about the complexity of LOAD [44]. In essence, they suggested that human and preclinical studies have provided convincing evidence that in the brains of many LOAD patients and rodents there is a decrease in energy metabolism and, in particular, a decrease in glucose utilization. As a consequence, that LOAD will represent a metabolic disease in which brain glucose utilization and energy production are altered is gaining attention [24–28,39]. Additional data by Grillo and co-workers reported in a very interesting study, that insulin resistance in the hippocampus would prevent the correct structuring of memory, which would be directly related to cognitive loss [42,52]. The administration of a lentiviral vector expressing an antisense sequence of the brain IRs to rats caused for cognitive loss. Using this experimental approach, the authors were able to decrease the number of IR in the hippocampus without affecting peripheral glucose homeostasis, thus generating a specific rat model of altered brain insulin signalling in the hippocampus [42]. This study demonstrated that insulin resistance in the hippocampus might induce a neuroplasticity deficit, including deficits in spatial learning and memory. In addition, the hippocampal levels of the phosphorylated GluN2B and GluA1 subunits were reduced, providing a possible molecular evidence on how the deficit in synaptic transmission occurs when there are alterations on the insulin signalling in the hippocampus [52].

Concurrently, the de Felice research group has demonstrated that Aβ oligomers bind to IR, causing for their removal from the neuronal surface membrane, causing its cellular internalization and, thereby providing an evidence for brain insulin resistance in LOAD [19,29]. In addition, some authors have reported that insulin prevents detrimental effects of Aβ oligomers on the inactivation of brain IR [53]. Furthermore, insulin promotes the release of intracellular synaptic Aβ, and regulates expression of insulin-degrading enzyme (IDE), a protease involved in clearance of Aβ (Table 1) [17].

A possible conclusion from the outcome of these studies might suggest that the presence of Aβ peptide may not be the only factor necessary for cognitive loss. However, Aβ paired with a process of obesity and hence, peripheral and central insulin resistance, may exacerbate the onset of LOAD and worsen cognitive loss. Then, LOAD should be considered globally as a brain expression of a metabolic disease of the whole organism, and correspondingly should not focus only on events that occur in the brain [32].

3. Molecular Bases of Insulin Receptor Modulation

Insulin is a peptide hormone of 5.8 KDa that is synthesized and secreted by the pancreatic β cells. Once released to the blood vessels, insulin is transported to the brain through the blood brain barrier (BBB) and binds to their cognate receptors [24,25]. The IR is a glycoprotein consisting of an extracellular α subunit (135 KDa) that inhibits the activity of the β-transmembrane subunit (95 KDa) [26–28]. The IRs belongs to the tyrosine kinase receptor superfamily. When insulin binds to the α subunit, it dimerizes to form the α2β2 complex in the cell membrane, it leads to autophosphorylation of the beta subunit on Tyr1158, Tyr1162, and Tyr1163, which constitutes the first step in IR activation.

It has been shown that the activation of the IR tyrosine kinase, leads to the recruitment and phosphorylation of several substrates, including IRS1-4, the adapter protein SHC, growth factor receptor-bound protein-2 (Grb-2 or GAB1), dedicator of cytokinesis (DOCK1), casitas B-lineage lymphoma (CBL) and an interacting protein called APS which are associated proteins, all of which provide specific binding sites for the recruitment of other proteins of the signalling cascade [49]. These phospho-tyrosine residues bind to IRS 1 and 2 in order to initiate several signalling pathways, including the PI3K-AKT pathway [54,55]. PI3K converts phosphatidylinositol-4,5-bisphosphate (PIP2) to phosphatidylinositol-3,4,5-trisphosphate (PIP3). This conversion favours the activation of the PKB/AKT through the 3-phosphoinositide dependent kinase (PDK). PIP3 recruits AKT to the plasma membrane, where it becomes phosphorylated by 3-phosphoinositide-dependent protein kinase 1 (PDK1), which regulates the translocation of glucose transporter type 4 (GLUT4) to the plasma membrane in the hippocampus.

In the brain, IR activation promotes neuronal survival through the phosphorylation of the FOXO transcription factor, favouring its way out of the nucleus of the cell [55–58]. FOXO is a transcription factor involved in the expression of pro-apoptotic mediators, thus contributing to the process of cell death. All this processes that are regulated by the signalling of the IR, result in deleterious effects on synaptic function and cognitive impairment. The activation of IR tyrosine kinase also results in the activation of the RAS/MAPKs pathway. The stress activated protein kinases (SAPK) or MAPK, include extracellular signal-regulated kinases 1 and 2 (ERK1 and ERK2), p38 and the c-Jun-N-terminal kinases (JNKs) [56]. The JNK family is made up by 3 genes that codify for 10 different products classified into 3 different isoforms: JNK1 (*Mapk8*), JNK2 (*Mapk9*) and JNK3 (*Mapk10*) and while JNK1 and JNK2 are ubiquitously expressed, JNK3 expression is principally restricted to regions of the brain, heart and testis. When activated, the JNK1 phosphorylates IRS-1 in the serine residues (IRS-1pSer) [29]. This alteration blocks the signalling of the insulin pathway and favours peripheral resistance to this hormone. Based on this activation sequence, JNK1 appears as a key protein to investigate novel therapeutic targets that prevent the development T2DM [54,56,58].

4. Relationship between Insulin Receptor Activation and TAU Phosphorylation

Recent studies have suggested a potential link between impaired insulin signalling and pathogenic alterations of TAU. As we stated before, the activation of IR, IRS1 and 2 initiates several signalling pathways, including the conversion of PIP2 into PIP3, which favours the activation of PKB/AKT and, consequently, leads to the translocation of GLUT4 to the plasma membrane [56,59–62]. Concurrently, AKT signalling affects other diverse cellular responses, like neuronal survival and TAU phosphorylation. Other important targets such as the GSK3β are also regulated by AKT, inhibiting its activation by phosphorylation. Insulin resistance reinforces the activation of GSK3β leading to increased phosphorylation levels of TAU protein and, the subsequent formation of neurofibrillary tangles, one of the hallmarks of AD neuropathology [59–62]. Schubert and co-workers investigate the biochemical processes associated with neurodegeneration in a brain specific IR knockout (NIRKO) mice model [63]. They reported that NIRKO mice presented decreased AKT activity thus, having the previously mentioned increases in GSK3β activation and TAU hyperphosphorylation at specific sites associated with LOAD. This data, along with other being produced in the same line on the study of metabolic alterations, confirm how altered insulin signalling in the brain leads to the appearance of classical hallmarks of LOAD and, demonstrates, how neuronal insulin resistance predisposes for the appearance of pathologies. Freude and co-workers reported that brain insulin receptor specifically modulates TAU phosphorylation at Ser202, a key site which predisposes for tangle formation after peripheral insulin injection in mice [64]. The effects of injected insulin on TAU were abolished in the NIRKO mice.

Studies performed in *post-mortem* brains from patients with tauopathies including AD, Pick's disease, corticobasal degeneration, and progressive supranuclear palsy, showed increases in phosphorylated IRS1 levels which, as we have already mentioned, is a specific marker of insulin resistance. Interestingly, two independent research groups published their research on alterations in brain insulin receptors and downstream pathway in LOAD. Liu and colleagues reported that the insulin-signalling pathway is decreased in LOAD brain and demonstrated that alteration in insulin signaling may contribute to LOAD through the hyperphosphorylation of TAU [59]. In addition, authors suggest that brain insulin resistance is also correlated with calpain activation, a protease involved in cyclin-dependent kinase (CDK5) activation, a kinase involved in the phosphorylation of TAU [35]. Similar results were reported by other authors:

- Talbot and co-workers reported that LOAD patients show impaired brain insulin-signaling transduction with reduced tyrosine kinase activity of the IR [35]. IR and its receptor analogous IGF1R form heterodimers (IR/IGF1R) that modulate the selectivity and affinity for insulin and IGF1 in the activation of signaling molecules [65].
- Yarchoan and co-workers reported an increase in serine phosphorylation of IRS1 (inactivation), the phosphorylation of IRS1 on multiple serine residues can inhibit IRS1 activity, leading to insulin resistance in the hippocampus in LOAD and other tauopathies [54].

Finally, recent data reported that insulin accumulates intraneuronally together with hyperphosphorylated TAU in LOAD and several other tauopathies suggesting that hyperphosphorylated TAU-bearing neurons is a causative factor involved in the brain insulin resistance observed in LOAD (Table 1) [66].

5. Role of the Glucose Transporter 4 in Cognition

Glucose transporter 4 (GLUT4) is found in peripheral tissues like the skeletal muscle, heart, and adipose tissue [67–69]. Its role in the physiology of the cell is mainly the transport from the extracellular space into the citosol for its metabolism. Thus, in response to the activation of the IR signaling cascade by insulin, GLUT4 is translocated to the plasma membrane to facilitate glucose entry into the cell. Moreover, GLUT4 is found in brain regions such as the cerebellum, and especially the hippocampus. At the hippocampal level, the cognitive improvement effects related to insulin may occur via upregulation in GLUT4-mediated glucose uptake [68]. Thus hippocampal GLUT4 overexpression could be a target to improve the cognitive process in AD. This could be the case of quercetin which improves cognitive dysfunction mediated by chronic unpredicted stress, through upregulation of GLUT4 expression in the hippocampus [69].

6. Effects of Aβ Oligomers on Brain Insulin and Peripheral Metabolic Tissues

Recent hypothesis suggests that since diabetes increases both Aβ production and TAU phosphorylation, both T2DM and Aβ may cooperate to induce neurodegeneration in LOAD [70,71]. It has been pointed out that soluble Aβ peptide oligomers would act as synaptotoxins [10–12]. Moreover, since Aβ and insulin are both amyloidogenic peptides sharing a common sequence recognition motif, it is possible that both molecules are able to bind to the IR. Given this assumption, Aβ may also potentiate insulin resistance through antagonistic effects, blocking the downstream pathway and facilitating the phosphorylation of GSK3β. Thus, the aging process associated with insulin resistance, jointly with Aβ production and hyperphosphorylation of TAU, can have a synergic effect leading to neuronal dysfunction.

In addition to the effects of Aβ oligomers on TAU phosphorylation, a recent study using a mice model of AD, reported peripheral metabolic changes in plasma and liver extracts [72]. Also, Zhang and co-workers demonstrated in APPswe/PS1E9 mice that the Aβ42 peptide induces hepatic insulin resistance in vivo through the activation of the Janus Kinase 2 (JAK2), suggesting that inhibition of Aβ42 peptide production in the brain may be a novel strategy for the treatment of insulin resistance and therefore T2DM [73–75].

As, an overview, we can state that LOAD has a multifactorial component and should be addressed as a disease affecting the whole organism [70,71]. Moreover, preclinical studies in rodents have established that the oligomers of Aβ administered directly to hippocampal neurons induce synaptic loss and neuronal dysfunction, which eventually leads to memory loss [11]. Likewise, intracerebroventricular (icv) administration of Aβ oligomers causes behavioral changes and AD-like pathology in primates, providing an excellent model for investigating AD-related mechanisms [72]. Furthermore, Clarke and co-workers reported that intracerebral injected Aβ causes peripheral glucose intolerance and insulin resistance, as well as, inflammatory processes in the hypothalamus and adipose tissue, along with alterations of GLUT-4 insulin-induced cell membrane translocation in skeletal muscle [76].

Accordingly, Aβ peptides generated in the brain reach the hypothalamus and alter the body's energy balance, favouring the apparition of a T2DM. In this line, Arietta-Cruz et al. demonstrated an increase in plasma glucose levels when injecting β25-35 into the hypothalamus of rat as a consequence of enhanced hepatic glucose production [77,78].

In addition, generated brain Aβ could accumulate in peripheral tissues such as the pancreas and skeletal muscle contributing to the negative effect on peripheral glucose metabolism [79]. Thus, when trying to explain this complicated bidirectional process between LOAD and T2DM, recent reported data suggests the existence of something called Factor X, a molecule or pathway that would be the bridge between Aβ as responsible of LOAD and T2DM. In addition, authors suggest that characterization of Factor X will be important in order to the development of a potential therapeutic target for LOAD prevention [70].

7. Is BACE1 a Potential Bridge between Aβ and T2DM?

BACE1 is involved in LOAD as the enzyme responsible for the rate-limiting step in Aβ production through the cleaving of the amyloid precursor protein (APP). It has been demonstrated that monomers of Aβ1-42 augment BACE1 gene transcription activation through the MAPK8/JNK1-MAPK9/JNK2 signalling pathway and by interfering with its lysosomal degradation leading to an amyloid vicious cycle [80–82].

Interestingly, recent data demonstrated at the preclinical level that neuronal expression of human BACE1 causes systemic diabetic complications via the induction of hypothalamic impairment, insulin resistance, hepatic deficits and global glucose alterations [79,80]. Using the PLB4 mouse it was demonstrated that the risk of diabetes when BACE1 is overexpressed in neurons increases, providing for a complex mechanistic interaction between T2DM and LOAD. Human (h) BACE1 neurogenic knockout has recently been shown to induce Aβ accumulation, promotes brain inflammation and generates LOAD-like phenotypes in mice in the absence of expression of mutant APP, suggesting that BACE1 represents a molecular risk factor for AD related to the aging process [83].

Pluciǹskaí and colleagues showed that the overexpression in neurons of the amyloidogenic enzyme, BACE1, is sufficient to increase the risk of developing T2DM [80]. Therefore, this study demonstrates that neuronal BACE1 causes metabolic dysregulation throughout the body along with brain inflammation and cognitive impairment related to the process of amyloidosis. The PLB4 mouse presents a diabetic profile, thus demonstrating that neuronal BACE1 is in part responsible for the appearance of these peripheral metabolic alterations [84].

Therefore, even though the hypothesis states that diabetic complications promote the onset and or progression of AD, the reverse scenario may also apply. This is also in agreement with the potential hypothesis that hyperglycaemia can also originate in the brain and affect the rest of the body (Figure 2). Meakin and colleagues demonstrated that knockout mice for BACE1$^{-/-}$ are thin, resistant to obesity induced by high fat diet and show an increase in insulin sensitivity in peripheral tissues with a regulation of improved glucose metabolism throughout the body [85]. These results outline a novel aspect of BACE1 function in the regulation of metabolic homeostasis and, provide a possible connection between T2DM and AD [85].

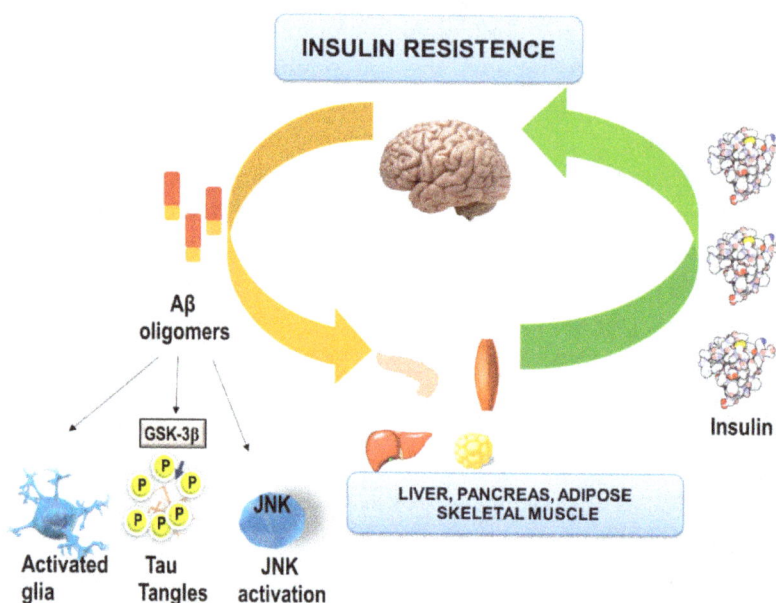

Figure 2. Aβ acting on the hypothalamus can dysregulate energy homeostasis in the human organism through a neuroinflammatory process. Furthermore, in the hippocampus, activation of glial reactivity could increase cytokine levels (such as TNF-α), activating c-Jun N-terminal Kinase and inducing IR resistance and TAU phosphorylation. Likewise, brain generated Aβ could accumulate in peripheral tissues such as the pancreas and skeletal muscle, favouring the appearance of T2DM.

8. Potential Pharmacological Approaches for Late Onset Alzheimer's Disease Treatment Related with the Regulation of Insulin Metabolism

For all of the above, development of LOAD would pivot on the loss of IR functionality, oxidative stress and loss of control of protein homeostasis [86–90]. In order to modulate these mechanisms, different pharmacological approaches are proposed which may act in a combined and, potentially, synergistic manner. On the one hand, it may be appropriate to combine the use of antidiabetic drugs such as pioglitazone, intranasal insulin, NMDAR antagonists such as memantine and inhibitors of mTOR activity such as rapamycin and its derivatives (rapalogs) [22,44,91–102]. In all cases, they are drugs that have been validated in different Phase II (pioglitazone) and III (rapamycin) clinical trials. Since in no case did these molecules improve the evolution of patients with LOAD (in the different Phase III studies), this allows for the possibility of studying their possible synergies when administered in combination.

8.1. Antidiabetic Drugs. Modulators of Proliferation of Activated Gamma Peroxisome Receptor. Pioglitazone

Pioglitazone is an orally active antidiabetic drug in the family of thioazolidinediones, also called "insulin sensitizers" [93,94]. Pioglitazone is a potent and selective receptor agonist for the proliferation of activated gamma peroxisomes receptor (PPARγ). These receptors regulate the transcription of a number of genes that respond to insulin [93]. PPARγs are found in most tissues in which insulin exerts its action: adipose tissue, skeletal muscle and liver. Activation of these receptors regulates the transcription of genes involved in the control of glucose production, transport and its utilization. In relationship to LOAD, the treatment with pioglitazone has been shown to reduce glial pro-inflammatory activity and, to decrease Aβ peptide levels due to the phagocytic activity of microglia [92]. In 3xTg-AD mice treated with pioglitazone for 4 months, this drug improves brain spatial learning impairment, TAU hyperphosphorylation, and neuroinflammation [93]. In a recent preclinical study Fernandez-Martos and co-workers reported that the association of pioglitazone with leptin showed beneficial effects on the preclinical APPswe/PS1dE9 mice model of familial AD improving cognition and decreasing Aβ levels [102]. Recent studies indicate a very relevant effect of the drug reversing the damage that neuroinflammation causes in the structural plasticity of the dendrites. Thus, it has been observed that treatment with pioglitazone can reverse the loss of synaptic density induced by Aβ peptide generation [91]. Although preclinical data gives support to the potential beneficial effects of pioglitazone in AD, clinical data reported until now shows conflicting results regarding efficacy due to the many limitations of these trials [100,101]. Therefore, further clinical trials on the potential use of pioglitazone for the treatment of LOAD are necessary. Phase II clinical trials of the drug demonstrate that it is a safe and well tolerated molecule. Two Phase III trials are currently under way, of which conclusions regarding their effectiveness against AD cannot yet be obtained [91,100,101].

8.2. Intranasal Insulin for LOAD Treatment

In previous preclinical studies, intranasal treatments with insulin or insulin analogues have afforded some degree of memory improvement or of protection against cognitive deterioration in mice models of AD [101–109]. However, in a recent reported study (NCT01595646), Craft and co-workers reported that intranasal-administered insulin improves memory for adults with mild cognitive impairment and LOAD [108–110]. Furthermore, authors suggest that insulin could improve and modify the AD-related pathophysiologic processes. Another interesting point is that the therapeutic effects of insulin are modulated by APOE genotype. Accordingly, the study gives support to the continued investigation on potential stimulation of insulin receptor as a therapy for LOAD [108].

8.3. Rapalogs

It is well known that the PI3K/AKT/mTOR dysregulation may decrease the autophagic process leading to the accumulation of Aβ42 deposition and protein aggregation [44]. Likewise, mTOR is involved in the modulation of IRS1 activity, representing one of the best-characterized events leading to insulin resistance [44]. Therefore, alteration or better activation of the mTOR pathway could represent an important link between Aβ and insulin signalling, providing new insights into the relationship between insulin resistance and incidence of AD.

mTOR is a kinase involved in energy and protein homeostasis in cells. Both rapamycin and its derivatives prevent the formation of the mTORC1 complex, acting as allosteric inhibitors [109–111]. However, the main limitations of rapamycin are its solubility, long half-life and the poor oral absorption making it necessary for the development of analog molecules, among them temsirolimus, which is an ester derived from rapamycin, soluble in water and suitable for administration both oral and intravenously. Its use was approved in 1977 by the FDA and the European Medicines Agency for the treatment of renal carcinoma [111]. Both drugs have the same mechanism of action. Jiang and co-workers recently reported that temsirolimus promotes autophagic clearance of Aβ, exerts protective effects accompanied by an improvement in spatial cognitive functions in APP/PS1 model of familial AD [102]. This study give support to the therapeutic potentials of temsirolimus in preclinical models of AD.

9. Conclusions

Given the amount of data of which we are in possession now, it can be concluded that the pathology hereby described as LOAD is very closely related to the alterations derived of insulin resistance. Effective energy metabolism is the base on the proper functioning of cellular types and, when disrupted, affects negatively their function. In the case of neurons, which are having glucose as its main energy source, this situation can be utterly disastrous leading to their ineffective activity and consequently cognitive decline. That is why the IR has such a prominent role.

It is now well established Aβ could bind to the IR in the hippocampus, revealing important cognitive loss, when the receptor is inhibited and enhancing the neurodegenerative process in this brain region. Moreover, Aβ bind to the liver IR in the preclinical APPswe/PS1E9 mice model of familial AD, suggesting the possibility that decreases of Aβ production may be a novel potential treatment for use in T2DM (Figure 2) [73,74,112]. Lastly, the therapeutic potential of Aβ inhibitors (for example BACE 1 inhibitors) has not yet been verified in clinical trials. However, antidiabetic therapies such as pioglitazone or intranasal insulin are more likely to be effective in individuals with LOAD. Therefore, we suggest that the future timing of a more effective LOAD therapy should be the key factor in determining if T2DM drugs shown beneficial actions in LOAD. Targeting the early stages of LOAD, before widespread cognitive loss due to synapses and neurons degeneration has occurred is likely to produce the best clinical outcome, but identification of individuals at this stage of LOAD is difficult. Accordingly, the modulation of brain IR preventing its inactivation could be a suitable strategy in a combinatory strategy therapy for LOAD.

Acknowledgments: This work was supported by the Spanish Ministry of Science and Innovation SAF2017-84283-R, PI2016/01, CB06/05/0024 (CIBERNED), the European Regional Development Founds and MAT 2014-59134-R project. Research team from UB and URV belongs to 2014SGR-525 from Generalitat de Catalunya. ESL and MLG belong to 2014SGR-1023 and ESL acknowledges the PhD scholarship FPI-MICINN (BES-2012-026083). CBZ is supported by grants from CONACyT Mexico (No. 0177594) and RDCT from Postdoctoral fellowship CONACYT No. 298337 and the Doctoral Program in Sciences in Molecular Biology in Medicine, LGAC Molecular Bases of Chronic Diseases-Degenerative and its Applications (000091, PNPC, CONACyT). PRM is supported by grants 2015/26084-1 and 2017/13224-5, São Paulo Research Foundation (FAPESP)—Brazil.

References

1.   Alzheimer's Association. 2016 Alzheimer's disease facts and figures. *Alzheimer's Dement.* **2016**, *12*, 459–509.

2.   Kamat, P.K.; Kalani, A.; Rai, S.; Swarnkar, S.; Tota, S.; Nath, C.; Tyagi, N. Mechanism of Oxidative Stress and Synapse Dysfunction in the Pathogenesis of Alzheimer's Disease: Understanding the Therapeutics Strategies. *Mol. Neurobiol.* **2016**, *53*, 648–661. [CrossRef] [PubMed]

3.   Alzheimer, A.; Stelzmann, R.A.; Schnitzlein, H.N.; Murtagh, F.R. An English translation of Alzheimer's 1907 paper, "Uber eine eigenartige Erkrankung der Hirnrinde". *Clin. Anat.* **1995**, *8*, 429–431. [PubMed]

4.   Vishal, S.; Sourabh, A.; Harkirat, S. Alois Alzheimer (1864–1915) and the Alzheimer syndrome. *J. Med. Biogr.* **2011**, *19*, 32–33. [CrossRef] [PubMed]

5.   Masters, C.L.; Bateman, R.; Blennow, K.; Rowe, C.C.; Spearling, R.A.; Cummings, J.L. Alzheimer's disease. *Nat. Rev. Dis. Primers* **2015**, *1*, 15056. [CrossRef] [PubMed]

6.   Craft, S. Alzheimer disease: Insulin resistance and AD: Extending the translational path. *Nat. Rev. Neurol.* **2012**, *8*, 360–362. [CrossRef] [PubMed]

7.   Ritchie, C.W.; Molinuevo, J.L.; Truyen, L.; Satlin, A.; Van der Geyten, S.; Lovestone, S. Development of interventions for the secondary prevention of Alzheimer's dementia: The European Prevention of Alzheimer's Dementia (EPAD) project. *Lancet Psychiatry* **2016**, *3*, 179–186. [CrossRef]

8.   Querfurth, H.W.; La Ferla, F.M. Alzheimer's disease. *N. Engl. J. Med.* **2010**, *362*, 329–344. [CrossRef] [PubMed]

9.   Mangialasche, F.; Solomon, A.; Winblad, B.; Mecocci, P.; Kivipelto, M. Alzheimer's disease: Clinical trials and drug development. *Lancet Neurol.* **2010**, *9*, 702–716. [CrossRef]

10. Selkoe, D.J. Resolving controversies on the path to Alzheimer's therapeutics. *Nat. Med.* **2011**, *17*, 1060–1065. [CrossRef] [PubMed]

11. Selkoe, D.J.; Hardy, J. The amyloid hypothesis of Alzheimer's disease at 25 years. *EMBO Mol. Med.* **2016**, *8*, 595–608. [CrossRef] [PubMed]

12. Viola, K.L.; Klein, W.L. Amyloid β oligomers in Alzheimer's disease pathogenesis, treatment, and diagnosis. *Acta Neuropathol.* **2015**, *129*, 183–206. [CrossRef] [PubMed]

13. Moser, V.A.; Pike, C.J. Obesity Accelerates Alzheimer-Related Pathology in APOE4but not APOE3Mice. *eNeuro* **2017**, *4*. [CrossRef] [PubMed]

14. Craft, S.; Peskind, E.; Schwartz, M.W.; Schellenberg, G.D.; Raskind, M.; Porte, D. Cerebrospinal fluid and plasma insulin levels in Alzheimer's disease: Relationship to severity of dementia and apolipoprotein E genotype. *Neurology* **1998**, *50*, 164–168. [CrossRef] [PubMed]

15. Liu, C.C.; Liu, C.C.; Kanekiyo, T.; Xu, H.; Bu, G. Apolipoprotein E and Alzheimer disease: Risk, mechanisms and therapy. *Nat. Rev. Neurol.* **2013**, *9*, 106–118. [CrossRef] [PubMed]

16. Zhao, N.; Liu, C.C.; Van Ingelgom, A.J.; Martens, Y.A.; Linares, C.; Knight, J.A.; Painter, M.M.; Sullivan, P.M.; Bu, G. Apolipoprotein E4 Impairs Neuronal Insulin Signaling by Trapping Insulin Receptor in the Endosomes. *Neuron* **2017**, *96*, 115–129. [CrossRef] [PubMed]

17. Neth, B.J.; Craft, S. Insulin Resistance and Alzheimer's Disease: Bioenergetic Linkages. *Front. Aging Neurosci.* **2017**. [CrossRef] [PubMed]

18. De la Monte, S.M. Insulin Resistance and Neurodegeneration: Progress towards the Development of New Therapeutics for Alzheimer's disease. *Drugs* **2017**, *77*, 47–65. [CrossRef] [PubMed]

19. De Felice, F.G.; Benedict, C. A Key Role of Insulin Receptors in Memory. *Diabetes* **2015**, *64*, 3653–3655. [CrossRef] [PubMed]

20. Chneider, L.S.; Mangialasche, F.; Andreasen, N.; Feldman, H.; Giacobini, E.; Jones, R.; Mantua, V.; Mecocci, P.; Pani, L.; Winblad, B.; et al. Clinical trials and late-stage drug development for Alzheimer's disease: An appraisal from 1984 to 2014. *J. Intern. Med.* **2014**, *275*, 251–283. [CrossRef] [PubMed]

21. Lipton, S.A. Paradigm shift in neuroprotection by NMDA receptor blockade: Memantine and beyond. *Nat. Rev. Drug Discov.* **2006**, *5*, 160–170. [CrossRef] [PubMed]

22. Allgaier, M.; Allgaier, C. An update on drug treatment options of Alzheimer's disease. *Front. Biosci.* **2014**, *19*, 1345–1354. [CrossRef]

23. Sevigny, J.; Chiao, P.; Bussière, T.; Weinreb, P.H.; Williams, L.; Maier, M.; Dunstan, R.; Salloway, S.; Chen, T.; Ling, Y.; et al. The antibody aducanumab reduces Aβ plaques in Alzheimer's disease. *Nature* **2016**, *537*, 50–56. [CrossRef] [PubMed]

24. Frolich, L.; Blum-Degen, H.G.; Bernstein, S.; Engelsberger, J.; Humrich, S.; Laufer, D.; Muschner, A.; Thalheimer, A.; Turk, S.; Hoyer, P.; et al. Insulin and insulin receptors in the brain in aging and in sporadic Alzheimer's disease. *J. Neural Transm.* **1998**, *105*, 423–438. [CrossRef] [PubMed]

25. Frolich, L.; Blum-Degen, D.; Riederer, P.; Hoyer, S. A disturbance of the neuronal insulin receptor signal transduction in sporadic Alzheimer's disease. *Ann. N. Y. Acad. Sci.* **1999**, *893*, 290–294. [CrossRef] [PubMed]

26. Hoyer, S. Glucose metabolism and insulin receptor signal transduction in Alzheimer disease. *Eur. J. Pharmacol.* **2004**, *490*, 115–125. [CrossRef] [PubMed]

27. Maurer, K.; Hoyer, S. Alois Alzheimer revisited: Differences in origin of the disease carrying his name. *J. Neural Transm.* **2006**, *113*, 1645–1658. [CrossRef] [PubMed]

28. Hoyer, S. Neurodegeneration, Alzheimer's disease, and beta-amyloid toxicity. *Life Sci.* **1994**, *55*, 1977–1983. [CrossRef]

29. De Felice, F.G.; Lourenco, M.V.; Ferreira, S.T. How does brain insulin resistance develop in Alzheimer's disease? *Alzheimer's Dement.* **2014**, *10*, S26–S32. [CrossRef] [PubMed]

30. De Felice, F.G.; Ferreira, S.T. Inflammation, defective insulin signaling, and mitochondrial dysfunction as common molecular denominators connecting type 2 diabetes to Alzheimer Disease. *Diabetes* **2014**, *63*, 2262–2272. [CrossRef] [PubMed]

31. De la Monte, S.M.; Wands, J.R. Review of insulin and insulin-like growth factor expresion, signaling, and malfunction in the central nervous system: Relevance to alzheimer's disease. *J. Alzheimer Dis.* **2005**, *7*, 45–61. [CrossRef]

32. De la Monte, S.M. Brain insulin resistance and deficiency as therapeutic targets in Alzheimer's disease. *Curr. Alzheimer Res.* **2012**, *9*, 35–66. [CrossRef] [PubMed]

33. Ott, A.; Stolk, R.P.; van Harskamp, F.; Pols, H.A.; Hofman, A.; Breteler, M.M. Diabetes mellitus and the risk of dementia: The Rotterdam Study. *Neurology* **1999**, *53*, 1937–1942. [CrossRef] [PubMed]

34. Schrijvers, E.M.; Witteman, J.C.; Sijbrands, E.J.; Hofman, A.; Koudstaal, P.J.; Breteler, M.M. Insulin metabolism and the risk of Alzheimer disease: The Rotterdam Study. *Neurology* **2010**, *75*, 1982–1987. [CrossRef] [PubMed]

35. Talbot, K.; Wang, H.; Kazi, H.; Han, L.; Bakshi, K.P.; Stucky, A.; Fuino, R.L.; Kawaguchi, K.R.; Samoyedny, A.J.; Wilson, R.S.; et al. Demonstrated brain insulin resistance in Alzheimer's disease patients is associated with IGF1 resistance, IRS1 dysregulation, and cognitive decline. *J. Clin. Investig.* **2012**, *122*, 1316–1338. [CrossRef] [PubMed]

36. Biessels, G.J.; Reagan, L.P. Hippocampal insulin resistance and cognitive dysfunction. *Nat. Rev. Neurosci.* **2015**, *16*, 660–671. [CrossRef] [PubMed]

37. Schwartz, M.W.; Porte, D., Jr. Diabetes, obesity, and the brain. *Science* **2005**, *307*, 375–379. [CrossRef] [PubMed]

38. McNay, E.C.; Recknagel, A.K. Brain insulin signaling a key component of cognitive processes and a potential basis for cognitive impairment in type 2 diabetes. *Neurobiol. Learn. Mem.* **2011**, *96*, 432–442. [CrossRef] [PubMed]

39. Schiöth, H.B.; Craft, S.; Brooks, S.K.; Frey, W.H.; Benedict, C. Brain insulin signaling and Alzheimer's disease: Current evidente and future direction. *Mol. Neurobiol.* **2011**, *46*, 4–10. [CrossRef] [PubMed]

40. Pearson-Leary, J.; McNay, E.C. Intrahippocampal administration of amyloid-β(1-42) oligomers acutely impairs spatial working memory, insulin signaling, and hippocampal metabolism. *J. Alzheimers Dis.* **2012**, *30*, 413–422. [PubMed]

41. Walker, J.M.; Harrison, F. Shared Neuropathological Characteristics of Obesity, Type 2 Diabetes and Alzheimer's Disease: Impacts on Cognitive Decline. *Nutrients* **2015**, *7*, 7332–7357. [CrossRef] [PubMed]

42. Grillo, C.A.; Piroli, G.G.; Lawrence, R.C.; Wrighten, S.A.; Green, A.J.; Wilson, S.P.; Sakai, R.R.; Kelly, S.J.; Wilson, M.A.; Mott, D.D.; et al. Hippocampal Insulin Resistance Impairs Spatial Learning and Synaptic Plasticity. *Diabetes* **2015**, *64*, 3927–3936. [CrossRef] [PubMed]

43. Craft, S. Insulin resistance syndrome and Alzheimer's disease: Age- and obesity-related effects on memory, amyloid, and inflammation. *Neurobiol. Aging* **2005**, *26*, 65–69. [CrossRef] [PubMed]

44. Di Domenico, F.; Barone, E.; Perluigi, M.; Butterfield, D.A. The Triangle of Death in Alzheimer's Disease Brain: The Aberrant Cross-Talk Among Energy Metabolism, Mammalian Target of Rapamycin Signaling, and Protein Homeostasis Revealed by Redox Proteomics. *Antioxid. Redox Signal.* **2017**, *26*, 364–387. [CrossRef] [PubMed]

45. Steen, E.; Terry, B.M.; Rivera, E.J.; Cannon, J.L.; Neely, T.R.; Tavares, R.; Xu, X.J.; Wands, J.R.; de la Monte, S.M. Impaired insulin and insulin-like growth factor expression and signaling mechanisms in Alzheimer's disease—Is this type 3 diabetes? *J. Alzheimer's Dis.* **2005**, *7*, 63–80. [CrossRef]

46. Nuzzo, D.; Picone, P.; Baldassano, S.; Caruana, L.; Messina, E.; Marino Gammazza, A.; Cappello, F.; Mulè, F.; Di Carlo, M. Insulin Resistance as Common Molecular Denominator Linking Obesity to Alzheimer's Disease. *Curr. Alzheimer Res.* **2015**, *12*, 723–735. [CrossRef] [PubMed]

47. Cholerton, B.; Baker, L.D.; Montine, T.J.; Craft, S. Type 2 Diabetes, Cognition, and Dementia in Older Adults: Toward a Precision Health Approach. *Diabetes Spectr.* **2016**, *29*, 210–219. [CrossRef] [PubMed]

48. McCrimmon, R.J.; Ryan, C.M.; Frier, B.M. Diabetes and cognitive dysfunction. *Lancet* **2012**, *379*, 2291–2299. [CrossRef]

49. Xu, H.; Moore, E.; Meiri, N.; Quon, M.J.; Alkon, D.L. Brain insulin receptors and spatial memory. *J. Biol. Chem.* **1999**, *274*, 34839–34842.

50. Chami, B.; Steel, A.J.; De La Monte, S.M.; Sutherland, G.T. The rise and fall of insulin signaling in Alzheimer's disease. *Metab Brain Dis.* **2016**, *31*, 497–515. [CrossRef] [PubMed]

51. Hokama, M.; Oka, S.; Leon, J.; Ninomiya, T.; Honda, H.; Sasaki, K.; Iwaki, T.; Ohara, T.; Sasaki, T.; LaFerla, F.M.; et al. Altered expression of diabetes-related genes in Alzheimer's disease brains: The Hisayama study. *Cereb. Cortex* **2014**, *24*, 2476–2488. [CrossRef] [PubMed]

52. De Felice, F.G. Connecting type 2 diabetes to Alzheimer's disease. *Expert Rev. Neurother.* **2013**, *13*, 1297–1299. [CrossRef] [PubMed]

53. Ma, Q.L.; Yang, F.; Rosario, E.R.; Ubeda, O.J.; Beech, W.; Gant, D.J.; Chen, P.P.; Hudspeth, B.; Chen, C.; Zhao, Y. Beta-amyloid oligomers induce phosphorylation of tau and inactivation of insulin receptor substrate via c-Jun N-terminal kinase signaling: Suppression by omega-3 fatty acids and curcumin. *J. Neurosci.* **2009**, *29*, 9078–9089. [CrossRef] [PubMed]

54. Yarchoan, M.; Toledo, J.B.; Lee, E.B.; Arvanitakis, Z.; Kazi, H.; Han, L.Y.; Louneva, N.; Lee, V.M.; Kim, S.F.; Trojanowski, J.Q.; et al. Abnormal serine phosphorylation of insulin receptor substrate 1 is associated with tau pathology in Alzheimer's disease and tauopathies. *Acta Neuropathol.* **2014**, *128*, 679–689. [CrossRef] [PubMed]

55. Havrankova, J.; Roth, J.; Brownstein, M. Insulin receptors are widely distributed in the central nervous system of the rat. *Nature* **1978**, *5656*, 827–829. [CrossRef]

56. Ribe, E.M.; Lovestone, S. Insulin signalling in Alzheimer's disease and diabetes: From epidemiology to molecular links. *J. Intern. Med.* **2016**, *280*, 430–442. [CrossRef] [PubMed]

57. Kandimalla, R.; Thirumala, V.; Reddy, P.H. Is Alzheimer's disease a Type 3 Diabetes? A critical appraisal. *Biochim. Biophys. Acta* **2017**, *1863*, 1078–1089. [CrossRef] [PubMed]

58. Diehl, T.; Mullins, R.; Kapogiannis, D. Insulin resistance in Alzheimer's disease. *Transl. Res.* **2017**, *183*, 26–40. [CrossRef] [PubMed]

59. Liu, Y.; Liu, F.; Grundke-Iqbal, I.; Iqbal, K.; Gong, C.X. Deficient brain insulin signalling pathway in Alzheimer's disease and diabetes. *J. Pathol.* **2011**, *225*, 54–62. [CrossRef] [PubMed]

60. Biessels, G.J.; Kappelle, L.J. Increased risk of Alzheimer's disease in Type II diabetes: insulin resistance of the brain or insulin-induced amyloid pathology? *Biochem. Soc. Trans.* **2005**, *33*, 1041–1044. [CrossRef] [PubMed]

61. Stanley, M.; Macauley, S.L.; Holtzman, D.M. Changes in insulin and insulin signaling in Alzheimer's disease: Cause or consequence? *J. Exp. Med.* **2016**, *213*, 1375–1385. [CrossRef] [PubMed]

62. Pardeshi, R.; Bolshette, N.; Gadhave, K.; Ahire, A.; Ahmed, S.; Cassano, T.; Gupta, V.B.; Lahkar, M. Insulin signaling: An opportunistic target to minify the risk of Alzheimer's disease. *Psychoneuroendocrinology* **2017**, *83*, 159–171. [CrossRef] [PubMed]

63. Schubert, M.; Gautam, D.; Surjo, D.; Ueki, K.; Baudler, S.; Schubert, D.; Kondo, T.; Alber, J.; Galldiks, N.; Küstermann, E.; et al. Role for neuronal insulin resistance in neurodegenerative diseases. *Proc. Natl. Acad. Sci. USA* **2004**, *101*, 3100–3105. [CrossRef] [PubMed]

64. Freude, S.; Plum, L.; Schnitker, J.; Leeser, U.; Udelhoven, M.; Krone, W.; Bruning, J.C.; Schubert, M. Peripheral hyperinsulinemia promotes tau phosphorylation in vivo. *Diabetes* **2005**, *54*, 3343–3348. [CrossRef] [PubMed]

65. Guan, J.; Bennet, L.; Gluckman, P.D.; Gunn, A.J. Insulin-like growth factor-1 and post-ischemic brain injury. *Prog. Neurobiol.* **2003**, *70*, 443–462. [CrossRef] [PubMed]

66. Rodriguez-Rodriguez, P.; Sandebring-Matton, A.; Merino-Serrais, P.; Parrado-Fernandez, C.; Rabano, A.; Winblad, B.; Ávila, J.; Ferrer, I.; Cedazo-Minguez, A. Tau hyperphosphorylation induces oligomeric insulin accumulation and insulin resistance in neurons. *Brain* **2017**, *140*, 3269–3285. [CrossRef] [PubMed]

67. Ashrafi, G.; Wu, Z.; Farrell, R.J.; Ryan, T.A. GLUT4 Mobilization Supports Energetic Demands of Active Synapses. *Neuron* **2017**, *93*, 606–615. [CrossRef] [PubMed]

68. Pearson-Leary, J.; McNay, E.C. Novel Roles for the Insulin-Regulated Glucose Transporter-4 in Hippocampally Dependent Memory. *J. Neurosci.* **2016**, *36*, 11851–11864. [CrossRef] [PubMed]

69. Mehta, V.; Parashar, A.; Sharma, A.; Singh, T.R.; Udayabanu, M. Quercetin ameliorates chronic unpredicted stress-mediated memory dysfunction in male Swiss albino mice by attenuating insulin resistance and elevating hippocampal GLUT4 levels independent of insulin receptor expression. *Horm. Behav.* **2017**, *89*, 13–22. [CrossRef] [PubMed]

70. Shinohara, M.; Sato, N. Bidirectional interactions between diabetes and Alzheimer's disease. *Neurochem. Int.* **2017**, *108*, 296–302. [CrossRef] [PubMed]

71. Kang, S.; Lee, Y.H.; Lee, J.E. Metabolism-Centric Overview of the Pathogenesis of Alzheimer's disease. *Yonsei Med. J.* **2017**, *58*, 479–488. [CrossRef] [PubMed]

72. Wu, J.; Fu, B.; Lei, H.; Tang, H.; Wang, Y. Gender differences of peripheral plasma and liver metabolic profiling in APP/PS1 transgenic AD mice. *Neuroscience* **2016**, *332*, 160–169. [CrossRef] [PubMed]

73. Zhang, Y.; Zhou, B.; Deng, B.; Zhang, F.; Wu, J.; Wang, Y.; Le, Y.; Zhai, Q. Amyloid-β induces hepatic insulin resistance in vivo via JAK2. *Diabetes* **2013**, *62*, 1159–1166. [CrossRef] [PubMed]

74. Zhang, Y.; Zhou, B.; Zhang, F.; Wu, J.; Hu, Y.; Liu, Y.; Zhai, Q. Amyloid-β induces hepatic insulin resistance by activating JAK2/STAT3/SOCS-1 signaling pathway. *Diabetes* **2012**, *61*, 1434–1443. [CrossRef] [PubMed]

75. Forny-Germano, L.; Lyra e Silva, N.M.; Batista, A.F.; Brito-Moreira, J.; Gralle, M.; Boehnke, S.E.; Coe, B.C.; Lablans, A.; Marques, S.A.; Martinez, A.M.; et al. Alzheimer's disease-like pathology induced by amyloid-β oligomers in nonhuman primates. *J. Neurosci.* **2014**, *34*, 13629–13643. [CrossRef] [PubMed]

76. Clarke, J.R.; Lyra, E.; Silva, N.M.; Figueiredo, C.P.; Frozza, R.L.; Ledo, J.H.; Beckman, D.; Katashima, C.K.; Razolli, D.; Carvalho, B.M.; et al. Alzheimer-associated Aβ oligomers impact the central nervous system to induce peripheral metabolic deregulation. *EMBO Mol. Med.* **2015**, *7*, 190–210.

77. Arrieta-Cruz, I.; Knight, C.M.; Gutiérrez-Juárez, R. Acute Exposure of the Mediobasal Hypothalamus to Amyloid-β25–35 Perturbs Hepatic Glucose Metabolism. *J. Alzheimers Dis.* **2015**, *46*, 843–848. [CrossRef] [PubMed]

78. Arrieta-Cruz, I.; Gutiérrez-Juárez, R. The Role of Insulin Resistance and Glucose Metabolism Dysregulation in the Development of Alzheimer's Disease. *Rev. Investig. Clin.* **2016**, *68*, 53–58.

79. Roher, A.E.; Esh, C.L.; Kokjohn, T.A.; Castaño, E.M.; Van Vickle, G.D.; Kalback, W.M.; Patton, R.L.; Luehrs, D.C.; Daugs, I.D.; Kuo, Y.M.; et al. Amyloid beta peptides in human plasma and tissues and their significance for Alzheimer's disease. *Alzheimers Dement.* **2009**, *5*, 18–29. [CrossRef] [PubMed]

80. Guglielmotto, M.; Monteleone, D.; Giliberto, L.; Fornaro, M.; Borghi, R.; Tamagno, E.; Tabaton, M. Amyloid-β42 activates the expression of BACE1 through the JNK pathway. *J. Alzheimers Dis.* **2011**, *27*, 871–883. [PubMed]

81. Guglielmotto, M.; Monteleone, D.; Boido, M.; Piras, A.; Giliberto, L.; Borgh, R.; Vercelli, A.; Fornaro, M.; Tabaton, M.; Tamagno, E. Aβ1–42-mediated downregulation of Uch-L1 is dependent on NF-κB activation and impaired BACE1 lysosomal degradation. *Aging Cell* **2012**, *11*, 834–844. [CrossRef] [PubMed]

82. Guglielmotto, M.; Monteleone, D.; Piras, A.; Valsecchi, V.; Tropiano, M.; Ariano, S.; Fornaro, M.; Vercelli, A.; Puyal, J.; Arancio, O.; et al. Aβ1–42 monomers or oligomers have different effects on autophagy and apoptosis. *Autophagy* **2014**, *10*, 1827–1843. [CrossRef] [PubMed]

83. Plucińska, K.; Crouch, B.; Koss, D.; Robinson, L.; Siebrecht, M.; Riedel, G.; Platt, B. Knock-in of human BACE1 cleaves murine APP and reiterates Alzheimer-like phenotypes. *J. Neurosci.* **2014**, *34*, 10710–10728. [CrossRef] [PubMed]

84. Plucińska, K.; Dekeryte, R.; Koss, D.; Shearer, K.; Mody, N.; Whitfield, P.D.; Doherty, M.K.L.; Mingarelli, M.; Welch, A.; Riedel, G.; et al. Neuronal human BACE1 knockin induces systemic diabetes in mice. *Diabetologia* **2016**, *59*, 1513–1523. [CrossRef] [PubMed]

85. Meakin, P.J.; Harper, A.J.; Hamilton, D.L.; Gallagher, J.; McNeilly, A.D.; Burgess, L.A.; Vaanholt, L.M.; Bannon, K.A.; Latcham, J.; Hussain, I.; et al. Reduction in BACE1 decreases body weight, protects against diet-induced obesity and enhances insulin sensitivity in mice. *Biochem. J.* **2012**, *441*, 285–296. [CrossRef] [PubMed]

86. De la Monte, S.M. Type 3 diabetes is sporadic Alzheimer's disease: Mini-review. *Eur. Neuropsychopharmacol.* **2014**, *24*, 1954–1960. [CrossRef] [PubMed]

87. Cardoso, S.; Correia, S.; Santos, R.X.; Carvalho, C.; Santos, M.S.; Oliveira, C.R.; Perry, G.; Smith, M.A.; Zhu, X.; Moreira, P.I. Insulin is a two-edged knife on the brain. *J. Alzheimers Dis.* **2009**, *18*, 483–507. [CrossRef] [PubMed]

88. De la Monte, S.M.; Tong, M.; Lester-Coll, N.; Plater, M., Jr.; Wands, J.R. Therapeutic rescue of neurodegeneration in experimental type 3 diabetes: Relevance to Alzheimer's disease. *J. Alzheimer's Dis.* **2006**, *10*, 89–109. [CrossRef]

89. Ott, V.; Benedict, C.; Schultes, B.; Born, J.; Hallschmid, M. Intranasal administration of insulin to the brain impacts cognitive function and peripheral metabolism. *Diabetes Obes. Metab.* **2012**, *14*, 214–221. [CrossRef] [PubMed]

90. De la Monte, S.M. Early intranasal insulin therapy halts progression of neurodegeneration: Progress in Alzheimer's disease therapeutics. *Aging Health* **2012**, *8*, 61–64. [CrossRef] [PubMed]

91. Galimberti, D.; Scarpini, E. Pioglitazone for the treatment of Alzheimer's disease. *Expert Opin. Investig. Drugs* **2017**, *26*, 97–101. [CrossRef] [PubMed]

92. Zhang, H.B.; Zhang, Y.; Chen, C.; Li, Y.Q.; Ma, C.; Wang, Z.J. Pioglitazone inhibits advanced glycation end product-induced matrix metalloproteinases and apoptosis by suppressing the activation of MAPK and NF-κB. *Apoptosis* **2016**, *21*, 1082–1093. [CrossRef] [PubMed]

93. Sato, T.; Hanyu, H.; Hirao, K.; Kanetaka, H.; Sakurai, H.; Iwamoto, T. Efficacy of PPAR-gamma agonist pioglitazone in mild Alzheimer disease. *Neurobiol. Aging* **2011**, *32*, 1626–1633. [CrossRef] [PubMed]

94. Hölscher, C. Drugs developed for treatment of diabetes show protective effects in Alzheimer's and Parkinson's diseases. *Sheng Li Xue Bao* **2014**, *66*, 497–510. [PubMed]

95. Lambert, M.P.; Barlow, A.K.; Chromy, B.A.; Edwards, C.; Freed, R.; Liosatos, M.; Morgan, T.E.; Rozovsky, I.; Trommer, B.; Viola, K.L.; et al. Diffusible, nonfibrillar ligands derived from Abeta1–42 are potent central nervous system neurotoxins. *Proc. Natl. Acad. Sci. USA* **1998**, *95*, 6448–6453. [CrossRef] [PubMed]

96. Pimplikar, S.W. Neuroinflammation in Alzheimer's disease: From pathogenesis to a therapeutic target. *J. Clin. Immunol.* **2014**, *34*, S64–S69. [CrossRef] [PubMed]

97. Zhu, X.C.; Yu, J.T.; Jiang, T.; Tan, L. Autophagy modulation for Alzheimer's disease therapy. *Mol. Neurobiol.* **2013**, *48*, 702–714. [CrossRef] [PubMed]

98. Jiang, T.; Yu, J.T.; Zhu, X.C.; Tan, M.S.; Wang, H.F.; Cao, L.; Zhang, Q.Q.; Shi, J.Q.; Gao, L.; Qin, H.; et al. Temsirolimus promotes autophagic clearance of amyloid-β and provides protective effects in cellular and animal models of Alzheimer's disease. *Pharmacol. Res.* **2014**, *81*, 54–63. [CrossRef] [PubMed]

99. Tramutola, A.; Lanzillotta, C.; Di Domenico, T. Targeting mTOR to reduce Alzheimer-related cognitive decline: From current hits to future therapies. *Expert Rev. Neurother.* **2017**, *17*, 33–45. [CrossRef] [PubMed]

100. Hanyu, H.; Sato, T.; Kiuchi, A.; Sakurai, H.; Iwamoto, T. Pioglitazone improved cognition in a pilot study on patients with Alzheimer's disease and mild cognitive impairment with diabetes mellitus. *J. Am. Geriatr. Soc.* **2009**, *57*, 177–179. [CrossRef] [PubMed]

101. Geldmacher, D.S.; Fritsch, T.; McClendon, M.J.; Landreth, G. A randomized pilot clinical trial of the safety of pioglitazone in treatment of patients with Alzheimer disease. *Arch. Neurol.* **2011**, *68*, 45–50. [CrossRef] [PubMed]

102. Fernandez-Martos, C.M.; Atkinson, R.A.K.; Chuah, M.I.; King, A.E.; Vickers, J.C. Combination treatment with leptin and pioglitazone in a mouse model of Alzheimer's disease. *Alzheimers Dement.* **2016**, *3*, 92–106. [CrossRef] [PubMed]

103. Gasparini, L.; Gouras, G.K.; Wang, R.; Gross, R.S.; Beal, M.F.; Greengard, P.; Xu, H. Stimulation of beta-amyloid precursor protein trafficking by insulin reduces intraneuronal beta-amyloid and requires mitogen-activated protein kinase signaling. *J. Neurosci.* **2001**, *21*, 2561–2570. [PubMed]

104. Rivera, E.J.; Goldin, A.; Fulmer, N.; Tavares, R.; Wands, J.R.; de la Monte, S.M. Insulin and insulin-like growth factor expression and function deteriorate with progression of Alzheimer's disease: Link to brain reductions in acetylcholine. *J. Alzheimers Dis.* **2005**, *8*, 247–268. [CrossRef] [PubMed]

105. Banks, W.A.; Farr, S.A.; Salameh, T.S.; Niehoff, M.L.; Rhea, E.M.; Morley, J.E.; Hanson, A.J.; Hansen, K.M.; Craft, S. Triglycerides cross the blood-brain barrier and induce central leptin and insulin receptor resistance. *Int. J. Obes.* **2017**. [CrossRef] [PubMed]

106. Baura, G.D.; Foster, D.M.; Porte, D.; Kahn, S.E.; Bergman, R.N.; Cobelli, C.; Schwartz, M.W. Saturable transport of insulin from plasma into the central-nervous-system of dogs in-vivo—A mechanism for regulated insulin delivery to the brain. *J. Clin. Investig.* **1993**, *92*, 1824–1830. [CrossRef] [PubMed]

107. Plum, L.; Schubert, M.; Brüning, J.C. The role of insulin receptor signaling in the brain. *Trends Endocrinol. Metab.* **2005**, *16*, 59–65. [CrossRef] [PubMed]

108. Craft, S.; Claxton, A.; Baker, L.D.; Hanson, A.J.; Cholerton, B.; Trittschuh, E.H.; Dahl, D.; Caulder, E.; Neth, B.; Montine, T.J.; et al. Effects of Regular and Long-Acting Insulin on Cognition and Alzheimer's Disease Biomarkers: A Pilot Clinical Trial. *J. Alzheimers Dis.* **2017**, *57*, 1325–1334. [CrossRef] [PubMed]

109. Craft, S.; Baker, L.D.; Montine, T.J.; Minoshima, S.; Watson, G.S.; Claxton, A.; Arbuckle, M.; Callaghan, M.; Tsai, E.; Plymate, S.R.; et al. Intranasal insulin therapy for Alzheimer disease and amnestic mild cognitive impairment: A pilot clinical trial. *Arch. Neurol.* **2012**, *69*, 29–38. [CrossRef] [PubMed]

110. Bergmann, L.; Maute, L.; Guschmann, M. Temsirolimus for advanced renal cellcarcinoma. *Expert Rev. Anticancer Ther.* **2014**, *14*, 9–21. [CrossRef] [PubMed]

111. Kwitkowski, V.E.; Prowell, T.M.; Ibrahim, A.; Farrell, A.T.; Justice, R.; Mitchell, S.S.; Sridhara, R.; Pazdur, R. FDA approval summary: Temsirolimus as treatment foradvanced renal cell carcinoma. *Oncologist* **2010**, *15*, 428–435. [CrossRef] [PubMed]

112. Wang, J.; Gu, B.J.; Masters, C.L.; Wang, Y.J. A systemic view of Alzheimer disease—Insights from amyloid-β metabolism beyond the brain. *Nat. Rev. Neurol.* **2017**, *13*, 612–623. [CrossRef] [PubMed]

7

Iron Absorption in Iron-Deficient Women, Who Received 65 mg Fe with an Indonesian Breakfast, Is Much Better from NaFe(III)EDTA than from Fe(II)SO$_4$, with an Acceptable Increase of Plasma NTBI

Eka Ginanjar [1], **Lilik Indrawati** [2], **Iswari Setianingsih** [3], **Djumhana Atmakusumah** [4],
Alida Harahap [3], **Ina S. Timan** [2] and **Joannes J. M. Marx** [5,*]

[1] Department of Internal Medicine, Faculty of Medicine, University of Indonesia/Dr Cipto Mangunkusumo Hospital, Jakarta 10430, Indonesia; ekginanjar@gmail.com

[2] Department of Clinical Pathology, Faculty of Medicine, University of Indonesia/Dr Cipto Mangunkusumo Hospital, Jakarta 10430, Indonesia; lilikindrawati.dr@gmail.com (L.I.); ina_sutanto@yahoo.com (I.S.T.)

[3] Eijkman Institute for Molecular Biology, Jakarta 10430, Indonesia; ning@eijkman.go.id (I.S.); alida@eijkman.go.id (A.H.)

[4] Division of Hematology and Medical Oncology, Department of Internal Medicine, Faculty of Medicine, University of Indonesia/Dr Cipto Mangunkusumo Hospital, Jakarta 10430, Indonesia; endjum@hotmail.com

[5] Department of Medical Microbiology, University Medical Centre Utrecht, Heidelberglaan 100, Utrecht 3584 CX, The Netherlands

* Correspondence: jjmmarx@me.com

Abstract: Plasma non-transferrin-bound iron (NTBI) is potentially harmful due to the generation of free radicals that cause tissue damage in vascular and other diseases. Studies in iron-replete and iron-deficient subjects, receiving a single oral test dose of Fe(II)SO$_4$ or NaFe(III)EDTA with water, revealed that FeSO$_4$ was well absorbed when compared with NaFeEDTA, while only the Fe(II) compound showed a remarkable increase of NTBI. As NaFeEDTA is successfully used for food fortification, a double-blind randomized cross-over trial was conducted in 11 healthy women with uncomplicated iron deficiency. All subjects received a placebo, 6.5 mg FeSO$_4$, 65 mg FeSO$_4$, 6.5 mg NaFeEDTA, and 65 mg NaFeEDTA with a traditional Indonesian breakfast in one-week intervals. Blood tests were carried out every 60 min for five hours. NTBI detection was performed using the fluorescein-labeled apotransferrin method. Plasma iron values were highly increased after 65 mg NaFeEDTA, twice as high as after FeSO$_4$. A similar pattern was seen for NTBI. After 6.5 mg of NaFeEDTA and FeSO$_4$, NTBI was hardly detectable. NaFeEDTA was highly effective for the treatment of iron deficiency if given with a meal, inhibiting the formation of nonabsorbable Fe-complexes, while NTBI did not exceed the range of normal values for iron-replete subjects.

Keywords: iron deficiency anemia; nutrient iron; oral iron therapy; FeSO$_4$; NaFeEDTA; non-transferrin-bound iron (NTBI); developing countries; Indonesia

1. Introduction

Iron deficiency anemia (IDA) is a worldwide health problem, affecting about 2 billion people, particularly in developing countries like Indonesia [1]. IDA has a large impact on productivity, mental performance, child growth, immunity, and pregnancy outcome. About 20 years ago in Indonesia, 25–30% of the population (50 to 70 million subjects) suffered from IDA [2]. The management of iron deficiency by oral iron salts and food iron fortification were effective for raising plasma hemoglobin concentration in Indonesia as demonstrated by large family life surveys on anemia prevalence, estimated in 1997, 2000, and 2008 [3]. The prevalence of anemia decreased in all groups studied, e.g., in women >15 years from 36.0 to 26.6%. Nevertheless, iron deficiency anemia remains a health problem in Indonesia due to insufficient nutrient daily intake [4].

Meanwhile, iron supplementation is commonly practiced by physicians in rural and urban areas. Furthermore, the community has easy access to oral iron supplements for their own consumption. Unfortunately, iron drugs are often consumed without a proper diagnosis of iron deficiency anemia, and are even used to combat lethargy or to gain strength and vitality. Measures to prevent iron deficiency should be specifically aimed at population groups at risk because actions to increase iron intake and bioavailability in the general population can be harmful for subjects with undiagnosed homozygous and heterozygous forms of iron overload diseases such as thalassemia intermedia [5].

Despite the fact that plasma-transferrin in iron-deficient patients has a large capacity of free iron-binding sites, treatment with a standard oral dose of 200 mg $FeSO_4$ (ferrous sulfate, containing 65 mg of elementary iron) was observed to generate potentially toxic amounts of non-transferrin-bound iron (NTBI) [6]. NTBI is the fraction of iron in plasma that is not tightly and safely bound to transferrin, including a heterogeneous mixture of labile and stable molecular species. NTBI is associated with oxygen radical formation and tissue damage in normal subjects and those with iron overload diseases [7]. In addition, NTBI and many other human iron-containing molecules can be utilized by microorganisms [8]. Therefore, the detection of NTBI after oral administration of regular iron medication, even in subjects with iron deficiency, needs further investigation. As iron-deficient subjects, with mainly free iron-binding sites on circulating transferrin, may be protected against iron-catalyzed reactive oxygen species, it is not clear whether the detection of NTBI after oral iron therapy can be harmful or is just associated with iron absorption physiology.

Not only should ferrous sulfate be investigated, being the standard treatment of iron deficiency, but also the Fe(III) compounds that have been used since 1950 for food iron fortification. In particular, NaFe(III)EDTA (Ferrazone, Akzo Nobel), recommended by the WHO as the preferred iron fortificant for wheat and maize flour, which are staple foods used by the whole population. Layrisse and co-workers described in 1977 that iron absorption from Fe(III)EDTA was about twice as high as that observed from ferrous sulfate [9].

NaFeEDTA is widely used in Indonesia, not only as a food fortificant, but also for the treatment of iron deficiency in children, which is recommended by the Pediatrician Association of Indonesia (IDAI). It is available as a syrup, Ferrostrane® (Teofarma S.r.l., Pavia, Italy), with one teaspoon (5 mL) containing 34 mg of iron. For adults, three to six teaspoons per day are recommended (102–204 mg of iron).

In previous studies that investigated the iron absorption and generation of NTBI in subjects receiving a single oral therapeutic dose of $Fe(II)SO_4$ or NaFe(III)EDTA with water, the absorption of iron from $FeSO_4$ was much better when compared with NaFeEDTA, while only the Fe(II) compound showed a remarkable increase of NTBI. This was found in iron-replete [10] and in iron-deficient subjects [11].

In the present clinical crossover study in iron-deficient women (without signs or symptoms of inflammation), the post-absorption values for plasma iron and NTBI were measured during five hours from both a therapeutic elementary iron dose (65 mg) and a dose relevant for iron fortification (6.5 mg) in the form of $Fe(II)SO_4$ and NaFe(III)EDTA, all presented after a traditional Indonesian breakfast.

2. Results

2.1. Selection of Participants and Data Collection

After screening 63 apparently healthy female candidates, 11 were selected for a randomized clinical trial as described in the Materials and Methods. All selected subjects fulfilled the criteria for iron deficiency anemia with low values for hemoglobin (Hb), mean cellular volume (MCV), mean cellular hemoglobin (MCH), low seum iron (SI), and high total iron binding capacity (TIBC). Mean transferrin saturation was 7.7% and serum ferritin was less than 20 µg/L These basic data were obtained from examination on minute 0 on the first day of the study when all subjects were only given the test meal: Group A received $FeSO_4$ first, and Group B received NaFeEDTA first. There was no significant difference between any of the laboratory characteristics of the subjects from both groups.

In some samples, taken before the consumption of the standard meal, a raised level of C-reactive protein (CRP) (>10 mg/L) was found, which was interpreted as a sign of inflammation. As iron absorption is decreased during inflammation [12], such episodes were removed from the final results. We also decided to remove investigation episodes if hemolytic blood samples were identified in the laboratory. The minimum number of episodes that could be analyzed, however, was never below six. In all three subjects with increased CRP, of whom the results were removed from the study, serum iron and NTBI curves after iron ingestion were flat, even after the administration of 65 mg Fe as NaFeEDTA, and were no different from the 0 mg Fe placebo dose.

The complete set of data collected during this investigation is available in the Appendix. One table indicates which data were excluded from further evaluation due to hemolysis of the blood sample or CRP-values > 10 mg/L as a nonspecific sign of inflammation. If a test subject's data for $FeSO_4$ had to be removed, data for NaFeEDTA for the same iron dose (6.5 or 65 mg) were also removed.

2.2. Results for Iron Absorption and NTBI Generation

Presented are the results of the increase of serum iron values (Figure 1A) and NTBI (Figure 1B) after donation of one meal only and a meal with the addition of 6.5 or 65 mg iron as either $FeSO_4$ or NaFeEDTA. Such simple values represent the dynamic processes after ingestion of the meal with the specified test dose during migration through the stomach and upper intestine (all with a distinct function in iron absorption), and the binding of iron to and the release from transferrin in plasma.

Accumulatively, the increase of serum iron and NTBI after the different oral doses of $FeSO_4$ and NaFeEDTA is demonstrated in Table 1 with the area under the curve (AUC) according to Conway et al. [13]. From the calculation of AUC, NTBI generation after 65 mg $FeSO_4$ and 65 mg NaFeEDTA was far higher when compared to the placebo and iron supplement of a lower dosage. NTBI generated after 65 mg NaFeEDTA was higher when compared to 65 mg $FeSO_4$.

Table 1. Area under the curve (AUC) of serum iron and NTBI during 300 min after ingestion.

Test Dose	AUC Serum Iron (µmol/L)	AUC NTBI (µmol/L)
Fe 0.0 mg (placebo)	100	3.0
6.5 mg $FeSO_4$	89	−10.5
65 mg $FeSO_4$	2017	203.7
6.5 mg NaFeEDTA	370	−1.8
65 mg NaFeEDTA	2968	324

With the method used, hardly any increase in serum iron and NTBI was observed after a meal only (placebo 0 mg Fe), or 6.5 mg iron as either $FeSO_4$ or NaFeEDTA. Additionally, no significant difference could be seen for both parameters for all time points after the donation of 6.5 mg iron between $FeSO_4$ and NaFeEDTA.

There was a significant difference, however, in the increment of both serum iron and NTBI levels ($p < 0.05$) in subjects given a standard therapeutic dose of 65 mg Fe of both $FeSO_4$ and NaFeEDTA. It was remarkable, however, that both iron absorption (estimated by an increase of plasma iron) and the appearance of potentially harmful NTBI were about twice as high after the donation of NaFeEDTA than after FeSO4.

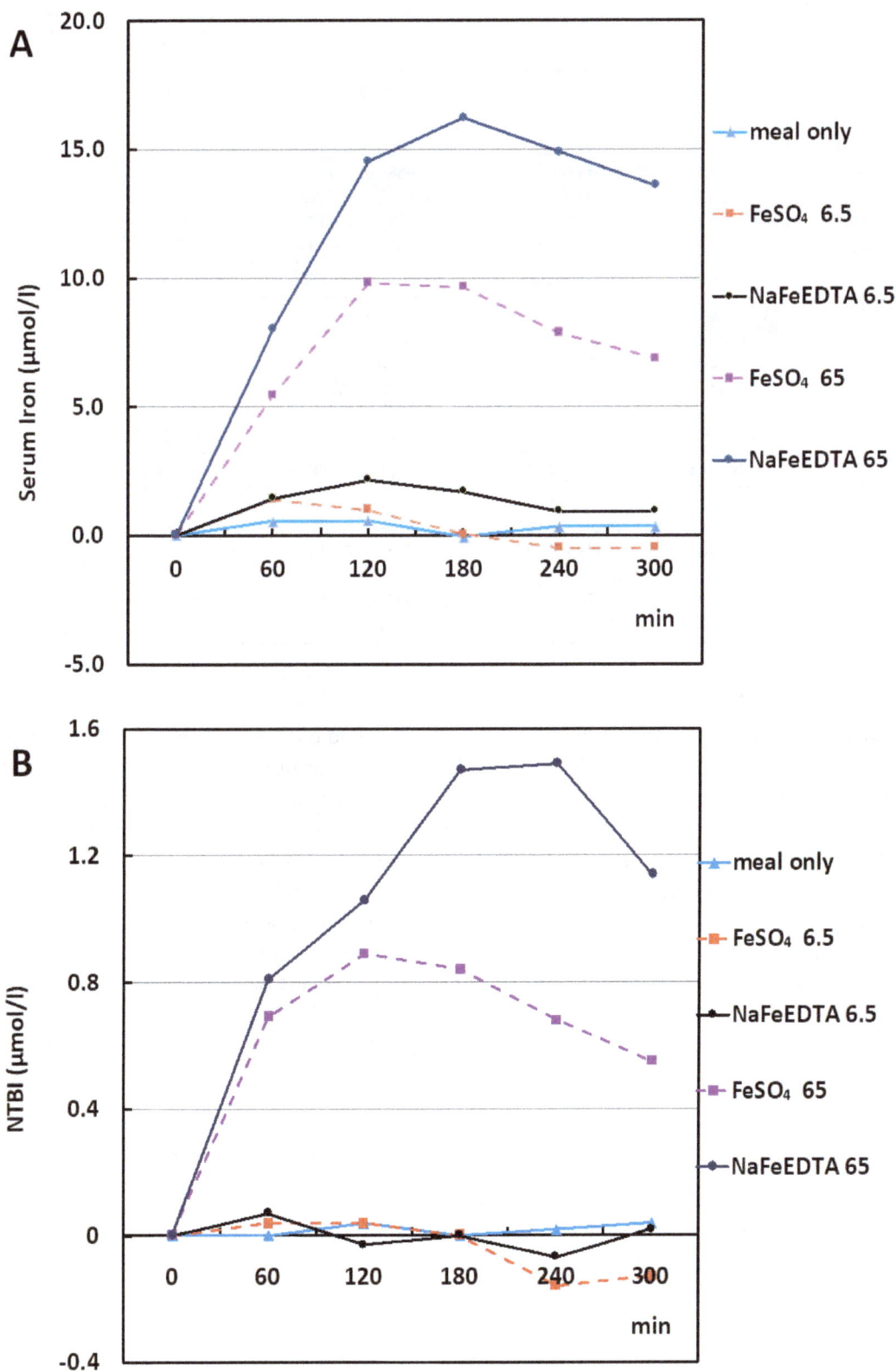

Figure 1. Increase of serum iron (**A**) and serum NTBI (**B**) after 6.5 and 65 mg iron administered after a standard meal as Fe(II)SO$_4$ or as NaFe(III)EDTA.

In Table 2, more detailed data are presented for the NTBI values after the administration of 0 mg (placebo) and the high, but therapeutically most relevant, dose of 65 mg FeSO$_4$ and NaFeEDTA. In both cases, a considerable increase of NTBI was observed.

Table 2. NTBI (μmol/L) generation after ingestion of a meal, followed by 0 mg Fe (placebo), 65 mg FeSO$_4$ and 65 mg NaFeEDTA.

Minute	Placebo	65 mg FeSO$_4$	p-Value
0	0	0	-
60	−0.0034 ± 0.1798	0.6866 ± 0.7498	0.002
120	0.0433 ± 0.1565	0.8886 ± 0.9156	0.012
180	−0.0031 ± 0.1781	0.8412 ± 0.7522	<0.001
240	0.0154 ± 0.2372	0.6795 ± 0.4329	0.001
300	0.0409 ± 0.2194	0.5531 ± 0.6003	0.020

Minute	Placebo	65 mg NaFeEDTA	p-Value
0	0	0	-
60	−0.0034 ± 0.1798	0.8106 ± 0.8073	0.007
120	0.0433 ± 0.1565	1.0566 ± 0.7181	0.002
180	−0.0031 ± 0.1781	1.4695 ± 0.7247	<0.001
240	0.0154 ± 0.2372	1.4922 ± 0.7523	<0.001
300	0.0409 ± 0.2194	1.1421 ± 0.7509	<0.001

Minute	65 mg FeSO$_4$	65 mg NaFeEDTA	p-Value
0	0	0	-
60	0.6866 ± 0.7498	0.8106 ± 0.8073	0.530
120	0.8886 ± 0.9156	1.0566 ± 0.7181	0.423
180	0.8412 ± 0.7522	1.4695 ± 0.7247	0.017
240	0.6795 ± 0.4329	1.4922 ± 0.7523	0.001
300	0.5531 ± 0.6003	1.1421 ± 0.7509	0.011

2.3. Complications and Side Effects

Blood loss. Due to this study protocol, all participants had considerable blood loss. During each of the five test episodes, there was 50 mL blood loss (10 mL at minute 0 min, then 5 times 8 mL) with a total of 250 mL. During the test period, hemoglobin concentration decreased around 0.7 g/dL. Therefore, at the end of the study protocol, all participants received iron supplement therapy.

Phlebitis in subject 11 after phlebotomy at the administration of 6.5 mg NaFeEDTA. Topical heparin (Thrombophob®) was applied and resolved the problem after three days.

Nausea in subject 1 after the administration of 6.5 mg NaFeEDTA, in subject 4 after the administration of 65 mg NaFeEDTA and in subject 10 after the administration of 6.5 mg FeSO$_4$. All three subjects were given one omeprazole 20 mg capsule and one domperidone 10 mg tablet. The symptoms were resolved after 30 min.

Other side effects or complications were not observed.

3. Discussion

3.1. Comparison with Results from Studies Using Similar and Different Methodologies

Numerous clinical studies on the absorption of iron for the treatment or prevention of iron deficiency have been published [14,15]. The method used in the present investigation is not able to provide absolute quantitative values, but iron uptake from the gut after presenting different compounds and amounts of iron can be compared. However, there is a limitation as small increases of non-radiolabelled iron in plasma are undetectable if low iron doses are given.

In this study, iron uptake and the appearance of potentially harmful non-transferrin-bound iron (NTBI) were investigated by administering doses relevant for iron therapy (65 mg Fe) and also for food iron fortification (6.5 mg) to healthy, iron-deficient Indonesian females after an Indonesian standard breakfast. The compounds were Fe(II)SO$_4$ (medication of choice for treatment of iron deficiency anemia) and NaFe(III)EDTA (supplement of choice for the fortification of food products and therefore for the prevention of iron deficiency anemia). Intestinal iron uptake was estimated by comparing the serum iron concentration during six hours, and increase of serum NTBI [6]. We compared our results with investigations from Guatemala, published in 2012 [10] and 2013 [11], to try to answer similar questions and use the same experimental approach, however, with a completely different outcome. In all three studies, NTBI tests were performed in the same laboratory in Utrecht.

In the 2012 study [10], an oral supplement of a 0 mg Fe placebo dose in 200 mL water, a therapeutic dose of 100 mg iron as $FeSO_4$ (as a commercial syrup dissolved in 200 mL water) or 100 mg of iron as 770 mg of NaFeEDTA powder dissolved in 200 mL of water, was administered to healthy, iron-replete males after at least eight hours of fasting. In this cross-over study, each subject served as his own control. Venepuncture was performed at 0, 90, 180, and 270 min. In the 2013 study [11], the design was identical, in particular, the donation of iron with water, but the test subjects were non-pregnant healthy women with low ferritin values (<30 ng/mL). After 100 mg iron as $FeSO_4$, a considerable increase of serum iron was seen in men with adequate iron stores and normal CRP, and a much higher increase in females with low iron stores and normal CRP. Iron uptake from 100 mg iron as NaFeEDTA in men was identical to that from water. Additionally, in iron-deficient females, the serum iron values were only a bit higher.

Troesch et al. [16] and Brittenham et al. [17] used stable isotopes to estimate the percentages of iron absorption in post-absorption curves, and iron utilization by circulating erythrocytes 14 days after ingestion of the labeled test doses. Troesch et al. investigated iron uptake from 6 mg iron as $FeSO_4$ with ascorbic acid (AA) and from 6 mg iron as NaFeEDTA. Hardly any increase was seen for both $FeSO_4$ and NaFeEDTA when the serum iron values were measured. When labeled with stable isotopes, the 6 mg iron uptake curves were almost identical with those found by us after the uptake of 65 mg iron. After 6 mg iron, the increase of serum iron was higher after $FeSO_4$ with AA than after NaFeEDTA.

Brittenham studied women with replete and reduced iron stores, receiving a 6 mg or a 60 mg iron dose as $FeSO_4$ with a standard meal. Red blood cell iron utilization was measured using stable isotopes. With this approach, the values for real iron absorption could be calculated, which were higher for iron-deficient than for iron-replete women. Of interest was the percentage of iron absorption in iron-deficient women from the test dose given with a meal, which was 1.22 mg (20.4%) from the 6 mg dose, and 8.82 mg (10.0%) from the 60 mg dose. Peak values for NTBI were 0.1 μmol/L after the 6 mg dose and 0.81 μmol/L after 60 mg Fe. These values were almost identical with those from the comparable doses in our study. After the donation of 65 mg Fe as NaFeEDTA, the mean peak NTBI values were twice as high, but remained below 1.5 μmol/L.

Although the design of our study was similar to the two from Guatemala, there were crucial differences. Most importantly, our iron test dose was not given after eight hours of fasting but directly after ingestion of a standard breakfast. This resulted in a high uptake from 65 mg iron as NaFeEDTA, even twice as high as that from 65 mg Fe as $FeSO_4$ (Figure 1A). The conclusion was that the absorption of iron was much better if given with a meal than with water. The pattern for NTBI in plasma was almost identical, suggesting that NaFeEDTA may be less safe than $FeSO_4$ (Figure 1B). In addition to a therapeutic dose of 65 mg Fe, we studied a fortification dose of 6.5 mg Fe. No NTBI could be detected in the serum for both iron compounds. Serum iron values were marginally higher for NaFeEDTA. The absolute NTBI values were low because all subjects were iron deficient.

3.2. Aspects of Iron Absorption

If iron is administered in an aqueous solution on an empty stomach, passage through the stomach and upper intestinal tract is rapid. This is an advantage for the uptake of iron from ferrous sulfate as Fe(II) is directly available for transport by the divalent metal transporter (DMT1) to the cytosol of duodenal mucosal cells by simple diffusion [18]. Complexed Fe(III) like in NaFeEDTA must first be reduced to Fe(II) by the reductase duodenal cytochrome B (DcytB) in direct proximity of DMT1. Fe(II) leaves the mucosal cells by ferroportin, mainly depending on the free iron binding sites for Fe(III) on transferrin. Oxidation of Fe(II) by hephestin (membrane) or ceruloplasmin (plasma) is needed for binding to transferrin. The mucosal cell function in processing absorbable iron is summarized in Figure 2.

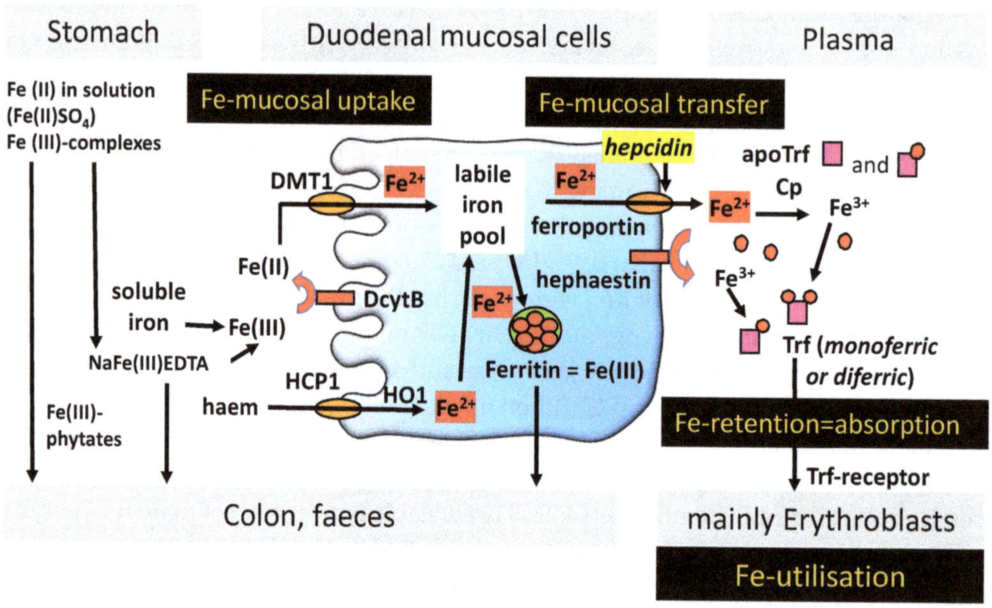

Figure 2. Processing of absorbable iron by the duodenal mucosal cells. DMT1 = divalent metal transporter 1; DcytB = duodenal cytochrome B; HCP1 = hem carrier protein 1; HO1 = hem oxygenase-1; Cp = ceruloplasmin; Trf = transferrin.

Plasma iron concentration is the resultant of iron transported to the plasma, free iron-binding sites on transferrin, and iron demand for erythropoiesis, which is increased in iron deficiency and in hemolytic anemias.

After the duodenum, the nonabsorbed Fe(II) is oxidized in the intestinal lumen and forms complexes with a variety of ligands in more distal parts of the intestinal tract before being removed with the feces. While the results for $FeSO_4$ in the Guatemalan studies can be explained by normal physiology, this was not the case with NaFeEDTA administered with water.

EDTA is a chelator that can combine with virtually every metal, depending on its stability constant with the metal. This is influenced by pH, the molar ratio of the chelator to the metal ion, and the presence of competing metal ions and other ligands. Ferric iron has the highest stability constant with EDTA at 25.1 (optimum pH = 1), followed by ferrous iron (14.6) (optimum pH = 5) [19]. The intraluminal pH is rapidly changed from acidic in the stomach (empty state pH 4–5, after meal pH 1.3) to about pH 6 in the duodenum. The pH gradually changes in the small intestine from pH 6 to about pH 7.4 in the terminal ileum, 5.7 in the cecum, and pH 6.7 in the rectum [20].

The binding of EDTA to iron is favored by the acidic environment of the stomach (due to the very high binding constant), but in the more alkaline surroundings of the duodenum, the iron is exchanged in part for other metals. EDTA protects iron in the stomach from inhibitory dietary ligands such as phytates and polyphenols and releases iron in the duodenum, where iron can be absorbed after reduction by DcytB and transport by DMT1. Phytates, present in many cereals and legumes, are powerful inhibitors of iron absorption. Some direct evidence of the ability of NaFeEDTA to prevent their action was obtained in an experiment where bran, a rich source of phytates, was shown to reduce the absorption of iron from ferrous sulfate eleven-fold. In contrast, no such inhibition occurred when bran was fed with NaFeEDTA [21].

Fe(III) reaches the cecum in complexed forms. With EDTA, however, it will form a stable complex. Nonabsorbed Fe as NaFeEDTA may reach the colon with a pH of 5.6 and a relatively low stability constant for NaFe(II)EDTA. Iron absorption from the colon is possible [22]. Some DcytB has been found to be expressed in the large intestine, while ferroportin and DMT1 are expressed at significant levels and are increased in iron deficiency [23].

3.3. Toxic Effects of NTBI in Plasma after Absorption of Iron

NTBI includes plasma iron that is not bound to transferrin or is a structural part of other proteins in plasma including ferritin. While transferrin-bound iron is redox-inactive and safe, many forms of NTBI are labile and able to exchange iron with other molecular species that can cause the formation of toxic oxygen species and tissue damage. NTBI was first identified in 1978 in patients with beta thalassemia major and intermedia [24]. For decades, NTBI was exclusively associated with (severe) iron overload, although it was also associated with other pathological conditions.

After a publication on the appearance of NTBI in plasma after oral treatment with $FeSO_4$ [6] and in hereditary hemochromatosis (HH) heterozygotes [25], the general view was that in these conditions, NTBI might also generate oxygen radicals. In a large epidemiological investigation, high mortality due to myocardial infarction and stroke was detected in female HH heterozygotes, but only in those reported with smoking and/or hypertension as combined risk factors [26]. In another large study investigating the relation of NTBI, serum iron, transferrin saturation, and serum ferritin with the risk of coronary heart disease (CHD) and acute myocardial infarction (AMI), the results did not show an excess risk of CHD or AMI within the highest NTBI tertile when compared with the lowest, but rather seemed to demonstrate a decreased risk [27]. The NTBI was measured with the same method as in the present study, and the total range of NTBI concentrations was -2.06 to 3.51 μmol/L.

As we wanted to compare the post-absorption curves of NTBI in this study, for all compounds and Fe-doses, the 0-min NTBI was set to 0 with the appropriate correction of all NTBI values. When reviewing the complete range of all time-points including the high dose of 65 mg Fe as $FeSO_4$ and NaFeEDTA, the range of all values of NTBI was between -0.59 and 0.37 μmol/L. This was very low, and in agreement with the iron-deficient state of the test subjects.

As can be seen in Figure 1, only about 10% of the absorbed iron was identified as NTBI. Many molecular species in plasma can bind iron, however, with a much lower affinity than apotransferrin. This was described in a review by Hider [28]. Most important are citrate and albumin. The citrate level in plasma is 100–120 μmol/L, representing a considerable iron binding capacity. In our test subjects, the total iron binding capacity (TIBC) of transferrin was 45–73 μmol/L. Citrate forms a wide range of oligomeric iron(III) species, which are stable complexes. Transfer of iron between an iron(III) citrate complex and desferrioxamine takes several hours to complete at pH 7.4 [29]. The rate-limiting step is the dissociation of iron from the polynuclear complex. Another molecule able to bind large amounts of iron in plasma is albumin [28]. Its concentration is 34–50 g/L plasma, and albumin possesses a large number of negative carboxylate sites on its surface that are able to bind Fe(III). Absorbed iron bound to citrate or albumin cannot be considered as toxic labile NTBI.

Our conclusion is that humans, after being exposed for a longer time to NTBI values in plasma that can be reached after treatment with highly absorbable iron compounds with a rather moderate increase of serum NTBI, remained healthy. These considerations may contribute to the discussion on the maximum acceptable daily intake of EDTA for iron fortification and iron therapy [30].

3.4. Iron Therapy in Developing Countries

Iron is needed for microbial proliferation [8]. There is enormous diversity in the mechanisms of iron uptake and of iron species that can be processed. A minority of pathogenic microorganisms are able to use plasma NTBI, one important species being malaria parasites. This is a huge health problem as malaria, together with iron deficiency anemia, is endemic in many regions of the world [31].

Thalassemia has a high prevalence along the Mediterranean coast, Africa, Middle East, India, Burma, Southeast Asia including Indonesia, and Melanesia up to the Pacific Islands [32,33]. A total of 3–10% of the world's population are β thalassemia carriers with the prevalence in Indonesia reaching 8% [34]. Thalassemia with iron overload and iron deficiency co-exists in the same population. Both are microcytic anemias, and clinical symptoms of iron deficiency and thalassemia heterozygotes are similar. Thalassemia patients frequently receive oral iron supplements for six months for up to two years. This practice is based on screening difficulties between iron deficiency anemia and anemia in

Thalassemia trait or intermedia. Apart from that, the public has access to hematinics that are sold freely over the counter.

The result of this study, showing an increment of NTBI generation after the administration of oral iron supplements may create awareness in healthcare providers to include sufficiently informative laboratory tests before providing oral iron supplements for iron deficiency only and to exclude iron-replete subjects and thalassemia heterozygotes.

4. Materials and Methods

This investigation was a randomized double-blind phase III clinical trial. After randomization, a cross-over design was used. The trial was carried out at the Eijkman Institute Jakarta from November 2008 to April 2009. Laboratory tests were performed at the University of Indonesia/Dr Cipto Mangunkusumo Hospital, Jakarta, Indonesia. NTBI values were measured in the laboratory of the Department of Medical Microbiology, University Medical Centre Utrecht, Utrecht, The Netherlands.

4.1. Selection of Test Subjects

Inclusion criteria: (1) Female; (2) Age 15–60 years old; (3) Iron deficiency (serum Ferritin < 20 µg/mL); and (4) Informed consent to be involved in the research.

Exclusion criteria: (1) Suffering from a chronic illness; (2) Currently having an acute or severe chronic infection; (3) Currently under drug therapy or receiving an iron supplement in any form, minimum one week prior to the clinical investigation; (4) Oral iron supplement allergy; (5) Suffering from a disease or disorder of the alimentary tract; and (6) Pregnancy.

Eleven females were selected after screening 63 apparently healthy women: (1) students of the Faculty of Medicine University of Indonesia who went for Thalassemia screening at the Eijkman Institute for Molecular Biology of Jakarta who were found to have microcytic hypochromic anemia; and (2) healthy women from several areas in Jakarta who were known to be iron deficiency patients at the Hematology and Medical Oncology outpatient clinic in the department of Internal Medicine RSCM. Eleven iron-deficient females were finally selected for this investigation.

The age range of the research subjects was between 15 and 34 years with a mean age of 24.18 years. A major portion of the study subjects were of a low education level (seven persons) and nine persons of low income, thus can be assumed to be of low socioeconomic level. A description of the selected test subjects is provided in Table 3.

Table 3. Distribution characteristics of the selected subjects.

Characteristic	Mean	Reference Value
Age	(n = 11) 24.18	
Education		
Low	7 subjects	
Medium	3 subjects	
High	1 subject	
Income		
Low	9 subjects	
Medium	2 subjects	
High	-	
Hemoglobin	10.9	12–14 gr/dL
MCV	74.9	82–92 fl
MCH	24.6	27–31 pg
MCHC	32.9	32–36 g/dL
Serum Iron	4.8	6.6–26.0 µmol/L
TIBC	76.9	44.6–73.4 µmol/L
Transferrin Saturation	7.7	<15% = Iron Deficiency
Ferritin	6.2	20–300 µg/L

4.2. *Procedure of the Investigation*

The selected subjects were asked to visit the Eijkman Institute five times with one-week intervals to undergo the test procedure.

The subjects were divided into two groups of six (A) and five (B) subjects. A cross-over procedure was used as shown in Scheme 1. The procedure sequence towards the subjects was determined by double-blind randomization using a voting technique. Randomization and crossing-over were performed to determine who would receive either $FeSO_4$ or NaFeEDTA first. Each subject needed to attend five times with a one-week interval as a wash-out period.

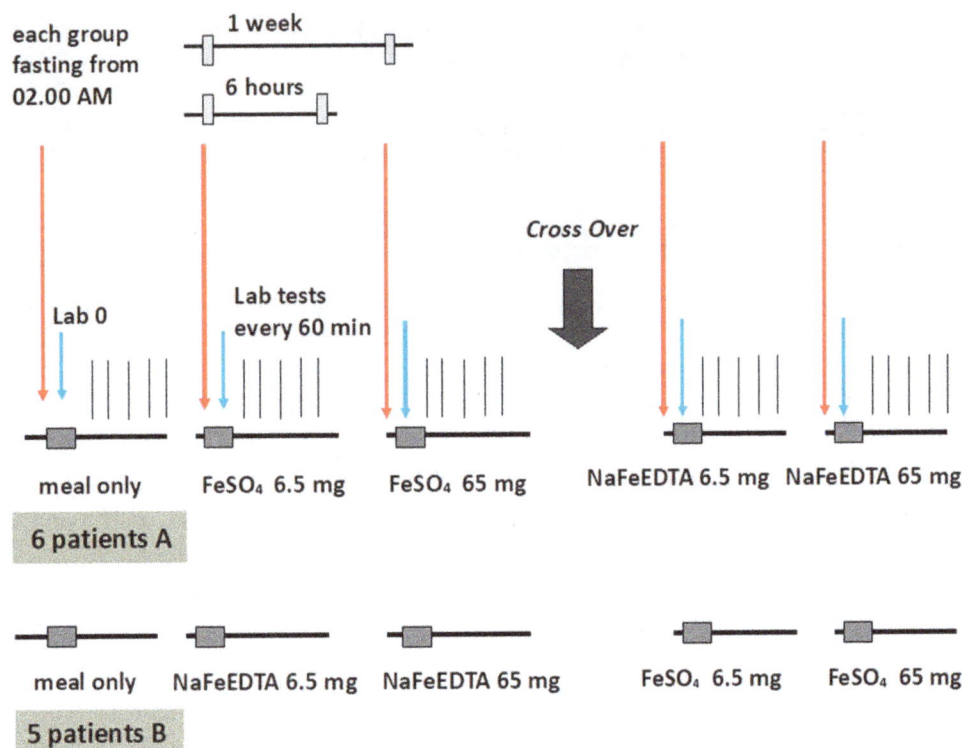

Scheme 1. Iron supplement administration schedule and iron doses.

Before any test episode (with or without receiving an iron dose), the test subjects were not allowed to take anything orally except plain water for at least six hours prior to the study. An intravenous catheter (Veinplon®) with a saline lock method was applied to enable multiple blood drawings in all subjects. A quantity of 10 mL blood was taken for the first venous blood drawing for Hb, MCV, MCH, MCHC, NTBI, Ferritin, SI, TIBC, transferrin saturation, CRP, and hepcidin.

Next, subjects were asked to consume a meal of rice with coconut milk (*nasi uduk*) and omelet, which is low in iron content, followed by the oral iron supplementation as shown in the table (see Scheme 2).

The mean reason why a meal prior to supplementation was included in the protocol was the reduction of side effects of oral iron supplementation like nausea, vomiting, epigastric pain, and burning sensation in the chest. A placebo dose was included to see the influence of the standard meal, and eventually circadian fluctuations of serum iron and NTBI.

After each test dose of oral iron supplement, 8 mL venous blood was taken at 60th, 120th, 180th, 240th, and 300th min for the measurement of NTBI, SI, TIBC, and transferrin saturation. Subjects were allowed to take anything orally after one hour of the test dose of oral iron supplement. Low iron snacks were provided during the whole procedure because subjects were at the research area for about six hours.

```
┌─────────────────────────────────────────────────────────────────┐
│        Screening of 63 clinically healthy women with iron deficiency  │
│                  Laboratory tests : CBC, ferritin                     │
└─────────────────────────────────────────────────────────────────┘
                               │
┌─────────────────────────────────────────────────────────────────┐
│       11 subjects selected according to inclusion and exclusion criteria │
└─────────────────────────────────────────────────────────────────┘
                               │
                    ┌──────────────────┐
                    │   Randomization  │
                    └──────────────────┘
        ┌──────────────┴───────────────────────────┐
┌───────────────────────────────┐          ┌───────────────────────────────┐
│ Group A: 6 subjects start with FeSO₄ │    │ Group B: 5 subjects start with NaFeEDTA │
└───────────────────────────────┘          └───────────────────────────────┘
        └──────────────┬───────────────────────────┘
┌─────────────────────────────────────────────────────────────────┐
│   Fasting starts at 02.00 am; arrival at Eijkman Institute Jakarta at 08.00 am │
└─────────────────────────────────────────────────────────────────┘
                               │
┌─────────────────────────────────────────────────────────────────┐
│                   Phlebotomy (10 ml) at minute 0 for:                 │
│ CBC, CRP, ferritin, NTBI, SI, TIBC, transferrin saturation, plasma Hb, haptoglobin, hepcidin │
└─────────────────────────────────────────────────────────────────┘
                               │
┌─────────────────────────────────────────────────────────────────┐
│   Directly after phlebotomy consumption of "nasi uduk" (Indonesian meal of cooked rice │
│     with coconut + fried egg) without or with test dose of iron supplement │
└─────────────────────────────────────────────────────────────────┘
                               │
┌─────────────────────────────────────────────────────────────────┐
│       Phlebotomy (8 ml) at minutes  60, 120, 180, 240 and 300 for:    │
│         NTBI, SI, TIBC, transferrin saturation, hepcidin              │
└─────────────────────────────────────────────────────────────────┘
                               │
              ┌──────────────────────────────────────┐
              │     Data recording and data analysis   │
              └──────────────────────────────────────┘
```

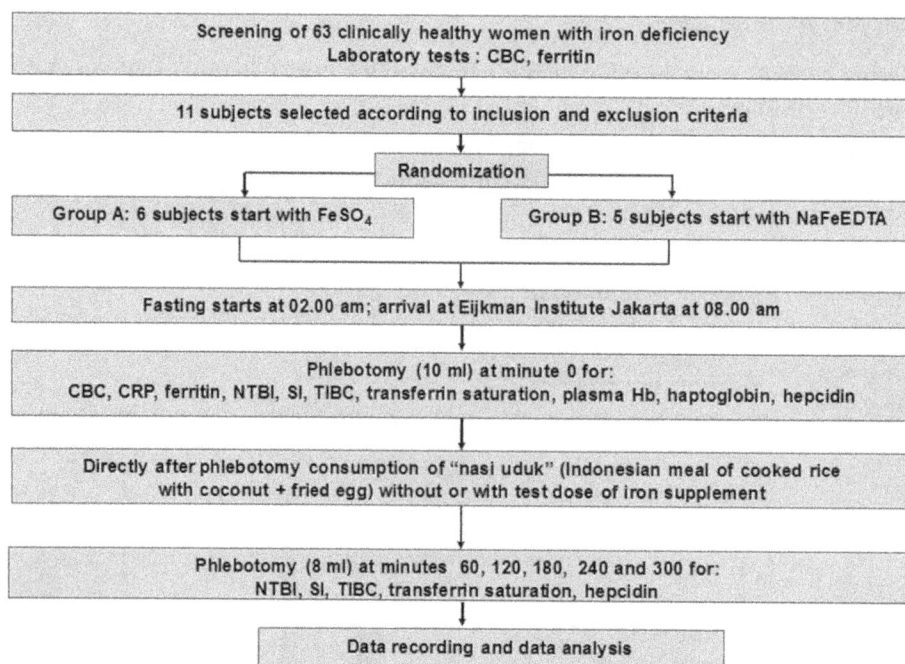

Scheme 2. Algorithm of the investigation.

4.3. Production of NaFeEDTA Capsules

Ferric sodium EDTA ($C_{10}H_{12}FeN_2NaO_8 3H_2O$) MW = 421.1 was provided by Akzo Nobel, The Netherlands, as Ferrazone®. The capsules were produced in the Pharmacy of Dr. Cipto Mangunkusumo Hospital, Jakarta, Indonesia. One capsule with 65 mg elementary iron was composed of 490 mg NaFeEDTA, and 110 mg lactose. One capsule with 6.5 mg elementary iron consisted of 49 mg NaFeEDTA and 600 mg lactose.

4.4. Composition of Test Meal

Before taking the test dose of the iron supplement, all subjects consumed *"nasi uduk"* (a standard Indonesian meal of cooked rice with coconut + fried egg). This meal is free from fortified iron and has a very low amount of natural iron. Composition of one portion of rice 100 g = 178 calories: protein: 6.8 g; fat: 0.7 g; carbohydrate: 78.9 g; and iron: 0.5 mg. One portion of fried egg (50 g) = 105.8 calories: protein: 9.3 g; fat: 14.6 g; carbohydrate: 1.5 g; and iron: 2.7 mg.

4.5. Laboratory Test Methods

Routine laboratory tests were performed by the Laboratory of Clinical Pathology, Faculty of Medicine, University of Indonesia/Dr Cipto Mangunkusumo Hospital.

Laboratory test methods included hemoglobin: cyanide-free sodium lauryl sulfate (SLS) Sysmex XT-2000i; erythrocytes, leukocytes, hematocrit, MCV, MCH, MCHC: flow cytometry with semiconductor laser hydrodynamic focusing (Sysmex XT-2000i); serum iron and total iron binding capacity: Ferrozine (Cobas Integra 400, Roche Diagnostics, Risch-Rotkreuz, Switzerland) Transferrin saturation %: SI/TIBC x %; C-reactive protein (CRP): turbidimetric (Cobas Integra 400)

Non-transferrin iron (NTBI): fluorescein-labeled apotransferrin (Fl-aTf) [35] was performed at the Eijkman-Winkler Institute for Microbiology, Infectious Diseases, and Inflammation, University Medical Centre Utrecht, The Netherlands. Frozen samples were sent from Jakarta to Utrecht.

4.6. Estimation of Iron Absorption

For the estimation of iron absorption from the gut, the most superior technique is a double isotope method where iron is labeled with Fe^{59} and a nonabsorbable substance ($^{51}CrCl$), while the accumulation of both radioactive isotopes in the body can be measured simultaneously with a whole-body counter (WBC) [36]. As such methods, using in vivo radioactive material and very expensive equipment, are no longer available, stable isotopes or chemical laboratory techniques are used for comparing iron uptake from two different compounds. For a comparison of iron absorption from two non-labeled different iron compounds, with or without a meal, in different iron-doses, either Fe(II) or Fe(III), a comparison of serum iron curves is considered a reliable and powerful tool [13,37]. Absolute values for total iron absorption, however, cannot be estimated with this method.

4.7. Data Management and Analysis

Research data were recorded in tested research questionnaires. Verified data were analyzed and organized in text format, tables, or figures using SPSS version 16.0 and NCSS 2007 research software. Multivariate analysis was carried out using one-way ANOVA parametric tests to see the difference in NTBI level generation in each test dose of iron supplement and placebo every hour. Normality tests were performed before using the Shapiro–Wilk method in view of the small number of subjects (11 persons with $n < 50$). The result of the normality tests showed a slightly abnormal distribution of data by which log10 transformation was carried out. However, in 6.5 mg $FeSO_4$ from the 240th min, the distribution was still abnormal, thus a nonparametric Kruskal–Wallis test was performed followed by a Mann–Whitney test to have a look at the significance between test doses in the 240th min. One-way ANOVA was performed followed by post hoc analysis.

4.8. Ethical Assessment

Signed, informed consent was obtained from all test subjects before participation in the study. The study was conducted in accordance with the Declaration of Helsinki. Ethical assessment of the study protocol was conducted by the Ethical Committee of the Faculty of Medicine, University of Indonesia/Dr Cipto Mangunkusumo Hospital and was approved on 13 October 2008. The Project Identification Number is 338/PT02.FK/ETIK/2008.

The original protocol also contained an investigation, similar to the iron-deficient subjects, in apparently healthy females with nontransfused alpha thalassemia intermedia. This part of the study was not approved as it implicated the donation of iron to a potentially endangered group of patients.

5. Conclusions

1. In healthy iron-deficient females, intestinal iron uptake from NaFe(III)EDTA, provided as a therapeutic dose of 65 mg Fe, was twice as high as that from Fe(II)SO_4 if ingested with a traditional Indonesian meal.

2. Measured in the same samples, non-transferrin-bound iron (NTBI) also increased with an almost identical time-related pattern.

3. When a 6.5 mg iron dose (representing iron fortification) was ingested, the post-absorption curves and increase of NTBI of NaFeEDTA and $FeSO_4$ were almost flat, being below the detection level of the method used. Such studies should be performed with stable isotopes, estimating red blood cell iron utilization.

4. For NTBI, the post-absorption concentration in plasma was representative for the whole circulation being the dilution volume. If the NTBI values remain within the range considered to be normal for iron-replete men after the therapeutic dose of 65 mg iron, then one should not fear pathological side effects.

5. Although iron absorption from NaFeEDTA was almost zero if given with water, as was demonstrated for iron-replete men and women, its absorption was excellent (and even much better than that from $FeSO_4$), if given with a meal as described in this study.

Author Contributions: Conceptualization, I.S. and J.J.M.M.; Data curation, E.G. and L.I.; Formal analysis, E.G. and L.I.; Funding acquisition, I.S. and J.J.M.M.; Investigation, E.G., L.I., A.H., and I.S.T.; Resources, D.A., A.H., and I.S.T.; Supervision, I.S., D.A., A.H., I.S.T., and J.J.M.M.; Visualization, E.G. and J.J.M.M.; Writing—original draft, E.G.; Writing—review & editing, I.S., D.A., and J.J.M.M.

Funding: This research was funded by Akzo Nobel Functional Chemicals, Singapore. The founding sponsors had no role in the design of the study, in the collection, analyses, or interpretation of data, in the writing of the manuscript, and in the decision to publish the results.

Acknowledgments: Nanis S. Marzuki cooperated in the clinical study; Ari W. Satyagraha and Georgina Tapiheru supervised the laboratory tests; Henny van Kats-Renaud supervised and performed the NTBI tests at the University Medical Centre, Utrecht, The Netherlands; Sangkot Marzuki supported this investigation and provided the facilities as Director of the Eijkman Institute in Jakarta.

Conflicts of Interest: The authors declare no conflicts of interest.

References

1. Zimmermann, M.B.; Hurrell, R.F. Nutritional iron deficiency. *Lancet* **2007**, *370*, 511–520. [CrossRef]
2. Kodyat, B.; Kosen, S.; de Pree, S. Iron deficiency in Indonesia: Current situation and intervention. *Nutr. Res.* **1998**, *18*, 1953–1963. [CrossRef]
3. Barkley, J.S.; Kendrick, K.L.; Codling, K.; Muslimatun, S.; Pachón, H. Anaemia prevalence over time in Indonesia: Estimates from the 1997, 2000, and 2008 Indonesia Family Life Surveys. *Asia Pac. J. Clin. Nutr.* **2015**, *24*, 452–455. [CrossRef] [PubMed]
4. Darmawan, M.A.; Karima, N.N.; Maulida, N.N. Potential of Iron Fortification Complex Compounds against Soybean Food for Anemia Problem Solution in Indonesia. *J. Adv. Agric. Technol.* **2017**, *4*, 185–189. [CrossRef]
5. Marx, J.J.M. Iron deficiency in developed countries: Prevalence, influence of lifestyle factors and hazards of prevention. *Eur. J. Clin. Nutr.* **1997**, *51*, 491–494. [CrossRef] [PubMed]
6. Hutchinson, C.; Al-Ashgar, W.; Liu, D.Y.; Hider, R.C.; Powell, J.J.; Geissler, C.A. Oral ferrous sulphate leads to a marked increase in pro-oxidant nontransferrin-bound iron. *Eur. J. Clin. Investig.* **2004**, *34*, 782–784. [CrossRef] [PubMed]
7. Voest, E.E.; Vreugdenhil, G.; Marx, J.J.M. Iron chelating agents in non-iron overload conditions. Current and future perspectives. *Ann. Intern. Med.* **1994**, *120*, 490–499. [CrossRef] [PubMed]
8. Marx, J.J.M. Iron and infection: Competition between host and microbes for a precious element. *Best Pract. Res. Clin. Haematol.* **2002**, *15*, 411–426. [CrossRef] [PubMed]
9. Layrisse, M.; Martinez-Torres, C. EDTA-Fe(III) complex as iron fortification. *Am. J. Clin. Nutr.* **1977**, *30*, 166–1174. [CrossRef] [PubMed]
10. Schuemann, K.; Solomons, N.W.; Romero-Abal, M.E.; Orozco, M.; Weiss, G.; Marx, J.J.M. Oral administration of ferrous sulfate, but not of iron polymaltose or NaFeEDTA, results in a substantial increase of NTBI in healthy iron-adequate men. *Food Nutr. Bull.* **2012**, *33*, 128–136. [CrossRef] [PubMed]
11. Schuemann, K.; Solomons, N.W.; Orozco, M.; Romero-Abal, M.E.; Weiss, G. Differences in circulating NTBI after oral administration of ferrous sulfate, NaFeEDTA, or iron polymaltose in women with marginal iron stores. *Food Nutr. Bull.* **2013**, *34*, 185–193. [CrossRef] [PubMed]
12. Weber, J.; Werre, J.M.; Julius, H.W.; Marx, J.J.M. Decreased iron absorption in patients with active rheumatoid arthritis, with and without iron deficiency. *Ann. Rheum. Dis.* **1988**, *47*, 404–409. [CrossRef] [PubMed]
13. Conway, R.W.; Geissler, C.A.; Hider, R.C.; Thompson, R.P.H.; Powell, J.J. Serum Iron Curves Can Be Used to Estimate Dietary Iron Bioavailability in Humans. *J. Nutr.* **2006**, *136*, 1910–1914. [CrossRef] [PubMed]
14. Marx, J.J.M. Iron absorption and its regulation. A review. *Haematologica* **1979**, *64*, 479–493. [PubMed]
15. Bothwell, T.H.; Mac-Phail, A.P. The potential role of NaFeEDTA as an iron fortificant. *Int. J. Vitam Nutr. Res.* **2004**, *74*, 421–434. [CrossRef] [PubMed]
16. Troesch, B.; Egli, I.; Zeder, C.; Richard, F.; Hurrell, R.F.; Zimmermann, M.B. Fortification Iron as Ferrous Sulfate Plus Ascorbic Acid Is More Rapidly Absorbed Than as Sodium Iron EDTA but Neither Increases Serum Nontransferrin-Bound Iron in Women. *J. Nutr.* **2011**, *141*, 822–827. [CrossRef] [PubMed]
17. Brittenham, G.M.; Andersson, M.; Egli, I.; Foman, J.T.; Zeder, C.; Westerman, M.E.; Hurrell, R.F. Circulating non-transferrin-bound iron after oral administration of supplemental and fortification doses of iron to healthy women: A randomized study. *Am. J. Clin. Nutr.* **2014**, *100*, 813–820. [CrossRef] [PubMed]

18. Marx, J.J.M.; Aisen, P. Uptake of iron by rabbit intestinal membrane vesicles. *Biochim. Biophys. Acta* **1981**, *649*, 297–304. [CrossRef]

19. West, T.S.; Sykes, A.S. Diamino-ethane-tetraacetic. In *Analytical Applications of Diamino-Ethane-Tetra-Acetic-Acid*, 2nd ed.; British Drug Houses, Laboratory Chemicals Divison: Poole, UK, 1960; pp. 9–22.

20. Fallingborg, J. Intraluminal pH of the human gastrointestinal tract. *Dan. Med. Bull.* **1999**, *46*, 183–196. [PubMed]

21. Gillooly, M.; Bothwell, T.H.; Charlton, R.E.; Torrance, J.D. Factors affecting the absorption of iron from cereals. *Br. J. Nutr.* **1984**, *51*, 37–46. [CrossRef] [PubMed]

22. Chernelch, M.; Fawwaz, R.; Sargent, T.; Winchell, H.S. Effect of phlebotomy and pH on iron absorption from the colon. *J. Nucl. Med.* **1969**, *11*, 25–27.

23. Takeushi, K.; Bjarnason, I.; Abas, H.; Laftah, A.H.; Latunde-Dada, G.O.; Simpson, R.J.; McKie, A.T. Expression of iron absorption genes in mouse large intestine. *Scand. J. Gastroenterol.* **2005**, *40*, 169–177. [CrossRef] [PubMed]

24. Hershko, C.; Graham, G.; Bates, G.W.; Rachmilewitz, E.A. Non-specific serum iron in thalassaemia: An abnormal serum iron fraction of potential toxicity. *Br. J. Haematol.* **1978**, *40*, 255–263. [CrossRef] [PubMed]

25. De Valk, B.; Addicks, M.A.; Gosriwatana, I.; Lu, S.; Hider, R.C.; Marx, J.J.M. Non-transferrin-bound iron is present in serum of hereditary haemochromatosis heterozygotes. *Eur. J. Clin. Investig.* **2000**, *30*, 248–251. [CrossRef]

26. Roest, M.; van der Schouw, Y.T.; de Valk, B.; Marx, J.J.M.; Tempelman, M.J.; de Groot, P.G.; Sixma, J.J.; Banga, J.D. Heterozygosity for a hereditary hemochromatosis gene is associated with cardiovascular death in women. *Circulation* **1999**, *100*, 1268–1273. [CrossRef] [PubMed]

27. Van der A, D.L.; Marx, J.J.M.; Grobbee, D.E.; Kamphuis, M.H.; Georgiou, N.A.; van Kats-Renaud, H.; Breuer, W.; Cabantchik, Z.I.; Mark Roest, M.; Voorbij, H.A.M.; et al. Non–Transferrin-Bound Iron and Risk of Coronary Heart Disease in Postmenopausal Women. *Circulation* **2006**, *113*, 1942–1949. [CrossRef] [PubMed]

28. Hider, R.C. Nature of nontransferrin-bound iron. *Eur. J. Clin. Investig.* **2002**, *32* (Suppl. 1), 50–54. [CrossRef]

29. Faller, B.; Nick, H. Kinetics and mechanism of iron (III) removal from citrate by desferrioxamine B and 3-hydroxy-1, 2-dimethyl-4 pyridone. *J. Am. Chem. Soc.* **1994**, *116*, 3860–3865. [CrossRef]

30. Wreesmann, C.T.J. Reasons for raising the maximum acceptable daily intake of EDTA and the benefits for iron fortification of foods for children 6–24 months of age. *Matem. Child Nutr.* **2014**, *10*, 481–495. [CrossRef] [PubMed]

31. Sangaré, L.; van Eijk, A.M.; ter Kuile, F.O.; Walson, J.; Stergachis, A. The Association between Malaria and Iron Status or Supplementation in Pregnancy: A Systematic Review and Meta-Analysis. *PLoS ONE* **2014**, *9*, e87743. [CrossRef] [PubMed]

32. Fucharoen, S.; Winichagoon, P. Haemoglobinopathies in Southeast Asia. *Indian J. Med. Res.* **2011**, *134*, 498–506. [PubMed]

33. Weatherall, D. Fortnightly review: The thalassaemias. *Br. Med. J.* **1997**, *314*, 1675–1679. [CrossRef]

34. Setianingsih, I. β thalassaemia in Indonesia: Molecular Basis and Phenotype-Genotype Correction. Ph.D. Thesis, University of Melbourne, Melbourne, Australia, 2000.

35. Breuer, W.; Cabantchik, Z.I. A fluorescence-based one-step assay for serum non-transferrin-bound iron. *Anal Biochem.* **2001**, *299*, 194–201. [CrossRef] [PubMed]

36. Marx, J.J.M. Mucosal uptake, mucosal transfer and retention of iron, measured by whole-body counting. *Scand. Haematol.* **1979**, *23*, 293–302. [CrossRef]

37. Dainty, J.R.; Roe, M.A.; Teucher, B.; Eagles, J.; Fairweather-Tait, S.J. Quantification of unlabeled non-haem iron absorption in human subjects: A pilot study. *Br. J. Nutr.* **2003**, *90*, 503–506. [CrossRef] [PubMed]

8

Evaluation of Anti-*Toxoplasma gondii* Effect of Ursolic Acid as a Novel Toxoplasmosis Inhibitor

Won Hyung Choi [1],* and In Ah Lee [2]

[1] Marine Bio Research & Education Center, Kunsan National University, 558 Daehak-ro, Gunsan-si, Jeollabuk-do 54150, Korea

[2] Department of Chemistry, College of Natural Science, Kunsan National University, 558 Daehak-ro, Gunsan-si, Jeollabuk-do 54150, Korea; leeinah@kunsan.ac.kr

* Correspondence: whchoi@kunsan.ac.kr or whchoi@khu.ac.kr

Abstract: This study was carried out to evaluate the anti-parasitic effect of ursolic acid against *Toxoplasma gondii* (*T. gondii*) that induces toxoplasmosis, particularly in humans. The anti-parasitic effects of ursolic acid against *T. gondii*-infected cells and *T. gondii* were evaluated through different specific assays, including immunofluorescence staining and animal testing. Ursolic acid effectively inhibited the proliferation of *T. gondii* when compared with sulfadiazine, and consistently induced anti-*T. gondii* activity/effect. In particular, the formation of parasitophorous vacuole membrane (PVM) in host cells was markedly decreased after treating ursolic acid, which was effectively suppressed. Moreover, the survival rate of *T. gondii* was strongly inhibited in *T. gondii* group treated with ursolic acid, and then 50% inhibitory concentration (IC_{50}) against *T. gondii* was measured as 94.62 μg/mL. The *T. gondii*-infected mice treated with ursolic acid indicated the same survival rates and activity as the normal group. These results demonstrate that ursolic acid causes anti-*T. gondii* action and effect by strongly blocking the proliferation of *T. gondii* through the direct and the selective *T. gondii*-inhibitory ability as well as increases the survival of *T. gondii*-infected mice. This study shows that ursolic acid has the potential to be used as a promising anti-*T. gondii* candidate substance for developing effective anti-parasitic drugs.

Keywords: zoonosis; parasites; *Toxoplasma gondii*; infectious disease

1. Introduction

Toxoplasmosis is caused in all age groups, including young children or adults globally, which is one of parasitic diseases as zoonosis infected through *Toxoplasma gondii* (*T. gondii*). *T. gondii* not only induces chronic infection in various sites of human body, but it also causes brain infection through the central nervous system as zoonotic parasitosis. In addition, *T. gondii* has unique infectious subcellular organelles, including apicoplast, conoid, rhoptries, dense granules, and micronemes [1]. In general, *T. gondii* forms a unique proliferative membrane, such as a parasitophorous vacuole membrane (PVM) including reticular network (RN) during its proliferation after invasion into host cells, and grows in it [2]. Until recently, several drugs were developed to inhibit *T. gondii*, and they are being used to treat toxoplasmosis' patients in the clinic. However, their side effects are still clear in the clinic, and it is also being exposed to drug-resistance gradually [3–5]. In these aspects, pyrimethamine used for treating toxoplasmosis blocks the synthesis of tetrahydrofolic acid from dihydrofolate reductase (DHFR) by effectively inhibiting the dihydrofolate reductase in *T. gondii*, which inhibits consistently synthesis of the DNA and/or RNA in the proliferation of protozoa species, including malaria.

Until recently, it was reported that various extracts and/or natural products derived from medicinal plants had the possibility of useful medical resources for treating infectious virus diseases, including middle east respiratory syndrome (MERS), dengue fever or Zika fever, as well as showed in vitro inhibitory effects against chronic diseases, such as hepatitis, cancer, and tuberculosis [6–11]. Although various extracts derived from traditional medicinal plants and its natural compounds were reported to indicate anti-*T. gondii* activities/effects [12–16], an effective drug of the next generation for the treatment of toxoplasmosis caused by *T. gondii* has not yet been developed through the clinical study. Furthermore, despite various efforts for developing anti-parasitic drugs, zoonotic parasitosis derived from parasites has been consistently worsening a crisis of the public health worldwide.

In this aspect, various researches for discovering effective drugs against toxoplasmosis, and studies on new substances of relatively low toxicity with safety are urgently required to inhibit zoonosis. Ursolic acid is a bioactive substance contained in various medicinal plants that are used as natural resources in oriental medicine and in folk medicine, and is also known to have a variety of effects and bioactivity, such as anxiolytic activity [17], anti-angiogenic activity [18], and antiepileptic effect [19]. Furthermore, ursolic acid effectively induces extensive bioactivities, including anti-inflammatory [20,21], anticancer [22–24], antioxidant [25], antimicrobial [26], and anti-tubercular effects [27], as well as causes strong inhibitory effects against arthritic [28] and autoimmune disease [29]. These studies show that ursolic acid not only induces various physiological activities in both "in vitro" and "in vivo", but also has the possibility as an anti-parasitic candidate drug. However, studies regarding anti-*T. gondii* activity of ursolic acid has not been reported yet. In addition, a novel and/or effective drug for the treatment of toxoplasmosis has not been developed yet, even though significant results regarding anti-*T. gondii* activity have been reported through various studies globally [30,31]. For this reason, this study started from the hypothesis that ursolic acid may effectively inhibit or modulate the proliferation/growth of *T. gondii,* causing toxoplasmosis in human. This study was carried out to evaluate the anti-*T. gondii* effect of ursolic acid which is known as a bioactive substance, and to determine its potential as a promising candidate substance for developing novel anti-toxoplasmosis drugs.

2. Results

2.1. Effect of Ursolic Acid on the Proliferation and Growth of T. gondii

T. gondii causes parasitic disease on both animals and human, as well as having unique micro network systems and a specific structure, including various micro-organelles, such as mitochondria, rhoptries, and micronemes. We evaluated the anti-parasitic activity and the effects of UA on the proliferation and growth of *T. gondii* using an MTT assay and UA showed the anti-*T. gondii* activity in the range of 25–200 μg/mL. *T. gondii*-infected cells were incubated with different concentrations (25–200 μg/mL) of UA for 24 h, and their viability was markedly decreased in a dose dependent manner (Tables 1 and 2). In addition, the UA effectively inhibited the proliferation and growth of *T. gondii*-infected cells as compared with SF. In particular, *T. gondi*-infected cells treated with UA (100 μg/mL) showed a significant decrease of *T. gondii* including *T. gondii* fragmentation as well as morphological changes such as cell shrinkage and cell fragmentation when compared with the untreated *T. gondii*-infected cells (Data not shown), which suggests that UA has anti-parasitic activity and the inhibitory effect against *T. gondi* in infected cells (Table 2). Furthermore, the UA effectively inhibited the viability of the parasite through the direct inhibition of *T. gondii* when compared with SF, which is to strongly demonstrate its selective inhibitory effect against *T. gondii*, and then the parasitic SR was measured at less than 45% at concentrations of 100 μg/mL (Figure 1). The 50% inhibitory concentration (IC$_{50}$) value of UA against *T. gondii* and *T. gondii*-infected cells was measured as 94.62 μg/mL and 162.25 μg/mL, respectively. These results demonstrate that UA strongly induced anti-proliferation activity of *T. gondii* in the infected host cells by effectively blocking *T. gondii* as well as the direct inhibitory action against *T. gondii*.

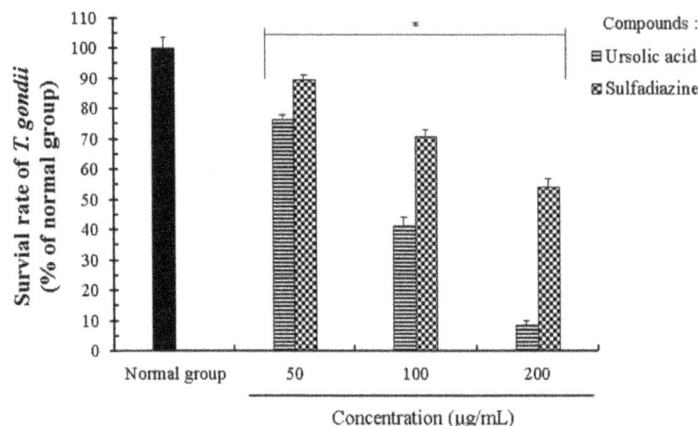

Figure 1. The *T. gondii*-inhibitory effect of ursolic acid regarding *T. gondii*. *T. gondii* was incubated with different concentrations (50–200 µg/mL) of ursolic acid and sulfadiazine for 24 h, respectively. The results were expressed as a percentage of the control group, and all of the results were presented as mean ± standard deviation (S.D.) of three independent experiments. * $p < 0.05$ was considered to be statistically significant.

Table 1. The 50% inhibitory concentration value of ursolic acid against the viability of *T. gondii* and *T. gondii*–infected cells measured by the MTT assay.

The Tested Compound	Structure ($C_{30}H_{48}O_3$)	The IC_{50} (µg/mL) of Ursolic Acid against *T. gondii*	The IC_{50} (µg/mL) of Ursolic Acid against *T. gondii*–Infected Cells
Ursolic acid (UA)		94.62	162.25

The anti-*T. gondii* effect of ursolic acid against the proliferation and the viability of *T. gondii* and *T. gondii*–infected cells was measured using the MTT assay. They were incubated with different concentrations (25–200 µg/mL) of the compound at 37 °C for 24 h respectively. IC_{50} (50% inhibitory concentration value of UA against the survival rate of *T. gondii* and *T. gondii*–infected cells). The results were carried out three times independently.

Table 2. The inhibitory effect of ursolic acid against the growth and the proliferation of *T. gondii*-infected cells.

Infection Ratio of *T. gondii* (MOI)	Incubation Time	Concentrations (µg/mL)	The Survival Rate (%) of *T. gondii*-Infected Cells	
			Ursolic Acid (UA)	Sulfadiazine (SF)
Cells:*T. gondii* = 1:5	24 h	0	100.00 ± 2.28	100.00 ± 3.46
		25	92.35 ± 2.74	94.26 ± 1.82
		50	85.52 ± 1.55	91.35 ± 1.64
		100	67.61 ± 1.87	77.58 ± 3.45
		200	38.42 ± 3.12	60.45 ± 1.68

T. gondii-infected cells were incubated with different concentrations (25–200 µg/mL) of ursolic acid (UA) and sulfadiazine (SF) for 24 h respectively, and their survival rates were measured using the MTT assay. The results were expressed as a percentage of the normal group, and all the results were presented as mean ± standard deviation (S.D.) of three independent experiments.

2.2. Anti-Parasitic Effect of Ursolic Acid on PVM Formed by T. gondii Proliferation

T. gondii induces anti-apoptotic steps and features through the inactivation of apoptotic proteins during its proliferative phase in host cells, which shows the unique parasitic life-cycle of *T. gondii*.

In particular, the formation of PVM is accelerated in a time-dependent manner after cell invasion of *T. gondii*. For this reason, we investigated the inhibition of PVM that is caused by the interaction between *T. gondii* and UA during the proliferation stage of *T. gondii* in host cells. As shown in Figure 2, the PVM formation and nucleus of *T. gondii* were markedly decreased in *T. gondii*-infected host cells when it was treated with 100 µg/mL of UA and SF, respectively, and their changes were clearly observed under a UV fluorescence. The results indicate the inhibitory effect of UA against PVM formation and the viability of *T. gondii*. Therefore, these results show substantial evidence that UA effectively inhibited or blocked the PVM formed by *T. gondii* during the proliferative stage as well as the proliferation of *T. gondii* in the infected host cells after cell invasion.

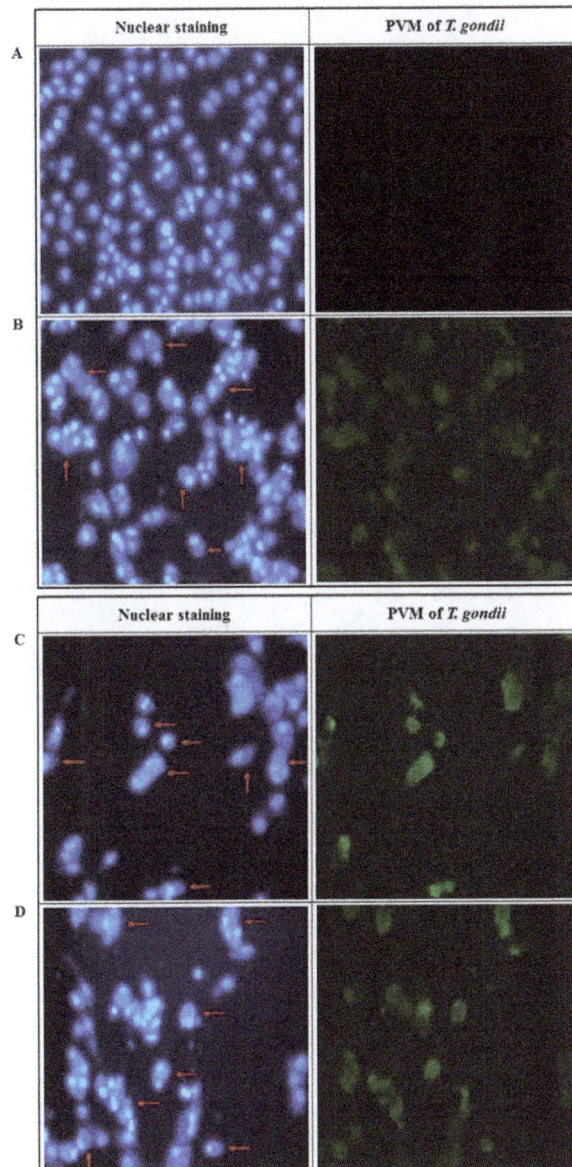

Figure 2. The changes of immunofluorescence of parasitophorous vacuole membrane (PVM) formed in *T. gondii*-infected cells and changes of nuclear staining. (**A**) Uninfected normal cells. (**B**) *T. gondii*-infected cells. (**C**) *T. gondii*-infected cells treated with 100 µg/mL of ursolic acid. (**D**) *T. gondii*-infected cells treated with 100 µg/mL of sulfadiazine. The cells were infected with *T. gondii* (host cells:*T. gondii* = 1:5), and *T. gondii*-infected cells were incubated with the compounds for 24 h. Green fluorescence shows morphology of PVM formed by *T. gondii* proliferation in host cells after *T. gondii* invasion. Blue fluorescence shows nucleus of *T. gondii* group proliferated in PVM, and nucleus of the host cells, respectively (the arrow shows the nucleus of *T. gondii* in PVM formed by *T. gondii* in the host cells).

2.3. Effect of Ursolic Acid through the Inhibition of T. gondii in T. gondii-Infected Mice

T. gondii induces infectious symptoms and diseases, such as lymphadenopathy and brain injury, particularly in human as a zoonotic parasite that is infected in both human and animals. In this aspect, we evaluated the anti-proliferative effect and the parasitic inhibitory activity of UA against the viability of *T. gondii* in *T. gondii*-infected mice. The mice were carefully observed during the experimental periods after the injection of *T. gondii* treated with 100, 200, and 400 μg/mL of UA for 24 h. As mentioned above, *T. gondii*-infected mice treated with different concentrations (200 and 400 μg/mL) of UA showed higher activity and viability than *T. gondii*-infected mice, and the mice indicated the dynamic and energetic activity as the normal group. In particular, it clearly confirmed a significant difference of the survival rate between *T. gondii*-infected mice and the infected mice treated with UA. However, *T. gondii*-infected mice treated with 100 μg/mL of UA showed that the effect of UA did not consistently maintain the survival of the infected mice by decreasing after 11.8 days. This result suggests that the death of mice may be owing to tissue damage and cytolysis by invasion of *T. gondii* than the loss of body weight of mice. Furthermore, symptoms and side effects, such as the loss of body weight, were not observed or induced in all of the groups treated with 200 and 400 μg/mL of UA for the experimental periods (Figure 3). The result shows effective and clear evidence regarding the effect of anti-*T. gondii* compounds, which indicates clarity regarding the results as a fusion method for both "in vitro" and "in vivo". These results demonstrate that UA has the selective anti-parasitic activity which strongly causes anti-*T. gondii* effects as well as suppressing their viability by effectively inhibiting *T. gondii*.

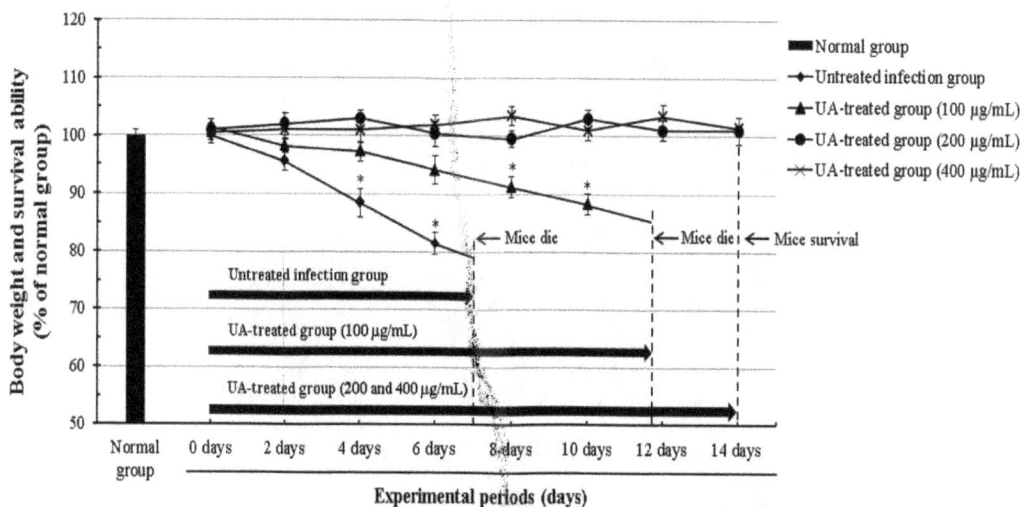

Figure 3. Changes of the body weight and the survival ability in *T. gondii*-infected mice. The mice were divided into normal group (*n* = 5), positive group (*T. gondii*-infected group, *n* = 5) and experimental groups (3 groups of UA, *n* = 15). The mice were infected with *T. gondii* treated by 100, 200, and 400 μg/mL of ursolic acid (UA) through the abdominal cavity of each mouse respectively. The mice were carefully observed during the experiment periods after *T. gondii* infection. The results were expressed as a percentage of the normal group, and presented as the mean ± S.D. * *p* < 0.05 was considered to be statistically significant.

3. Discussion

Until recently, the efforts for the treatment of neglected infectious diseases have been attempted at various fields. In particular, the global supporting organizations, including WHO, Bill & Melinda Gates Foundation, and the global pharmaceuticals are supporting the study for developing novel drugs and for effectively treating or blocking zoonosis such as malaria and tuberculosis, as well as infectious diseases, including AIDS, Zika, Ebola, MERS, and SARS. We should carefully focus on the neglected infectious diseases that are consistently caused through various pathways and infection factors. From these perspectives, *T. gondii* causes to fetus serious infectious diseases such as retinochoroiditis, hydrocephalus, and cerebral calcification through fetus infection during pregnancy, as well as induces symptoms, such as lymphadenopathy and meningoencephalitis in brain through acquired infection as a zoonotic parasite that is infected in both human and animals. It also induces serious complications in immune deficient patients and HIV patients as one of the infectious parasites that induce parasitic zoonosis, which may induce the interaction for parasitic proliferation and growth through parasitic relationship such as symbiosis in the host. In this aspect, *T. gondii* not only inhibits defensive mechanisms of cytokines, such as IL-2, -4, -6, -8, and IFN-γ released from host cells after invasion, but also suppresses the production of protective systems that are activated through the immune-response. Furthermore, it is known to block the signaling transport pathways that activate anti-parasitic system and the resistance to *T. gondii* invasion in host cells, as well as to suppress the apoptotic signals and cell arrest pathways during the early apoptotic stage of host cells after cell invasion [32,33]. Moreover, *T. gondii* promotes inactivation of cell cycle initiators and apoptotic mediators during the proliferative phase of *T. gondii* by forming PVM of *T. gondii* in host cells, which rapidly accelerates the proliferation of *T. gondii* in PVM [34].

In this study, we evaluated the anti-parasitic activity/effect of UA which inhibits the proliferation of *T. gondii*, and confirmed the viability of *T. gondii* after the parasite infection through *T. gondii*-infected in vitro system and animal testing. In the present study, the expression of PVM in the infected host cells was significantly increased when compared with *T. gondii*-infected cells treated with UA and SF, and uninfected cells. On the other hand, the proliferation of *T. gondii* and PVM were markedly inhibited in *T. gondii*-infected cells treated with UA compared with *T. gondii*-infected cells. In addition, we evaluated the anti-*T. gondii* activity of UA through *T. gondii*-infected mice. After the injection of *T. gondii* treated with UA (200 and 400 μg/mL), the mice showed the vitality and the viability such as the uninfected control group without the loss of body weight and the cytotoxicity during the experiment. In particular, it was recently reported that UA has the anti-protozoa effects against *Leishmania amazonesis* and *Leishmania infantums*, causing leishmaniasis among the neglected tropical diseases, and its mechanism of action is associated with programmed cell death and nitric oxide (NO) production [35,36]. In this aspect, the anti-*T. gondii* effect of UA suggests that UA may induce the anti-proliferation and the growth inhibitory action of *T. gondii* through the mechanism of action that is caused by nitric oxide (NO) production or programmed cell death in *T. gondii* and the infected host cells.

Taken together, these results indicate that the expression of PVM in *T. gondii*-infected cells was selectively inhibited or blocked in the host cells treated with UA, as well as significantly increased in infected cells. Furthermore, the *T. gondii*-infected mice treated with UA showed a stable life-cycle and survival rates when compared with infected positive group during the experimental period. The results clearly provide the inhibitory effect and activity of the compound against *T. gondii*, and indicate whether UA induces the direct inhibition of *T. gondii* or increase the survival of mice by effectively blocking and inhibiting the viability of *T. gondii*.

4. Materials and Methods

4.1. Materials

Fetal bovine serum (FBS), antibiotics, and trypsin-EDTA were purchased from Invitrogen Corporation (Gibco®, Waltham, MA, USA). MTT (3-(4,5-dimethylthiazol-2-yl)-2,5-diohenyl-2H-tetrazolium bromide; Thiazolyl blue), RPMI medium 1640, sulfadiazine, dimethyl sulfoxide (DMSO), phosphate buffered saline (PBS), 0.4% trypan blue solution, and Hoechst 33342 were purchased from Sigma-Aldrich Chemical Co., Ltd. (St. Louis, MO, USA). All the other chemicals and reagents were purchased from Merck Chemical Co., Ltd. (Darmstadt, Germany) and Sigma-Aldrich Chemical Co., Ltd. (St. Louis, MO, USA).

4.2. Animals

BALB-c/mice (six weeks, $n = 25$) were purchased from DaeHan Bio-Link Co., Ltd. (Chungcheongbuk-do, Korea), and all animals were kept at 23 ± 0.5 °C and 12 h-light/dark cycle in a controlled environment of a central animal care facility. Food and water were provided ad libitum to all animals. The facility was strictly maintained in accordance with the guidelines of the National Institutes of Health for the Care and Use of Laboratory Animals.

4.3. Preparation of Anti-T. gondii Drugs

The anti-*T. gondii* drug, sulfadiazine (SF), was dissolved in DMSO and ursolic acid (UA) was also dissolved in DMSO to a concentration of 50 mg/mL, according to the manufacturer's instruction. Sulfadiazine was used as a standard drug to evaluate whether or not ursolic acid has an anti-parasitic effect and activity against *T. gondii*. All of the compounds were filtered using 0.2 μm membrane syringe filters (Roshi Kaisha, Ltd., Tokyo, Japan) before use, and were stored at −80 °C deep-freezer until use.

4.4. Cell Lines and Culture Conditions of T. gondii

Glioma cells (C6 cells) were purchased from Korean Cell Line Bank at Seoul National University. C6 cells were cultured in RPMI medium 1640 containing 2 mM L-glutamine, supplemented with 10% fetal bovine serum (FBS), 100 units/mL penicillin, and 100 μg/mL streptomycin (Biofluids, Rockville, MD, USA) in a humidified atmosphere containing 5% CO_2 in air at 37 °C. The RH strain of *T. gondii* was suspended with 1X PBS, which was injected in the abdominal cavity of each BALB-c/mouse. Five days after the injection, *T. gondii* was collected from the peritoneal fluids of each mouse kept in the abdominal cavities of the mice before use in the studies. In the in vitro study, cells were infected with *T. gondii* (cells:*T. gondii* = 1:5).

4.5. Evaluation of The Viability of T. gondii

To evaluate the inhibitory effects of UA against the viability of *T. gondii*, we investigated the viability of *T. gondii* exposed to UA and SF. Briefly, after *T. gondii* was seeded in a 24 well plate (1×10^7/well), *T. gondii* was incubated with different concentrations (50–200 μg/mL) of UA and SF for 24 h, respectively, and their viabilities were determined by MTT assay. It is to determine whether or not UA has direct anti-parasitic activity and/or effect against *T. gondii*. The survival rate (SR) of *T. gondii* was calculated, as follows: % of SR = ($OD_{\text{drug-tested wells}} - OD_{\text{blank}}$)/($OD_{\text{control}} - OD_{\text{blank}}$) $\times$ 100. The optical density (OD) was measured at a wavelength of 570 nm using an ELISA leader.

4.6. Microscopic Observation of T. gondii in Infected Cells

The cells were seeded in a 24 well plate (1×10^5/well), which were incubated at 37 °C for 24 h. The cells were infected with *T. gondii* (5×10^5 tachyzoites/well), and then *T. gondii*-infected cells were treated with 100 μg/mL of UA and SF for 24 h, respectively. The morphological changes of *T. gondii*-infected host cells were observed under a light microscope (Nikon Eclipse TE 2000-U, Tokyo, Japan).

4.7. Nuclear Staining of T. gondii-Infected Host Cells

The anti-*T. gondii* effect of UA against *T. gondii*-infected cells was evaluated using Hoechst 33342, according to the nuclear staining method described previously [37]. The cells were seeded onto cover slips in a 24 well plate (1×10^5 cells/well), which were infected with *T. gondii* (5×10^5 tachyzoites/well) after 24 h. The *T. gondii*-infected cells were incubated with 100 μg/mL of UA and SF for 24 h respectively. After washing with 1X PBS, the *T. gondii*-infected cells were fixed in 1X PBS containing 5% formaldehyde for 30 min, and then washed with 1X PBS and stained with a final concentration of 20 μM (Hoechst 33342, St. Louis, MO, USA) for 30 min in the dark. After nuclear staining, the cells were washed with 1X PBS three times, and their nuclear changes were observed under a UV fluorescent microscope (Nikon Eclipse TE 2000-U, Tokyo, Japan).

4.8. PVM Formation in T. gondii-Infected Cells

The cells were seeded onto cover slips in a 24 well plate (1×10^5 cells/well), which were infected with *T. gondii* (5×10^5 tachyzoites/well). *T. gondii*-infected cells were incubated with 100 µg/mL of UA and SF for 24 h, respectively. After washing with 1X PBS, they were fixed with 5% formaldehyde for 10 min and 0.05% (v/v) Triton X-100 for 5 min. The cells were blocked with 1X PBS containing 1% BSA for 1 h at room temperature after washing. A mouse monoclonal anti-PVM antibody was diluted with 1:100 (v/v) using 1% BSA/PBS, and then the cells were incubated with anti-PVM antibody solution at room temperature for 1 h. After washing, goat anti-mouse IgG-FITC-conjugated secondary antibody was diluted with 1:100 (v/v) using 1X PBS, which was added to each well. The cells were incubated at room temperature for 1 h, and were washed with 1X PBS every 15 min, four times. Their fluorescence was observed under a UV fluorescent microscope (Nikon Eclipse TE 2000-U, Tokyo, Japan).

4.9. The Survival Rate of T. gondii-Infected Mice

Twenty-five animals (mouse/6 weeks, $n = 25$) were divided into normal ($n = 5$) and experimental groups (four groups, $n = 20$). *T. gondii* was seeded in a 12 well plate (4×10^6/well), which was incubated with different concentrations (100, 200, and 400 µg/mL) of UA for 24 h, respectively. *T. gondii* treated with the compounds was harvested before the injection in the abdominal cavity of each mouse in the experiment group, which was washed with 1X PBS three times. The pellets were suspended with 1X PBS, which were injected in the abdominal cavity of each BALB-c/mouse in the experimental groups. *T. gondii*-infected mice untreated with UA were used as an infected positive group, and the animals were kept in a central animal care facility during the experiment.

4.10. Statistical Analysis

All of the results were expressed as mean $\pm$ S.D. Statistical analysis of the data was performed using Student's *t*-test and analysis of variance (ANOVA). * $p < 0.05$ was considered to be statistically significant.

5. Conclusions

The results of this study demonstrate that UA not only has anti-*T. gondii* activity causing the direct inhibition of *T. gondii*, but also causes anti-parasitic effect against *T. gondii* by strongly inhibiting the proliferation and growth of *T. gondii* in infected host cells. In addition, our results show clearly for the first time that UA has anti-*T. gondii* effect which consistently induces the survival of *T. gondii*-infected mice. Therefore, this study provides substantial results and the potential that UA can be utilized as a promising candidate substance for anti-*T. gondii* drug development of next-generation through *T. gondii*-infected cells and infected-mice model. In addition, UA suggests novel perspectives of the approach for anti-*T. gondii* drug development, which shows the need of further study regarding the safety and/or efficacy against toxoplasmosis through preclinical study in the near future.

Author Contributions: W.H.C. designed and carried out the "in vivo" experiments related to the parasitic work, and wrote a draft of the manuscript. I.A.L. and W.H.C. measured anti-parasitic activity of the compound and performed the cell culture related to the parasite work. The data was analyzed by W.H.C. and I.A.L. The manuscript was finally written and revised by W.H.C. All authors have read and approved the final manuscript.

Acknowledgments: The authors would like to express sincere gratitude to the staffs of Kunsan National University and Kyung Hee University School of Medicine for providing laboratory facilities and research equipment during the experiment. This work was supported by C&K pharmaceuticals (CKP, 2015003002), Korea, and the authors thank the company.

Conflicts of Interest: The authors declare no conflict of interest.

References

1. Joiner, K.A.; Roos, D.S. Secretory traffic in the eukaryotic parasite *Toxoplasma gondii*: Less is more. *J. Cell Biol.* **2002**, *157*, 557–563. [CrossRef] [PubMed]

2. Bonhomme, A.; Bouchot, A.; Pezzella, N.; Gomez, J.; Le, M.H.; Pinon, J.M. Signaling during the invasion of host cells by *Toxoplasma gondii*. *FEMS Microbiol. Rev.* **1999**, *23*, 551–561. [CrossRef] [PubMed]

3. Meneceur, P.; Bouldouyre, M.A.; Aubert, D.; Villena, I.; Menotti, J.; Sauvage, V.; Garin, J.F.; Derouin, F. In vitro susceptibility of various genotypic strains of Toxoplasma gondii to pyrimethamine, sulfadiazine, and atovaquone. *Antimicrob. Agents Chemother.* **2008**, *52*, 1269–1277. [CrossRef] [PubMed]

4. Doliwa, C.; Xia, D.; Escotte-Binet, S.; Newsham, E.L.; Sanya, J.S.; Aubert, D.; Randle, N.; Wastling, J.M.; Villena, I. Identification of differentially expressed proteins in sulfadiazine resistant and sensitive strains of Toxoplasma gondii using difference-gel electrophoresis (DIGE). *Int. J. Parasitol. Drugs Drug Resist.* **2013**, *3*, 35–44. [CrossRef] [PubMed]

5. Aspinall, T.V.; Joynson, D.H.; Guy, E.; Hyde, J.E.; Sims, P.F. The molecular basis of sulfonamide resistance in Toxoplasma gondii and implications for the clinical management of toxoplasmosis. *J. Infect. Dis.* **2002**, *185*, 1637–1643. [CrossRef] [PubMed]

6. Choi, W.H.; Lee, I.A. The anti-tubercular activity of *Melia azedarach* L. and *Lobelia chinensis* Lour. and their potential as effective anti-*Mycobacterium tuberculosis* candidate agents. *Asian Pac. J. Trop. Biomed.* **2016**, *6*, 830–835. [CrossRef]

7. Qiu, L.; Chen, K.P. Anti-HBV agents derived from botanical origin. *Fitoterapia* **2013**, *84*, 140–157. [CrossRef] [PubMed]

8. Wycoff, K.; Maclean, J.; Belle, A.; Yu, L.; Tran, Y.; Roy, C.; Hayden, F. Anti-infective immunoadhesins from plants. *Plant Biotechnol. J.* **2015**, *13*, 1078–1093. [CrossRef] [PubMed]

9. De Oliveira, L.H.G.; Silva de Sousa, P.A.P.; Hilario, F.F.; Nascimento, G.J.; Morais, J.P.S.; de Medeiros, E.P.; de Sousa, M.F.; da Cruz Nunes, F. Agave sisalana extract induces cell death in Aedes aegypti hemocytes increasing nitric oxide production. *Asian. Pac. J. Trop. Biomed.* **2016**, *6*, 396–399. [CrossRef]

10. Wang, M.; Tao, L.; Xu, H. Chinese herbal medicines as a source of molecules with anti-enterovirus 71 activity. *Chin. Med.* **2016**, *11*, 2. [CrossRef] [PubMed]

11. Choi, W.H. Novel pharmacological activity of artesunate and artemisinin: Their potential as anti-tubercular agents. *J. Clin. Med.* **2017**, *6*, 30. [CrossRef] [PubMed]

12. Kavitha, N.; Noordin, R.; Chan, K.L.; Sasidharan, S. In vitro anti-*Toxoplasma gondii* activity of root extract/fractions of Eurycoma longifolia Jack. *BMC Complement. Altern. Med.* **2012**, *12*, 91. [CrossRef] [PubMed]

13. Alomar, M.L.; Rasse-Suriani, F.O.; Ganuza, A.; Coceres, V.M.; Cabrerizo, F.M.; Angel, S.O. In vitro evaluation of b-carboline alkaloids as potential anti-Toxoplasma agents. *BMC Res. Notes* **2013**, *6*, 193. [CrossRef] [PubMed]

14. Dzitko, K.; Grzybowski, M.M.; Pawełczyk, J.; Dziadek, B.; Gatkowska, J.; Stączek, P.; Długonska, H. Phytoecdysteroids as modulators of the *Toxoplasma gondii* growth rate in human and mouse cells. *Parasites Vectors* **2015**, *8*, 422. [CrossRef] [PubMed]

15. Gasparotto Junior, A.; Cosmo, M.L.; Reis Mde, P.; Dos Santos, P.S.; Gonçalves, D.D.; Gasparotto, F.M.; Navarro, I.T.; Lourenço, E.L. Effects of extracts from *Echinacea purpurea* (L.) MOENCH on mice infected with different strains of *Toxoplasma gondii*. *Parasitol. Res.* **2016**, *115*, 3999–4005. [CrossRef] [PubMed]

16. Zhang, X.; Jin, L.; Cui, Z.; Zhang, C.; Wu, X.; Park, H.; Quan, H.; Jin, C. Antiparasitic effects of oxymatrine and matrine against *Toxoplasma gondii* in vitro and in vivo. *Exp. Parasitol.* **2016**, *165*, 95–102. [CrossRef] [PubMed]

17. Colla, A.R.; Rosa, J.M.; Cunha, M.P.; Rodrigues, A.L. Anxiolytic-like effects of ursolic acid in mice. *Eur. J. Pharmacol.* **2015**, *758*, 171–176. [CrossRef] [PubMed]

18. Kanjoormana, M.; Kuttan, G. Antiangiogenic activity of ursolic acid. *Integr. Cancer Ther.* **2010**, *9*, 224–235. [CrossRef] [PubMed]

19. Kazmi, I.; Afzal, M.; Gupta, G.; Anwar, F. Antiepileptic potential of ursolic acid stearoyl glucoside by GABA receptor stimulation. *CNS Neurosci. Ther.* **2012**, *18*, 799–800. [CrossRef] [PubMed]

20. Lu, J.; Wu, D.M.; Zheng, Y.L.; Hu, B.; Zhang, Z.F.; Ye, Q.; Liu, C.M.; Shan, Q.; Wang, Y.J. Ursolic acid attenuates D-galactose-induced inflammatory response in mouse prefrontal cortex through inhibiting AGEs/RAGE/NF-κB pathway activation. *Cereb. Cortex* **2010**, *20*, 2540–2548. [CrossRef] [PubMed]

21. Checker, R.; Sandur, S.K.; Sharma, D.; Patwardhan, R.S.; Jayakumar, S.; Kohli, V.; Sethi, G.; Aggarwal, B.B.; Sainis, K.B. Potent anti-inflammatory activity of ursolic acid, a triterpenoid antioxidant, is mediated through suppression of NF-κB, AP-1 and NF-AT. *PLoS ONE* **2012**, *7*, e31318. [CrossRef] [PubMed]

22. Zhang, Y.X.; Kong, C.Z.; Wang, L.H.; Li, J.Y.; Liu, X.K.; Xu, B.; Xu, C.L.; Sun, Y.H. Ursolic acid overcomes Bcl-2-mediated resistance to apoptosis in prostate cancer cells involving activation of JNK-Induced Bcl-2 phosphorylation and degradation. *J. Cell. Biochem.* **2010**, *109*, 764–773. [CrossRef] [PubMed]

23. Choi, W.H.; Chu, J.P.; Jiang, M.H.; Baek, S.H.; Park, H.D. Effects of fraction obtained from Korean Corni Fructus extracts causing anti-proliferation and p53-dependent apoptosis in A549 lung cancer cells. *Nutr. Cancer* **2011**, *63*, 121–129. [CrossRef] [PubMed]

24. Prasad, S.; Yadav, V.R.; Sung, B.; Gupta, S.C.; Tyagi, A.K.; Aggarwal, B.B. Ursolic acid inhibits the growth of human pancreatic cancer and enhances the antitumor potential of gemcitabine in an orthotopic mouse model through suppression of the inflammatory microenvironment. *Oncotarget* **2016**, *7*, 13182–13196. [CrossRef] [PubMed]

25. Ramos, A.A.; Pereira-Wilson, C.; Collins, A.R. Protective effects of ursolic acid and luteolin against oxidative DNA damage include enhancement of DNA repair in Caco-2 cells. *Mutat. Res.* **2010**, *692*, 6–11. [CrossRef] [PubMed]

26. Do Nascimento, P.G.; Lemos, T.L.; Bizerra, A.M.; Arriaga, A.M.; Ferreira, D.A.; Santiago, G.M.; Braz-Filho, R.; Costa, J.G. Antibacterial and antioxidant activities of ursolic acid and derivatives. *Molecules* **2014**, *19*, 1317–1327. [CrossRef] [PubMed]

27. Jimenez-Arellanes, A.; Luna-Herrera, J.; Cornejo-Garrido, J.; Lopez-Garcia, S.; Castro-Mussot, M.E.; Meckes-Fischer, M.; Mata-Espinosa, D.; Marquina, B.; Torres, J.; Hernández-Pando, R. Ursolic and oleanolic acids as antimicrobial and immunomodulatory compounds for tuberculosis treatment. *BMC Complement. Altern. Med.* **2013**, *13*, 258. [CrossRef] [PubMed]

28. Kang, S.Y.; Yoon, S.Y.; Roh, D.H.; Jeon, M.J.; Seo, H.S.; Uh, D.K.; Kwon, Y.B.; Kim, H.W.; Han, H.J.; Lee, H.J.; et al. The anti-arthritic effect of ursolic acid on zymosan-induced acute inflammation and adjuvant-induced chronic arthritis models. *J. Pharm. Pharmacol.* **2008**, *60*, 1347–1354. [CrossRef] [PubMed]

29. Xu, H.; Zhang, M.; Li, X.L.; Li, H.; Yue, L.T.; Zhang, X.X.; Wang, C.C.; Wang, S.; Duan, R.S. Low and high doses of ursolic acid ameliorate experimental autoimmune myasthenia gravis through different pathways. *J. Neuroimmunol.* **2015**, *281*, 61–67. [CrossRef] [PubMed]

30. Borges, I.P.; Castanheira, L.E.; Barbosa, B.F.; de Souza, D.L.; da Silva, R.J.; Mineo, J.R.; Tudini, K.A.; Rodrigues, R.S.; Ferro, E.A.; de Melo, R.V. Anti-parasitic effect on *Toxoplasma gondii* induced by BnSP-7, a Lys49-phospholipase A2 homologue from Bothrops pauloensis venom. *Toxicon* **2016**, *119*, 84–91. [CrossRef] [PubMed]

31. Sanfelice, R.A.; da Silva, S.S.; Bosqui, L.R.; Miranda-Sapla, M.M.; Barbosa, B.F.; Silva, R.J.; Ferro, E.A.V.; Panagio, L.A.; Navarro, I.T.; Bordignon, J.; et al. Pravastatin and simvastatin inhibit the adhesion, replication and proliferation of Toxoplasma gondii (RH strain) in HeLa cells. *Acta Trop.* **2017**, *167*, 208–215. [CrossRef] [PubMed]

32. Carmen, J.C.; Southard, R.C.; Sinai, A.P. The complexity of signaling in host-pathogen interactions revealed by the Toxoplasma gondii-dependent modulation of JNK phosphorylation. *Exp. Cell Res.* **2008**, *314*, 3724–3736. [CrossRef] [PubMed]

33. Laliberte, J.; Carruthers, V.B. Host cell manipulation by human pathogen *Toxoplasma gondii*. *Cell. Mol. Life Sci.* **2008**, *65*, 1900–1915. [CrossRef] [PubMed]

34. Gubbels, M.J.; White, M.; Szatanek, T. The cell cycle and *Toxoplasma gondii* cell division: Tightly knit or loosely stitched. *Int. J. Parasitol.* **2008**, *38*, 1343–1358. [CrossRef] [PubMed]

35. Jesus, J.A.; Fragoso, T.N.; Yamamoto, E.S.; Laurenti, M.D.; Silva, M.S.; Ferreira, A.F.; Lago, J.H.; Santos-Gomes, G.; Passero, L.F. Therapeutic effect of ursolic acid in experimental visceral leishmaniasis. *Int. J. Parasitol. Drugs Drug Resist.* **2017**, *7*, 1–11. [CrossRef] [PubMed]

36. Yamamoto, E.S.; Campos, B.L.; Jesus, J.A.; Laurenti, M.D.; Ribeiro, S.P.; Kallas, E.G.; Rafael-Fernandes, M.; Santos-Gomes, G.; Silva, M.S.; Sessa, D.P.; et al. The Effect of Ursolic Acid on *Leishmania* (*Leishmania*) *amazonensis* is Related to Programed Cell Death and Presents Therapeutic Potential in Experimental Cutaneous Leishmaniasis. *PLoS ONE* **2015**, *10*, e0144946. [CrossRef] [PubMed]

37. Latt, S.A.; Stetten, G. Spectral studies on 33258 Hoechst and related bisbenzimidazole dyes useful for fluorescent detection of deoxyribonucleic acid synthesis. *J. Histochem. Cytochem.* **1976**, *24*, 24–33. [CrossRef] [PubMed]

9

Creatinine-Based Renal Function Estimates and Dosage of Postoperative Pain Management for Elderly Acute Hip Fracture Patients

Morten Baltzer Houlind [1,2,3,*][iD], Kristian Kjær Petersen [4], Henrik Palm [5],
Lillian Mørch Jørgensen [1], Mia Aakjær [1,2,3], Lona Louring Christrup [3][iD],
Janne Petersen [1,6], Ove Andersen [1,7] and Charlotte Treldal [1,2,3]

[1] Optimed, Clinical Research Centre, Copenhagen University Hospital Hvidovre, Kettegård Alle 30,
     Department 056, 2650 Hvidovre, Denmark; lillian.moerch.joergensen@regionh.dk (L.M.J.);
     mia.aakjaer@sund.ku.dk (M.A.); petersen.janne@gmail.com (J.P.); ove.andersen@regionh.dk (O.A.);
     charlotte.treldal.02@regionh.dk (C.T.)
[2] The Capital Region Pharmacy, Marielundvej 25, 2730 Herlev, Denmark
[3] Section of Pharmacotherapy, Department of Drug Design and Pharmacology, University of Copenhagen,
     Universitetsparken 2, 2100 København Ø, Denmark; llc@sund.ku.dk
[4] Center for Sensory-Motor Interaction (SMI), Department of Health Science and Technology, Faculty of
     Medicine, Aalborg University, Fredrik Bajers Vej 7, building A2-206, 9220 Aalborg Ø, Denmark;
     kkp@hst.aau.dk
[5] Orthopedic Department, Copenhagen University Hospital Bispebjerg, Bispebjerg Bakke 23,
     2400 København, Denmark; Henrik.palm@regionh.dk
[6] Section of Biostatistics, Department of Public Health, University of Copenhagen, Øster Farimagsgade 5,
     Enterance B, 2nd floor, 1014 København, Denmark
[7] Emergency Department, Copenhagen University Hospital Hvidovre, Kettegård Alle 30, Department 436,
     2650 Hvidovre, Denmark
*   Correspondence: morten.baltzer.houlind@regionh.dk

Abstract: Many analgesics and their metabolites are renally excreted. The widely used Chronic Kidney Disease Epidemiology Collaboration (CKD-EPI)-estimated glomerular filtration rate (eGFR) equations are not developed for use in the elderly, while the recent Berlin Initiative Study (BIS), Full Age Spectrum (FAS), and Lund-Malmö revised (LMR) equations are. This observational study investigated differences between creatinine-based eGFR equations and how the choice of equation influences dosage of analgesics in elderly ($\geq$70 years) patients admitted with acute hip fracture. eGFR was calculated by the CKD-EPI, BIS, Cockcroft-Gault (CG), FAS, LMR, and Modification of Diet in Renal Disease (MDRD) equations. Standard daily dose for postoperative pain medications ibuprofen, morphine and gabapentin was simulated for each equation according to dosage recommendations in Renbase®. For 118 patients, mean eGFR from the CKD-EPI, BIS, CG, FAS, LMR, and MDRD equations was 67.3 mL/min/1.73 m², 59.1 mL/min/1.73 m², 56.9 mL/min/1.73 m², 60.3 mL/min/1.73 m², 58.9 mL/min/1.73 m², and 79.1 mL/min/1.73 m², respectively ($p < 0.0001$). Mean difference to CKD-EPI was -10.4 mL/min/1.73 m² to 11.8 mL/min/1.73 m². Choice of eGFR equation significantly influenced the recommended dose ($p < 0.0001$). Shifting to BIS, FAS, or LMR equations led to a lower recommended dose in 20% to 31% of patients. Choice of eGFR equation significantly influenced dosing of ibuprofen, morphine, and gabapentin.

Keywords: renal function; kidney function; glomerular filtration rate; elderly; analgesic; pain management; drug dose adjustment; drug dosing; patient safety; clinical pharmacy

1. Introduction

Optimization of postoperative pain management in elderly patients is essential for fast-track surgery and patient-related outcomes [1,2]. Several medication regimens have been proposed to optimize postoperative pain recovery [3–5]. Unfortunately, many of these most frequently used medications and their metabolites are renally excreted and therefore a challenge to dose in patients with renal impairment [6,7]. Postoperative analgesics to patients with hip fractures, are often prescribed in standard doses, but must be adjusted according to renal function [7]. Renal function declines with age, and this decline is further accelerated by co-morbidities such as hypertension, diabetes mellitus, and chronic inflammation [8–10]. Because of their high age, high comorbidity and reduced kidney function, most acute hip fracture patients are categorized as fragile patients [11–16]. Elderly patients are also more likely to experience unpredictable pharmacokinetic and pharmacodynamic variations, making them more susceptible to dosing errors [17]. Several renally excreted analgesics in particular are known to cause adverse drug reactions when they or their active metabolites accumulate in the body or to cause nephrotoxicity [6,7,18]. These so-called "renal risk medications" include the first line choices in postoperative pain management, such as ibuprofen, morphine, and gabapentin. Ibuprofen is, like other Nonsteroidal Anti-Inflammatory Drugs (NSAIDs), nephrotoxic [19]. Morphine is metabolized to morphine-3-glucuronide and morphine-6-glucuronide, which are both excreted renally [18]. Gabapentin is almost exclusively eliminated unchanged by renal excretion [20]. The adverse reactions of ibuprofen, morphine, and gabapentin are dose-dependent, stressing the importance of prescribing these drugs at doses individually adjusted for the actual kidney function [6,7].

Glomerular filtration rate (GFR) is considered the best indicator of renal function and is commonly used to guide optimal dosing of medications [21]. Exogenous gold standard markers such as inulin and iohexol give accurate measures of GFR, but these are practically infeasible and too expensive to routinely use in hospital settings [22,23]. Instead, GFR is typically estimated based on serum concentration of an endogenous biomarker such as creatinine, which is fast and cheap to obtain [23]. The Chronic Kidney Disease Epidemiology Collaboration (CKD-EPI) equation based on creatinine [24] is commonly used in clinical practice worldwide and recommended both by "Kidney Disease: Improving Global Outcomes" (KDIGO) [25] and the Danish Society of Nephrology. Other widely used estimated GFR (eGFR) equations include the Modification of Diet in Renal Disease (MDRD) [26] and Cockcroft-Gault (CG) [27] equations. Unfortunately, the CKD-EPI and MDRD equations from North America are not developed for use among patients ≥70 years and are known to overestimate GFR in these patients [28–30]. Conversely, it is well known that the CG equation systematically underestimates GFR [31,32], but the equation is often used in drug development studies. The more recently developed European eGFR equations, including the Berlin Initiative Study (BIS) [29], Full Age Spectrum (FAS) [33], and Lund-Malmö revised (LMR) [34] equations, were adapted to more accurately estimate GFR in the elderly. However, so far, no studies have been conducted to directly compare how these equations perform in elderly hip fracture patients, and there is little research discussing the implications of switching between equations for dosing of analgesics. The aims of this study are: (1) to compare renal function estimates and CKD classification between the BIS, CG, FAS, LMR, and MDRD equations and the standard CKD-EPI equation in elderly hip fracture patients receiving postoperative pain management, and (2) to demonstrate how choice of eGFR equation influences dose recommendations for ibuprofen, morphine, and gabapentin.

2. Results

One hundred and eighty-three patients were hospitalized with acute hip fracture during the study period. Patients were excluded due to <70 years (n = 52), potential AKI on third postoperative day (n = 6), or death before the third postoperative day (n = 7). Patient characteristics for included patients (n = 118) are shown in Table 1. Among included patients, 68% were female and the median age was 82.6 years.

Table 1. Demographic data (n = 118), median values with range.

Variable	Value
Female sex, n (%)	80 (67.8)
Age (years)	82.6 (70.1–100.8)
Actual body weight (kg)	63.0 (32.0–98.0)
Height (cm)	167 (144–191)
Body Mass Index (kg/m^2)	22.4 (14.2–33.3)
Body Mass Index (kg/m^2) $\leq$ 18.5, n (%)	14 (11.9)
Body Mass Index (kg/m^2) > 30.0, n (%)	3 (2.50)
Body surface area (m^2)	1.71 (1.19–2.19)
Body surface area > 1.9 m^2, n (%)	25 (21.2)
Body surface area < 1.6 m^2, n (%)	40 (33.9)
Serum creatinine (µmol/L)	71.0 (25.0–430)
Comorbidities and medication	
Hypertension, n (%)	56 (47.5)
Osteoporosis, n (%)	34 (28.8)
Dementia, n (%)	21 (17.8)
Ischemic heart disease, n (%)	19 (16.1)
Diabetes, n (%)	18 (15.2)
Number of medication at admission	6 (0–21)

2.1. Estimated Glomerular Filtration Rate

Mean eGFR from the CKD-EPI, BIS, CG, FAS, LMR, and MDRD equations are given in Table 2. Mixed models with renal function estimate values showed that the BIS, CG, FAS, LMR, and MDRD equations were all significantly different from CKD-EPI ($p < 0.0001$). The BIS, CG, FAS, and LMR equations yield significantly lower eGFR than CKD-EPI, with a mean difference ranging from -7.0 mL/min/1.73 m^2 to -10.4 mL/min/1.73 m^2. The MDRD equation yields significantly higher eGFR than CKD-EPI, with a mean difference of 11.8 mL/min/1.73 m^2 ($p < 0.0001$).

No differences in eGFR were found by comparison of the BIS, FAS and LMR equations ($p \geq 0.142$). The CG equation yields significantly lower eGFR than all other equations, with a mean difference of -2.0 mL/min/1.73 m^2 to -22.2 mL/min/1.73 m^2 $p \leq 0.030$). Finally, the MDRD equation yields an eGFR significantly higher than all other equations, with a mean difference of 11.8 mL/min/1.73 m^2 to 22.2 mL/min/1.73 m^2 ($p < 0.0001$).

Table 2. Estimated eGFR (mL/min/1.73 m^2) and mean difference in eGFR values between the CKD-EPI standard equation and the five alternative eGFR equations (n = 118). *p*-values illustrate differences compared with the CKD-EPI equation.

Source of Equation	eGFR (Mean $\pm$ SD)	Estimated Difference in eGFR	95% CI	*p*-Value
CKD-EPI	67.3 $\pm$ 22.3	-	-	-
BIS	59.1 $\pm$ 21.3	-8.2	-10.0–-6.4	<0.0001
CG	56.9 $\pm$ 25.7	-10.4	-12.2–-8.6	<0.0001
FAS	60.3 $\pm$ 24.6	-7.0	-8.8–-5.2	<0.0001
LMR	58.9 $\pm$ 20.1	-8.4	-10.2–-6.6	<0.0001
MDRD	79.1 $\pm$ 33.6	$+11.8$	10.0–13.6	<0.0001

eGFR estimated Glomerular Filtration Rate, *CKD-EPI* Chronic Kidney Disease Epidemiology Collaboration, *BIS* Berlin Initiative Study, *CG* Cockcroft-Gault, *FAS* Full Age Spectrum, *LMR* Lund-Malmö revised, *MDRD* Modification of Diet in Renal Disease.

2.2. CKD Re-Classification Compared with the CKD-EPI

The distributions of CKD stages based on the eGFR equations are shown in Table 3. The CKD-EPI equation classified 79 patients (66.9%) in CKD stages 1–2, and only 39 patients (n = 33.1) in CKD stages 3–5. The BIS, FAS, and LMR equations classified between 53 patients and 59 patients (44.9% to 50.0%) in CKD stages 1–2, and between 59 patients and 65 patients (50.0% to 55.1%) in CKD stages 3–5.

The CG equation showed similar classification patterns as BIS, FAS, and LMR, but 70 patients (59.3%) were classified in CKD stages 3–5. In contrast, the MDRD equation only classified 32 patients (27.1%) in CKD stages 3–5. Table 4 shows the agreement of CKD classification between the eGFR equations. The MDRD equation had the highest agreement with CKD-EPI (κ = 0.70), while the CG equation had the lowest agreement (κ = 0.57). The BIS, FAS, and LMR equations all had almost perfect agreement with each other ($\kappa \geq 0.85$).

Table 3. Classification of chronic kidney disease stages based on the six different creatinine-based eGFR equations. Data are represented as the number (percentage) of participants in each chronic kidney disease stage (n = 118).

Source of Equation	CKD I eGFR ≥ 90	CKD II eGFR 60–89	CKD III eGFR 30–59	CKD IV eGFR 15–29	CKD V eGFR < 15
CKD-EPI	15 (12.7)	64 (54.2)	31 (26.3)	6 (5.1)	2 (1.7)
BIS	7 (5.9)	46 (39.0)	58 (49.2)	5 (4.2)	2 (1.7)
CG	6 (5.1)	42 (35.6)	56 (47.4)	12 (10.2)	2 (1.7)
FAS	10 (8.5)	43 (36.4)	54 (45.8)	9 (7.6)	2 (1.7)
LMR	4 (3.4)	55 (46.6)	47 (39.8)	10 (8.5)	2 (1.7)
MDRD	41 (34.8)	45 (38.1)	25 (21.2)	5 (4.2)	2 (1.7)

CKD Chronic Kidney Disease classification, *eGFR* estimated Glomerular Filtration Rate, *CKD-EPI* Chronic Kidney Disease Epidemiology Collaboration, *BIS* Berlin Initiative Study, *CG* Cockcroft-Gault, *FAS* Full Age Spectrum, *LMR* Lund-Malmö revised, *MDRD* Modification of Diet in Renal Disease.

Table 4. The agreement of chronic kidney disease (CKD) stage among the six different creatinine-based eGFR equations in relative values. Weighted kappa coefficient (95% CI), (number of patients with agreement in CKD stage; percentage patients with agreement in CKD stage).

	BIS	CG	FAS	LMR	MDRD
CKD-EPI	0.65 (0.54–0.76) (83; 70.4%)	0.57 (0.46–0.68) (75; 63.6%)	0.68 (0.57–0.78) (84; 71.2%)	0.65 (0.54–0.75) (83; 70.4%)	0.70 (0.60–0.79) (84; 71.2%)
BIS		0.78 (0.68–0.87) (97; 76.2%)	0.93 (0.87–0.98) (111; 94.0%)	0.85 (0.77–0.92) (104; 88.1%)	0.45 (0.34–0.56) (59; 50.0%)
CG			0.82 (0.74–0.90) (100; 84.7%)	0.80 (0.71–0.89) (100; 84.7%)	0.38 (0.28–0.49) (60; 50.8%)
FAS				0.87 (0.80–0.94) (105; 89.0%)	0.46 (0.36–0.56) (50; 42.4%)
LMR					0.44 (0.34–0.54) (49; 41.5%)

CKD-EPI Chronic Kidney Disease Epidemiology Collaboration, *BIS* Berlin Initiative Study, *CG* Cockcroft-Gault, *FAS* Full Age Spectrum, *LMR* Lund-Malmö revised, *MDRD* Modification of Diet in Renal Disease.

2.3. Shift in Recommended Prescription Dose of Ibuprofen, Morphine, and Gabapentin

Figure 1 and Table 5 show the potential changes in doses for ibuprofen, morphine, and gabapentin when switching between the CKD-EP, BIS, CG, FAS, LMR, or MDRD equations. Recommended doses for all three analgesics were statistically significantly different with CKD-EPI compared to the other eGFR equations ($p \leq 0.0078$). No differences in recommended ibuprofen and morphine doses were found between BIS, FAS and LMR equations ($p \geq 0.125$). However, gabapentin dose recommendations were significantly lower with the LMR equation compared to the BIS and FAS equations ($p \leq 0.0001$). All recommended doses for all three analgesics were statistically significantly lower with CG compared to the other eGFR equations ($p \leq 0.0287$), except for gabapentin based on the LMR equation ($p = 0.1082$). Finally, all recommended doses for all three analgesics were statistically significantly higher with MDRD compared to the other eGFR equations ($p \leq 0.0078$).

Overall, shifting from CKD-EPI to BIS, FAS, or LMR would result in a lower recommended dose of gabapentin and morphine for 34 to 35 patients (29% to 30%) and 24 to 29 patients (20% to 25%) for ibuprofen (Table 5). Recommended doses for ibuprofen, morphine, and gabapentin would be reduced according to renal function in over half of patients by using BIS, CG, FAS, or LMR, while they would be reduced in only one quarter of patients when using CKD-EPI or MDRD. Furthermore, ibuprofen and morphine would be contraindicated in about twice as many patients by using CG, FAS, or LMR instead of CKD-EPI, BIS, or MDRD.

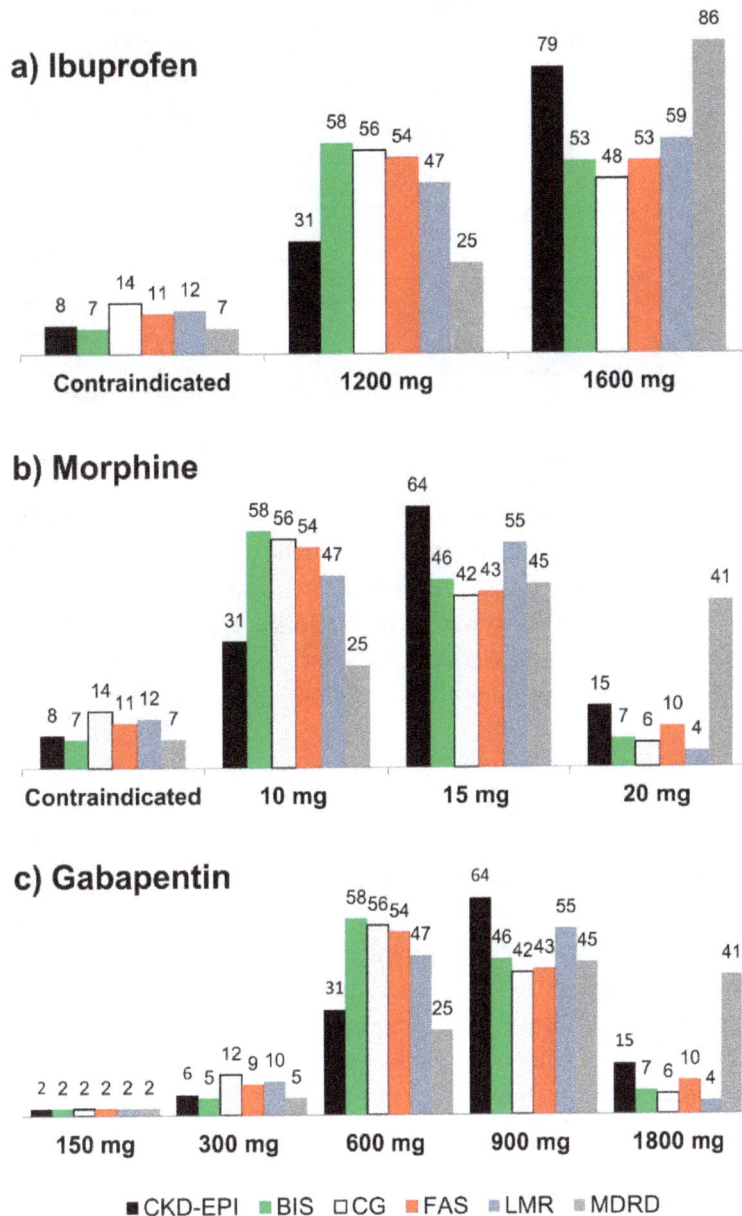

Figure 1. (a–c) Simulated recommended doses of ibuprofen (a), morphine (b), and gabapentin (c) according to the six different creatinine-based eGFR equations (n = 118). *CKD-EPI* Chronic Kidney Disease Epidemiology Collaboration, *BIS* Berlin Initiative Study, *CG* Cockcroft-Gault, *FAS* Full Age Spectrum, *LMR* Lund-Malmö revised, *MDRD* Modification of Diet in Renal Disease

Table 5. The agreement of simulated recommended doses of ibuprofen, morphine, and gabapentin among the six different creatinine-based eGFR equations in relative values (n = 118). Number of patients with agreement in dosage (number of patients where y doses higher than x/number of patients where y doses lower than x). Ibuprofen is marked with cursive font. Morphine and gabapentin are marked with bold font.

	BIS	CG	FAS	LMR	MDRD
CKD-EPI	*91 (26/1)* **83 (34/1)**	*81 (37/0)* **72 (46/0)**	*89 (29/0)* **84 (34/0)**	*94 (24/0)* **83 (35/0)**	*110 (0/8)* **84 (0/34)**
BIS		*100 (15/3)* **97 (17/4)**	*114 (4/0)* **111 (4/3)**	*107 (5/6)* **104 (6/8)**	*85 (0/33)* **51 (0/67)**
CG			*104 (3/11)* **100 (3/15)**	*101 (2/15)* **99 (4/15)**	*73 (0/45)* **41 (0/77)**
FAS				*111 (1/6)* **105 (7/6)**	*81 (0/37)* **50 (0/68)**
LMR					*86 (0/32)* **49 (0/69)**

CKD-EPI Chronic Kidney Disease Epidemiology Collaboration, *BIS* Berlin Initiative Study, *CG* Cockcroft-Gault, *FAS* Full Age Spectrum, *LMR* Lund-Malmö revised, *MDRD* Modification of Diet in Renal Disease.

3. Discussion

In the current study, estimates of renal function obtained with six equations were compared and the impact of their use for postoperative pain management in elderly hip fracture patients was assessed. It was found that the CG, BIS, FAS, and LMR equations estimated GFR significantly lower than CKD-EPI, while the MDRD equation estimated GFR significantly higher. These differences between GFR estimates based on the six equations led to significant differences in standard dosing of ibuprofen, morphine, and gabapentin according to renal function in 20–31% in elderly hip fracture patients.

3.1. eGFR Equations Based on Creatinine and Elderly

As expected, the recently developed BIS, FAS and LMR equations estimated GFR lower than CKD-EPI and classified considerably more patients in CKD stage III or below (<60 mL/min/1.73 m^2) [29,33,34]. The CKD-EPI equation based on creatinine is recommended by KDIGO [25] and used internationally in clinical practice. However, there are several drawbacks to using this equation in elderly acutely hospitalized patients. First, the CKD-EPI equation was not developed to estimate GFR in the elderly; rather, it developed to improve GFR estimation >60 mL/min/1.73 m^2 in adults [24], but optimization of prescription is primarily relevant at low renal function (<60 mL/min/1.73 m^2). A possible explanation for CKD-EPI performing poorly in elderly patients with low renal function is that the cohort in which CKD-EPI was developed only contained 4% (n = 217) over 70 years [24]. The more recent BIS, LMR and FAS equations were, however, developed in populations with a higher percentage of elderly patients. BIS was developed in a cohort where all patients were above 70 years (n = 610) [29]. LMR included 27% (n = 230) of patients over 70 years and was developed with the explicit goal of improving eGFR at lower levels of renal function [34]. FAS included 26% (n = 1764) patients over 70 years and was developed based on average GFR and age-normalized serum creatinine [33].

Recent studies have found that the BIS, FAS and LMR equations based on creatinine have a higher percentage of estimates within 30% of the measured GFR (P30 accuracy) than CKD-EPI in elderly patients [35–37]. However, there is no consensus about which of these alternative equations is best. The MDRD equation overestimates GFR in the elderly [28–30]. Heldal et al. found that BIS, CG, FAS, and LMR were more accurate than CKD-EPI in stable elderly kidney transplant patients [38], while results from several other studies have proven that CG underestimates GFR in the elderly [31,32]. The BIS equation was developed specifically in elderly patients and seems to be the most promising alternative to CKD-EPI. An in-depth review supports that BIS is most accurate in patients with GFR < 60 mL/min/1.73 m^2 [39], and a direct comparison by Oscanoa et al. of BIS and CKD-EPI in elderly patients suggests that BIS is more accurate [40]. However, no studies have directly compared these creatinine-based equations among elderly acutely hospitalized patients. The findings in the current study highlight the high degree of variability among the equations and emphasize the importance of considering how this variability could affect prescribing of renal risk medications.

A general challenge of using creatinine to estimate renal function in elderly patients is the biomarker's dependence on age, sex, race, muscle mass, and nutritional status [41,42]. The eGFR equations try to account for age, sex, and race. However, the association to muscle mass is particularly problematic in patients with low muscle mass, such as elderly, who will tend to have low baseline creatinine production. Segarra et al. studied the accuracy of CKD-EPI in hospitalized patients and found that CKD-EPI overestimates eGFR with a median bias of 2.7 mL/min/1.73 m^2 in patients over 70 years and 5.9 mL/min/1.73 m^2 in malnourished patients [43]. Median BMI among our acute hip fracture patients was only 22.4%, and 12% of the patients were underweight (BMI $\leq$ 18.5). Acute hip fracture patients are likely to be even more fragile than patients in the Segarra et al. cohort, so it is reasonable to expect that CKD-EPI also over-estimates eGFR in the current patient cohort presented here. Future studies should investigate which eGFR biomarker(s) and equation are most accurate for elderly frail hospitalized patients. These types of studies are needed to perform accurate pharmacokinetic studies in the elderly in drug development and for optimizing medication prescribing in the clinic

3.2. Renal Risk Medications and How to Meet the Challenge Clinical Practice

Inappropriate prescribing based on a patient's renal function is a well-known challenge. A study in Sweden by Helldén et al. found that 4.7% of all acutely hospitalized elderly patients were admitted due to adverse drug reactions related to impaired renal function [44]. Furthermore, it has been reported that 14% of elderly in primary care [45,46] and 23% of elderly in the hospital [47] lack proper dose adjustment according to renal function. Since approximately 40% of all medications must be dosed according to renal function [21], this clinical challenge applies to most medications used in postoperative pain management [7]. However, few studies have investigated how choice of eGFR equation influences dose recommendations in the elderly, and most of these studies only consider high-risk medications such as novel oral anticoagulants (NOACs). Results from two European studies in elderly patients showed that use of CG compared to CKD-EPI or MDRD results in lower eGFR values and lower recommended doses of NOACs [48,49]. On the other hand, a third study from Canada found that CG gave higher eGFR values than both CKD-EPI and MDRD, although this patient cohort had a mean BMI of 28 kg/m^2 [50]. There is evidently still debate about which eGFR equation is best among elderly patients, and our own results emphasize that choice of eGFR equation has a direct influence on medication prescribing for postoperative pain management in elderly patients.

Postoperative pain management is essential for patient quality and patient related outcomes in fast track surgery, and careful dosing is required to avoid complications and hospital readmission. Overdosing of morphine, for example, can lead to serious adverse reactions such as CNS and respiratory depression as well as narcosis [7,18]. Ibuprofen, morphine and gabapentin should all be avoided in patients with AKI due to the risk of accumulation of the substances, their metabolites and/or toxicity. To address this challenge in the clinic, dialogue with patients about their pain and medication dosing must be an integrated part of hospital ward rounds. Clinical-decision platforms or medication reviews should also be used in combination with patient dialogue to optimize prescribing practice. Lastly, clinicians treating elderly patients should consider use of pain medications with pharmacokinetic properties that make their effects less dependent on renal function. One example is oxycodone, which is metabolized in the liver to noroxycodone and oxymorphone [51], while 14% of the initial dose is excreted through the kidneys unchanged [52]. The major metabolite noroxycodone its inactive [53], and the active metabolite oxymorphone is formed only in minor amounts [51,54]. Oxymorphone is excreted mainly as the inactive oxymorphone-3-glucuronide conjugate [55]. Taken together, this makes oxycodone a safer alternative to morphine in patients with reduced renal function. Gabapentinoids is excreted unchanged renally and should be doses strictly according to the renal function [20]. Alternatively, tricyclic antidepressants are often used to treat neuropathic pain and are also independent of renal function. Unfortunately, there are no such alternatives to ibuprofen, since nephrotoxicity is a problem for the entire NSAID class [19].

3.3. Strengths and Limitations

The main strength of this study is that it identifies a daily clinical challenge of dosing renal risk medications in an unselected group of elderly hip fracture patients. This study also has several limitations. First, the current study lacks a gold standard for measuring GFR. Therefore, we compare the relative accuracies of each GFR equation and discuss how medication dosing would change by switching between equations. Second, this is a data simulation study and does not investigate clinical outcomes related to the simulation. Third, we simulate prescribing of NSAID to all patients in this study to show the clinical challenge of prescribing NSAID isolated to the choice of eGFR equation. In general, all NSAIDs should be used with caution in elderly patients due to the risk of ulcers, bleeding, and heart failure [56]. Some patients in this study would probably not be candidates to receive ibuprofen postoperatively in clinical practice due to co-morbidities. Fourth, we only calculate the normalization of GFR to a standardized body-surface area of 1.73 m^2. In drug development, the US Food and Drug Administration recommends the consideration of eGFR in relative or absolute values [57], while the European Medicines Agency only recommends eGFR in absolute values [58].

However, the finding of high variability between GFR equations should serve as a caution to clinicians who rely on only one equation in daily practice. Finally, this study is limited by the use of creatinine on the third postoperative day to define potential AKI. KDIGO guidelines suggest that a follow-up creatinine measurement should be taken at a later day to confirm AKI diagnosis [59].

4. Materials and Methods

4.1. Ethics Approval

Registry-based studies do not need prior ethical approval in Denmark [60]. The study was approved by the Danish Data Protection Agency (j.no. 2014-41-3001). All data was anonymized prior to access for this study.

4.2. Design and Setting

This was an observational registry study performed in the acute hip fracture ward, orthopaedic department, Copenhagen University Hospital, Hvidovre, Denmark from 1 January to 1 April 2015. Inclusion criteria were: acute hip fracture. Exclusion criteria were: age below 70 years or acute kidney injury (AKI) on the third postoperative day.

In accordance with standard practice, pain management from pre-operation to the morning of fourth postoperative day consisted of epidural infusion of 4 mL/h bupivacaine, 0.125%, with 50 μg/mL morphine as well as oral paracetamol 4 g per day. The daily dose of paracetamol was reduced to 2 g in case of: mild to moderate hepatic impairment (Child-Pugh Class A or B), severe malnutrition, anorexia, BMI ≤ 18.5 kg/m^2, chronic alcohol use or sepsis. Paracetamol was considered contraindicated in case of severe impairment (Child-Pugh Class C). During morning rounds of the third postoperative day, a pharmacological pain treatment was chosen to replace the epidural infusion. This pharmacological pain treatment consisted of ibuprofen, morphine or gabapentin, or a combination of the three in standard doses according to renal function and comobilities. Treatment was initiated immediately after the ward round to have an effect before discontinuation of epidural infusion on the following day. Oral paracetamol was continued in all patients. In this study, a suggested dose was simulated for each analgesic according to renal function on a patient-by-patient basis. The main outcome measures were

GFR estimated with CKD-EPI, BIS, CG, FAS, LMR, and MDRD; differences between GFR estimates by CKD-EPI and estimates by BIS, CG, FAS, LMR, and MDRD; and suggested doses for ibuprofen, morphine, and gabapentin according to each eGFR equation.

4.3. Study Data and Measurement

Information concerning hospital admission as well as comorbidities registered with ICD10 (International Statistical Classification of Diseases and Related Health Problems) is available in the National Patient Registry. Data concerning height and weight is available in the Danish Interdisciplinary Register for Hip Fractures. Information about dispensation of medication prescriptions prior to admission is available in The Danish Register of Medicinal Product Statistics. Finally, data about renal function is available in the Register of Laboratory Results for Research.

Serum creatinine values were available for the first, second, and third postoperative day, as well as the highest and lowest values between admission and discharge. Serum creatinine was measured at the Clinical Biochemical Department at Hvidovre University Hospital, Denmark, on a Roche Cobas® c 8000 701/702 (Roche Diagnostics International Ltd., Rotkreuz ZG, Switzerland) with a module instrument using the Roche Creatinine Plus version 2 IDMS-traceable enzymatic assay (coefficient of variation 1.4%) as recommended in KDIGO 2012 Guideline [25].

eGFR was calculated using six creatinine-based equations: CKD-EPI [24], BIS [29], CG [27], FAS [33], LMR [34], and MDRD [26] (see Appendix A). All equations account for age and sex. CKD-EPI and MDRD also adjust for race [24,26], while CG adjusts for body weight [27]. All GFR estimates were calculated relative to body surface area ($mL/min/1.73\ m^2$), where standard body surface area (BSA) is set to $1.73\ m^2$. For comparison with the other equations, creatinine clearance by CG was normalized per $1.73\ m^2$ of BSA using the DeBois and DeBois equation for calculating BSA [61]. The severity of renal impairment was determined for each equation and classified according to the 2003 National Kidney Foundation Kidney Disease Outcomes Quality Initiative Classification [62]. This classification system uses the following GFR value cutoffs as prescribing guidelines for renal risk medications: "normal GFR (CKD stage 1)" (eGFR $\geq 90\ mL/min/1.73\ m^2$), "mildly decreased GFR (CKD stage 2)" (eGFR 60–89 $mL/min/1.73\ m^2$), "moderately decreased GFR (CKD stage 3)" (eGFR 30–59 $mL/min/1.73\ m^2$), "severely decreased GFR (CKD stage 4)" (eGFR 15–29 $mL/min/1.73\ m^2$), or "kidney failure (CKD stage 5)" (eGFR < 15 ($mL/min/1.73\ m^2$).

4.4. Acute Kidney Injury (AKI)

For the purposes of this study, renal function had to stable on the third postoperative day. Renal function was considered unstable in patients with AKI according to 2012 KDIGO guidelines. Ased on the 2012 KDIGO criteria, AKI was determined by the first KDIGO criterion, which is an increase in serum creatinine of $\geq$50% from baseline or $\geq$26.5 µmol/L within 48 h [59]. The lowest serum creatinine value from admission to discharge was used as baseline. Two time intervals were used to determine creatinine change within 48 h: first to second postoperative day, and second to third postoperative day. Patients meeting this definition of AKI were excluded.

4.5. Medications

For all patients, we simulated the total daily doses of oral formulated ibuprofen, morphine, and gabapentin the participants would be prescribed based on their renal function according to the six eGFR equations. In patients with eGFR $\geq 90\ mL/min/1.73\ m^2$ standard doses of ibuprofen, morphine, and gabapentin, are 1600, 20, and 1200 mg, respectively.

In case of eGFR < 90 $mL/min/1.73\ m^2$ recommendations for dose reduction according to renal function were determined for each GFR equation by recommendations in Renbase® according to renal function [47,63]. Renbase® offers medication-specific dose adjustments for each stage of renal impairment. For ibuprofen, the dose recommendations are: 1600 mg for eGFR $\geq$ 60; 1200 mg for eGFR 30–59; and contraindicated for eGFR $\leq$ 29. For morphine, the dose recommendations are: 20 mg for eGFR $\geq$ 90; 15 mg for eGFR 60–89; 10 mg for eGFR 30–59; and contraindicated for eGFR $\leq$ 29. For gabapentin, the dose recommendations are: 1800 mg for eGFR $\geq$ 90; 900 mg for eGFR 60–89; 600 mg for eGFR 30–59; 300 mg for eGFR 16–29; and 150 mg for eGFR $\leq$ 15.

4.6. Statistical Analyses

A mixed linear model was used with patient ID modelled as a random effect and type of equation as fixed effect to evaluate differences in eGFR between the equations. Goodness of fit was checked by visual inspection of the following plots: histogram of residuals to inspect normal distribution, scatter plot of residuals versus predicted values to inspect variance homogeneity. To test the agreement between the five CKD stages calculated from the eGFR equations, a weighted kappa statistic (κ) was used. A kappa statistic of 0.21–0.40 was considered fair agreement; 0.41–0.60 moderate agreement; 0.61–0.80 substantial agreement, and 0.81–1.00 almost perfect agreement [64]. To test whether the dosage of ibuprofen, morphine, and gabapentin was dependent on eGFR equation, a Wilcoxon Matched-Pairs Signed Ranks Test was performed. For all statistical tests, $p \leq 0.05$ was considered statistically significant and data are presented as mean and standard deviation (SD). All calculations and statistical analyses were performed in SAS Enterprise Guide 7.1.

5. Conclusions

In the current study, significant differences in eGFR based on the BIS, CG, FAS, LMR, and MDRD equations were found when compared with the CKD-EPI equation in elderly acute hip fracture patients. The CG, BIS, FAS, and LMR equations estimated GFR to be lower than CKD-EPI, while the MDRD equation estimated GFR to be higher. The BIS, FAS, and LMR estimates had a high level of agreement. Choice of eGFR equation in elderly acute hip fracture patients would have a significant impact on the dosing of ibuprofen, morphine, and gabapentin according to the renal function. Future research should focus on which eGFR equations and biomarkers are most accurate in the elderly population, and it is recommended that clinicians take caution when using creatinine-based equations to estimate the dose of renally excreted analgesics to elderly patients.

Author Contributions: M.B.H., K.K.P., H.P., M.A., L.L.C., O.A., and C.T. contributed to conception of the study design. M.B.H. collected the data. M.B.H., K.K.P., L.M.J., J.P., M.A. and C.T. analyzed data. All others interpreted the data. M.B.H. drafted the manuscript. All others revised the manuscript. All authors read and approved the final manuscript.

Funding: This research received no external funding.

Acknowledgments: We thank Kari Laine for providing free access to Renbase®. We also thank Beata Malmquist and Mia Gemmer for their commentary on the study.

Conflicts of Interest: The authors have no conflicts of interest regarding to the study.

Appendix A

GFR estimating equations based on creatinine. For all the GFR estimating equations below, age is expressed in years and eGFR in mL/min/1.73 m^2 body surface area. Ln = natural logarithm.

CKD-EPI equation [24]: Serum creatinine (SCr) is expressed in mg/dL, $141 \times \min(SCr/\kappa,1)^{\alpha} \times \max(SCr/\kappa,1)^{-1.209} \times 0.993^{Age} \times 1.018$ (if female) $\times 1.159$ (if black), κ is 0.7 for females and 0.9 for males, α is 0.329 for females and 0.411 for males, min is the minimum of SCr/κ and 1 and max is the maximum of SCr/κ and 1.

BIS equation [29]: Serum creatinine (SCr) is expressed in mg/dL, $3.736 \times SCr \times Age^{-0.95} \times 0.82$ (if female).

CG equation [27]: Serum creatinine (SCr) is expressed in mg/dL, $(140 - Age) \times$ weight (kg)$/72 \times SCr \times 0.85$ (of female) $\times (1.73/BSA)$, body surface area was calculated using DuBois formula: $0.007184 \times$ weight (kg)$^{0.425} \times$ height (cm)$^{0.725}$.

FAS equation [33]: Serum creatinine (SCr) is expressed in mg/dL, $107.3/(SCr/QCr) \times 0.988^{(Age - 40)}$ (if 40 years or older), QCr is 0.7 mg/dL for females and QCr is 0.9 mg/dL for males.

LMR equation [34]: Serum creatinine (SCr) is expressed in mmol/L, $e^x = -0.0158 \times Age + 0.438 \times Ln(Age)$, x = if female and SCr < 150: x = 2.50 + 0.0121 x(150 − SCr), x = if female and SCr ≥ 150: x = 2.50 − 0.926 × In(SCr/150), x = if male and SCr < 180: x = 2.56 + 0.00968 × (180 − SCr), x = if male and SCr ≥ 180: x = 2.56 − 0.926 × In(SCr − 180).

MDRD equation [26]: Serum creatinine (SCr) is expressed in mg/dL, $175 \times SCr^{-1.154} \times Age^{-0.203} \times 0.742$ (if female).

References

1. White, P.F.; Kehlet, H. Improving postoperative pain management: What are the unresolved issues? *Anesthesiology* **2010**, *112*, 220–225. [CrossRef] [PubMed]

2. Jones, J.; Southerland, W.; Catalani, B. The Importance of Optimizing Acute Pain in the Orthopedic Trauma Patient. *Orthop. Clin. USA* **2017**, *48*, 445–465. [CrossRef] [PubMed]

3. Garimella, V.; Cellini, C. Postoperative Pain Control. *Clin. Colon Rectal Surg.* **2013**, *26*, 191–196. [CrossRef] [PubMed]

4. Chou, R.; Gordon, D.B.; de Leon-Casasola, O.A.; Rosenberg, J.M.; Bickler, S.; Brennan, T.; Carter, T.; Cassidy, C.L.; Chittenden, E.H.; Degenhardt, E.; et al. Management of Postoperative Pain: A Clinical Practice Guideline from the American Pain Society, the American Society of Regional Anesthesia and Pain Medicine, and the American Society of Anesthesiologists' Committee on Regional Anesthesia, Executive Committee, and Administrative Council. *J. Pain* **2016**, *17*, 131–157. [CrossRef] [PubMed]

5. Kehlet, H. Multimodal approach to control postoperative pathophysiology and rehabilitation. *Br. J. Anaesth.* **1997**, *78*, 606–617. [CrossRef] [PubMed]

6. Tawfic, Q.A.; Bellingham, G. Postoperative pain management in patients with chronic kidney disease. *J. Anaesthesiol. Clin. Pharmacol.* **2015**, *31*, 6–13. [CrossRef] [PubMed]

7. Parmar, M.S.; Parmar, K.S. Management of acute and post-operative pain in chronic kidney disease. *F1000Research* **2013**, *2*. [CrossRef]

8. Denic, A.; Glassock, R.J.; Rule, A.D. Structural and functional changes with the aging kidney. *Adv. Chronic Kidney Dis.* **2016**, *23*, 19–28. [CrossRef] [PubMed]

9. Zhou, X.J.; Rakheja, D.; Yu, X.; Saxena, R.; Vaziri, N.D.; Silva, F.G. The aging kidney. *Kidney Int.* **2008**, *74*, 710–720. [CrossRef] [PubMed]

10. Mallappallil, M.; Friedman, E.A.; Delano, B.G.; McFarlane, S.I.; Salifu, M.O. Chronic kidney disease in the elderly: Evaluation and management. *Clin. Pract.* **2014**, *11*, 525–535. [CrossRef] [PubMed]

11. Leung, F.; Blauth, M.; Bavonratanavech, S. Surgery for fragility hip fracture—Streamlining the process. *Osteoporos. Int.* **2010**, *21*, 519–521. [CrossRef] [PubMed]

12. Kronborg, L.; Bandholm, T.; Palm, H.; Kehlet, H.; Kristensen, M.T. Feasibility of Progressive Strength Training Implemented in the Acute Ward after Hip Fracture Surgery. *PLoS ONE* **2014**, *9*, e93332. [CrossRef] [PubMed]

13. Nitsch, D.; Mylne, A.; Roderick, P.J.; Smeeth, L.; Hubbard, R.; Fletcher, A. Chronic kidney disease and hip fracture-related mortality in older people in the UK. *Nephrol. Dial. Transplant.* **2009**, *24*, 1539–1544. [CrossRef] [PubMed]

14. Fried, L.F.; Biggs, M.L.; Shlipak, M.G.; Seliger, S.; Kestenbaum, B.; Stehman-Breen, C.; Sarnak, M.; Siscovick, D.; Harris, T.; Cauley, J.; et al. Association of kidney function with incident hip fracture in older adults. *J. Am. Soc. Nephrol.* **2007**, *18*, 282–286. [CrossRef] [PubMed]

15. Nickolas, T.L.; McMahon, D.J.; Shane, E. Relationship between Moderate to Severe Kidney Disease and Hip Fracture in the United States. *J. Am. Soc. Nephrol.* **2006**, *17*, 3223–3232. [CrossRef] [PubMed]

16. Marsh, D.; Palm, H. Rising to the challenge of fragility fractures. *Injury* **2018**, *49*, 1392. [CrossRef] [PubMed]

17. Hanlon, J.T.; Schmader, K.E. The Medication Appropriateness Index at 20: Where it Started, Where it has been and Where it May be Going. *Drugs Aging* **2013**, *30*, 893–900. [CrossRef] [PubMed]

18. Dean, M. Opioids in renal failure and dialysis patients. *J. Pain Symptom Manag.* **2004**, *28*, 497–504. [CrossRef] [PubMed]

19. Hörl, W.H. Nonsteroidal Anti-Inflammatory Drugs and the Kidney. *Pharmaceuticals* **2010**, *3*, 2291–2321. [CrossRef] [PubMed]

20. Raouf, M.; Atkinson, T.J.; Crumb, M.W.; Fudin, J. Rational dosing of gabapentin and pregabalin in chronic kidney disease. *J. Pain Res.* **2017**, *10*, 275–278. [CrossRef] [PubMed]

21. *Age-Associated General Pharmacological Aspects, Drug Therapy for the Elderly*; Martin, W. (Ed.) Springer: Berlin, Germany, 2013.

22. Macedo, E.; Mehta, R.L. Measuring renal function in critically ill patients: Tools and strategies for assessing glomerular filtration rate. *Curr. Opin. Crit. Care* **2013**, *19*, 560–566. [CrossRef] [PubMed]

23. Stevens, L.A.; Coresh, J.; Schmid, C.H.; Feldman, H.I.; Froissart, M.; Kusek, J.; Rossert, J.; Van Lente, F.; Bruce, R.D.; Zhang, Y.; et al. Estimating GFR using Serum Cystatin C Alone and in Combination with Serum Creatinine: A Pooled Analysis of 3418 Individuals with CKD. *Am. J. Kidney Dis.* **2008**, *51*, 395–406. [CrossRef] [PubMed]

24. Levey, A.S.; Stevens, L.A.; Schmid, C.H.; Zhang, Y.L.; Castro, A.F.; Feldman, H.I.; Kusek, J.W.; Eggers, P.; Van Lente, F.; Greene, T.; et al. CKD-EPI (Chronic Kidney Disease Epidemiology Collaboration) A new equation to estimate glomerular filtration rate. *Ann. Intern. Med.* **2009**, *150*, 604–612. [CrossRef] [PubMed]

25. KDIGO. 2012 Clinical Practice Guideline for the Evaluation and Management of Chronic Kidney Disease. *Int. Soc. Nephrol.* **2013**, 3.

26. Levey, A.S.; Coresh, J.; Greene, T.; Stevens, L.A.; Zhang, Y.L.; Hendriksen, S.; Kusek, J.W.; Van Lente, F. Chronic Kidney Disease Epidemiology Collaboration Using standardized serum creatinine values in the modification of diet in renal disease study equation for estimating glomerular filtration rate. *Ann. Intern. Med.* **2006**, *145*, 247–254. [CrossRef] [PubMed]

27. Cockcroft, D.W.; Gault, M.H. Prediction of creatinine clearance from serum creatinine. *Nephron* **1976**, *16*, 31–41. [CrossRef] [PubMed]

28. Björk, J.; Jones, I.; Nyman, U.; Sjöström, P. Validation of the Lund–Malmö, Chronic Kidney Disease Epidemiology (CKD-EPI) and Modification of Diet in Renal Disease (MDRD) equations to estimate glomerular filtration rate in a large Swedish clinical population. *Scand. J. Urol. Nephrol.* **2012**, *46*, 212–222. [CrossRef] [PubMed]

29. Schaeffner, E.S.; Ebert, N.; Delanaye, P.; Frei, U.; Gaedeke, J.; Jakob, O.; Kuhlmann, M.K.; Schuchardt, M.; Tölle, M.; Ziebig, R.; et al. Two novel equations to estimate kidney function in persons aged 70 years or older. *Ann. Intern. Med.* **2012**, *157*, 471–481. [CrossRef] [PubMed]

30. Dowling, T.C.; Wang, E.-S.; Ferrucci, L.; Sorkin, J.D. Glomerular filtration rate equations overestimate creatinine clearance in older individuals enrolled in the Baltimore Longitudinal Study on Aging: Impact on renal drug dosing. *Pharmacotherapy* **2013**, *33*, 912–921. [CrossRef] [PubMed]

31. Péquignot, R.; Belmin, J.; Chauvelier, S.; Gaubert, J.-Y.; Konrat, C.; Duron, E.; Hanon, O. Renal function in older hospital patients is more accurately estimated using the Cockcroft-Gault formula than the modification diet in renal disease formula. *J. Am. Geriatr. Soc.* **2009**, *57*, 1638–1643. [CrossRef] [PubMed]

32. Michels, W.M.; Grootendorst, D.C.; Verduijn, M.; Elliott, E.G.; Dekker, F.W.; Krediet, R.T. Performance of the Cockcroft-Gault, MDRD, and New CKD-EPI Formulas in Relation to GFR, Age, and Body Size. *Clin. J. Am. Soc. Nephrol.* **2010**, *5*, 1003–1009. [CrossRef] [PubMed]

33. Pottel, H.; Hoste, L.; Dubourg, L.; Ebert, N.; Schaeffner, E.; Eriksen, B.O.; Melsom, T.; Lamb, E.J.; Rule, A.D.; Turner, S.T.; et al. An estimated glomerular filtration rate equation for the full age spectrum. *Nephrol. Dial. Transplant.* **2016**, *31*, 798–806. [CrossRef] [PubMed]

34. Björk, J.; Grubb, A.; Sterner, G.; Nyman, U. Revised equations for estimating glomerular filtration rate based on the Lund-Malmö Study cohort. *Scand. J. Clin. Lab. Investig.* **2011**, *71*, 232–239. [CrossRef] [PubMed]

35. Werner, K.; Pihlsgård, M.; Elmståhl, S.; Legrand, H.; Nyman, U.; Christensson, A. Combining Cystatin C and Creatinine Yields a Reliable Glomerular Filtration Rate Estimation in Older Adults in Contrast to β-Trace Protein and β2-Microglobulin. *Nephron* **2017**, *137*, 29–37. [CrossRef] [PubMed]

36. Björk, J.; Grubb, A.; Gudnason, V.; Indridason, O.S.; Levey, A.S.; Palsson, R.; Nyman, U. Comparison of glomerular filtration rate estimating equations derived from creatinine and cystatin C: Validation in the Age, Gene/Environment Susceptibility-Reykjavik elderly cohort. *Nephrol. Dial. Transplant.* **2017**, *33*, 1380–1388. [CrossRef] [PubMed]

37. Fan, L. Comparing GFR estimating equations using cystatin C and creatinine in elderly individuals. *J. Am. Soc. Nephrol.* **2015**, *26*, 1982–1989. [CrossRef] [PubMed]

38. Heldal, K.; Midtvedt, K.; Hartmann, A.; Reisæter, A.V.; Heldal, T.F.; Bergan, S.; Salvador, C.L.; Åsberg, A. Estimated glomerular filtration rate in stable older kidney transplant recipients—Are present algorithms valid? A national cross-sectional cohort study. *Transplant Int.* **2018**, *31*, 629–638. [CrossRef] [PubMed]

39. Raman, M.; Middleton, R.J.; Kalra, P.A.; Green, D. Estimating renal function in old people: An in-depth review. *Int. Urol. Nephrol.* **2017**, *49*, 1979–1988. [CrossRef] [PubMed]

40. Oscanoa, T.J.; Amado, J.P.; Romero-Ortuno, R.; Hidalgo, J.A. Estimation of the glomerular filtration rate in older individuals with serum creatinine-based equations: A systematic comparison between CKD-EPI and BIS1. *Arch. Gerontol. Geriatr.* **2018**, *75*, 139–145. [CrossRef] [PubMed]

41. Inker, L.A.; Levey, A.S.; Coresh, J. Estimated Glomerular Filtration Rate From a Panel of Filtration Markers-Hope for Increased Accuracy Beyond Measured Glomerular Filtration Rate? *Adv. Chronic Kidney Dis.* **2018**, *25*, 67–75. [CrossRef] [PubMed]

42. Hornum, M.; Feldt-Rasmussen, B. Drug Dosing and Estimated Renal Function—Any Step Forward from Effersoe? *Nephron* **2017**, *136*, 268–272. [CrossRef] [PubMed]

43. Segarra, A.; de la Torre, J.; Ramos, N.; Quiroz, A.; Garjau, M.; Torres, I.; Azancot, M.A.; López, M.; Sobrado, A. Assessing glomerular filtration rate in hospitalized patients: A comparison between CKD-EPI and four cystatin C-based equations. *Clin. J. Am. Soc. Nephrol.* **2011**, *6*, 2411–2420. [CrossRef] [PubMed]

44. Helldén, A.; Bergman, U.; von Euler, M.; Hentschke, M.; Odar-Cederlöf, I.; Ohlén, G. Adverse drug reactions and impaired renal function in elderly patients admitted to the emergency department: A retrospective study. *Drugs Aging* **2009**, *26*, 595–606. [CrossRef] [PubMed]

45. Gheewala, P.A.; Peterson, G.M.; Curtain, C.M.; Nishtala, P.S.; Hannan, P.J.; Castelino, R.L. Impact of the pharmacist medication review services on drug-related problems and potentially inappropriate prescribing of renally cleared medications in residents of aged care facilities. *Drugs Aging* **2014**, *31*, 825–835. [CrossRef] [PubMed]

46. Sönnerstam, E.; Sjölander, M.; Gustafsson, M. Inappropriate Prescription and Renal Function Among Older Patients with Cognitive Impairment. *Drugs Aging* **2016**, *33*, 889–899. [CrossRef] [PubMed]

47. Nielsen, A.L.; Henriksen, D.P.; Marinakis, C.; Hellebek, A.; Birn, H.; Nybo, M.; Søndergaard, J.; Nymark, A.; Pedersen, C. Drug dosing in patients with renal insufficiency in a hospital setting using electronic prescribing and automated reporting of estimated glomerular filtration rate. *Basic Clin. Pharmacol. Toxicol.* **2014**, *114*, 407–413. [CrossRef] [PubMed]

48. MacCallum, P.K.; Mathur, R.; Hull, S.A.; Saja, K.; Green, L.; Morris, J.K.; Ashman, N. Patient safety and estimation of renal function in patients prescribed new oral anticoagulants for stroke prevention in atrial fibrillation: A cross-sectional study. *BMJ Open* **2013**, *3*, e003343. [CrossRef] [PubMed]

49. Helldén, A.; Odar-Cederlöf, I.; Nilsson, G.; Sjöviker, S.; Söderström, A.; von Euler, M.; Öhlén, G.; Bergman, U. Renal function estimations and dose recommendations for dabigatran, gabapentin and valaciclovir: A data simulation study focused on the elderly. *BMJ Open* **2013**, *3*, e002686. [CrossRef] [PubMed]

50. Andrade, J.G.; Hawkins, N.M.; Fordyce, C.B.; Deyell, M.W.; Er, L.; Djurdjev, O.; Macle, L.; Virani, S.A.; Levin, A. Variability in Non-Vitamin K Antagonist Oral Anticoagulants Dose Adjustment in Atrial Fibrillation Patients With Renal Dysfunction: The Influence of Renal Function Estimation Formulae. *Can. J. Cardiol.* **2018**, *34*, 1010–1018. [CrossRef] [PubMed]

51. Andreassen, T.N.; Klepstad, P.; Davies, A.; Bjordal, K.; Lundström, S.; Kaasa, S.; Dale, O. Influences on the pharmacokinetics of oxycodone: A multicentre cross-sectional study in 439 adult cancer patients. *Eur. J. Clin. Pharmacol.* **2011**, *67*, 493–506. [CrossRef] [PubMed]

52. Pöyhiä, R.; Seppälä, T.; Olkkola, K.T.; Kalso, E. The pharmacokinetics and metabolism of oxycodone after intramuscular and oral administration to healthy subjects. *Br. J. Clin. Pharmacol.* **1992**, *33*, 617–621. [CrossRef] [PubMed]

53. Kummer, O.; Hammann, F.; Moser, C.; Schaller, O.; Drewe, J.; Krähenbühl, S. Effect of the inhibition of CYP3A4 or CYP2D6 on the pharmacokinetics and pharmacodynamics of oxycodone. *Eur. J. Clin. Pharmacol.* **2011**, *67*, 63–71. [CrossRef] [PubMed]

54. Smith, H.S. Opioid Metabolism. *Mayo Clin. Proc.* **2009**, *84*, 613–624. [CrossRef]

55. Davis, M.P.; Homsi, J. The importance of cytochrome P450 monooxygenase CYP2D6 in palliative medicine. *Support. Care Cancer* **2001**, *9*, 442–451. [CrossRef] [PubMed]

56. O'Mahony, D.; O'Sullivan, D.; Byrne, S.; O'Connor, M.N.; Ryan, C.; Gallagher, P. STOPP/START criteria for potentially inappropriate prescribing in older people: Version 2. *Age Ageing* **2014**, *44*, 213–218. [CrossRef] [PubMed]

57. US Food and Drug Administration. *Guidance for Industry: Pharmacokinetics in Patients with Impaired Renal Function—Study Design, Data Analysis and Impact on Dosing and Labeling, Revision 1*; US Food and Drug Administration: Silver Spring, MD, USA, 2010. Available online: https://www.fda.gov/downloads/drugs/guidances/ucm204959.pdf (accessed on 12 September 2018).

58. European Medicines Agency. *Guideline on the Evaluation of the Pharmacokinetics of Medicinal Products in Patients with Decreased Renal Function*; European Medicines Agency: London, UK, 2014. Available online: http://www.ema.europa.eu/docs/en_GB/document_library/Scientific_guideline/2016/02/WC500200841.pdf (accessed on 12 September 2018).

59. KDIGO. Clinical Practice Guideline for Acute Kidney Injury. *Int. Soc. Nephrol.* **2012**, *2*, 8.

60. The Danish Council on Ethics Research with Health Data and Biological Material in Denmark Statement. Available online: http://www.etiskraad.dk/~/media/Etisk-Raad/en/Publications/Research-with-health-data-and-biological-material-in-Denmark-Statement-2015.pdf?la=da (accessed on 12 September 2018).

61. Du Bois, D.; Du Bois, E.F. A formula to estimate the approximate surface area if height and weight be known, 1916. *Nutrition* **1989**, *5*, 303–311. [PubMed]

62. Levey, A.S.; Coresh, J.; Balk, E.; Kausz, A.T.; Levin, A.; Steffes, M.W.; Hogg, R.J.; Perrone, R.D.; Lau, J.; Eknoyan, G. National Kidney Foundation National Kidney Foundation practice guidelines for chronic kidney disease: Evaluation, classification, and stratification. *Ann. Intern. Med.* **2003**, *139*, 137–147. [CrossRef] [PubMed]

63. Medbase, Ltd. *Renbase—Drug Dosing in Renal Failure*; Medbase, Ltd.: Turku, Finland, 2018.

64. McHugh, M.L. Interrater reliability: The kappa statistic. *Biochem. Med.* **2012**, *22*, 276–282. [CrossRef]

10

Improved Syntheses of the mGlu5 Antagonists MMPEP and MTEP Using Sonogashira Cross-Coupling

Boshuai Mu [1], **Linjing Mu** [1,2], **Roger Schibli** [1,2], **Simon M. Ametamey** [1] and
Selena Milicevic Sephton [1,2,3,*] (iD)

[1] Center of Radiopharmaceutical Sciences of ETH, PSI and USZ, Department of Chemistry and Applied
    Biosciences, Swiss Federal Institute of Technology, Vladimir-Prelog-Weg 4, 8093 Zurich, Switzerland;
    boshuai_mu@163.com (B.M.); linjing.mu@pharma.ethz.ch (L.M.); roger.schibli@psi.ch (R.S.);
    simon.ametamey@pharma.ethz.ch (S.M.A.)

[2] Department of Nuclear Medicine, University Hospital Zurich, Ramistrasse 101, 8003 Zurich, Switzerland

[3] Molecular Imaging Chemistry Laboratory, Wolfson Brain Imaging Centre, Department of Clinical
    Neurosciences, University of Cambridge, Box 65 Cambridge Biomedical Campus, Cambridge CB2 0QQ, UK

*   Correspondence: sms96@wbic.cam.ac.uk

Abstract: The Sonogashira cross-coupling, a key step in the syntheses of the mGlu5 antagonists
MMPEP and MTEP, provided an improved three-step method for the preparation of MMPEP in
62% overall yield. Using Spartan molecular modeling kit an explanation for the failure to employ
analogues method in the synthesis of MTEP was sought. The DFT calculations indicated that
meaningful isolated yields were obtained when the HOMO energy of the aryl halide was lower than
the HOMO energy of the respective alkyne.

Keywords: Sonogashira cross-coupling; MMPEP; MTEP; mGlu5 antagonist

---

1. Introduction

   Metabotropic glutamate receptor subtype 5 (mGlu5) [1–3] is a 7-member transmembrane
G-protein coupled receptor, which based on its pharmacology belongs to the group I of
metabotropic receptors and regulates glutamate, a major neurotransmitter in the mammalian
brain. Consequently, mGlu5 is associated with numerous central nervous system (CNS) disorders
such as Parkinson's [1,4] and Alzheimer's [5,6] disease. For this reason mGlu5 has been studied
extensively as a potential therapeutic target [7], resulting in the identification of 2-methyl-
6-(phenylethynyl)pyridine (MPEP, **1**, Figure 1) [8,9] as a potent mGlu5 antagonist which presented
the basis for further Structure Activity Relationship (SAR) studies. Additionally, significant
efforts have been made in establishing positron emission tomography (PET) [10] radiotracers for
non-invasive imaging of mGlu5 [11] with the aim of further assisting drug development and
also as a potential diagnostic tools of CNS impairments. As a part of the on-going program
on the development of fluorine-18 labelled mGlu5 radiotracer based on the structural scaffold of
(E)-3-[(6-methylpyridin-2-yl)ethynyl]cyclohex-2-enone O-[^{11}C]methyl oxime ([^{11}C]-ABP688) [12,13]
we recently required the two mGlu5 antagonists 2-((3-methoxy-phenyl)ethynyl)-6-methylpyridine
(MMPEP, **2**) [14] and 2-methyl-4-(pyridine-3-ylethynyl)thiazole (MTEP, **3**, Figure 1) [15–17]. The key
transformation in the syntheses of both mGlu5 antagonists was a Sonogashira cross-coupling [18].

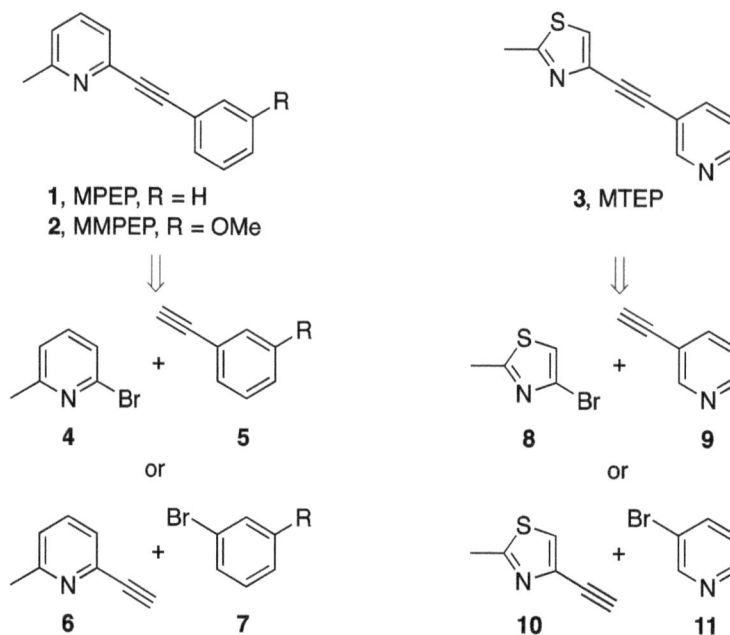

Figure 1. Structures of MPEP (**1**), MMPEP (**2**) and MTEP (**3**) and their assembly via the Sonogashira cross-coupling.

The Sonogashira cross-coupling reaction has been used for other analogous molecules [19,20] and is characterized by the ease of synthetic manipulation required to perform the reaction, generally mild reaction conditions, including ambient temperature and relatively short reaction times, and the versatility of substrates amenable to these conditions [21]. Extensive studies on the mechanism of the Sonogashira cross-coupling allowed for postulations about the effect of electronegativity of coupling partners, where electron-donating substituents on the aryl or alkyl halide lead to a higher activation barrier and electron-withdrawing substituents on the aryl or alkyl halide lower the barrier [22]. It was hypothesized that turnover-determining step in which aryl halides participate is preceded by the end-on ligation of the halogen atom to palladium making it therefore an electron-donating step [21]. Thus, electron-donating groups with higher HOMO energy of the substrate form more stable complexes and as a consequence have higher rate determining activation barrier. On the other hand, electron-withdrawing groups with low HOMO energy, hence lower the activation barrier and facilitate oxidative insertion. Herein we report our findings about the application of the Sonogashira coupling in the syntheses of two mGlu$_5$ antagonists resulting in a shorter synthetic route to MMPEP than that previously described. Rationale for the reactivity of Sonogashira partners was found through HOMO energy calculations using Density Functional Theory (DFT).

2. Results and Discussion

The previously reported synthesis of MMPEP involved a four step route starting with commercially available bromide **4** (Scheme 1) and giving 31% overall yield [14]. In the first step, **4** was converted to alkyne **12** employing Sonogashira cross-coupling, and the trimethylsilyl functionality was then removed under basic conditions (compound **6**) and the trimethyltin group introduced onto the terminal alkyne in **13**, and **13** then reacted with aryl bromide **7A** under Stille cross-coupling reaction conditions to afford MMPEP (**2**). Due to the total number of transformations as well as the toxicity of tin, an alternative direct route to access **2** was sought. Use of the same bromide **7A** with either TMS alkyne **12** in the presence of TBAF·THF for in situ deprotection, or the deprotected equivalent **6**, formed in one step from 2-bromopyridine (see Supplementary Materials), failed to furnish MMPEP (Scheme 1). The latter had precedent in the synthesis of ABP688 [23]. In this case, 3-bromocyclohex-2-enone was coupled with **6** in 60% yield but the reaction mixture required heating to 55 °C (not shown).

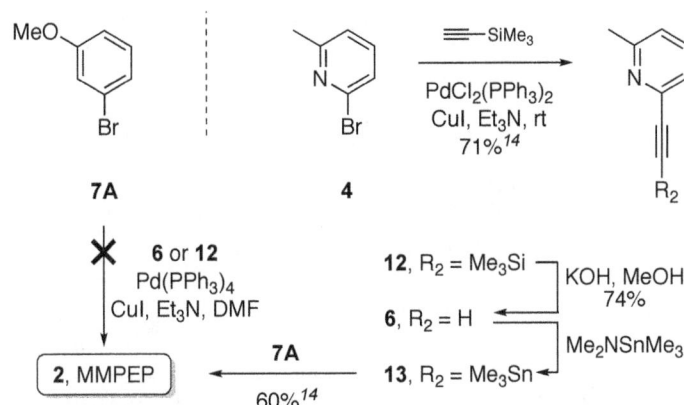

Scheme 1. 1-Bromo-3-methoxybenezene (**7A**) as reacting partner in Sonogashira coupling to access MMPEP (**2**).

The failure to form the desired cross-coupling product between bromide **7A** and alkynes **12** or **6** prompted us to further explore an alternative synthetic route towards **2** (Scheme 2). For this, alkyne **5A** was obtained from 3-methoxyanisole (**14**) in two steps employing classical Corey-Fuchs reaction in 66% overall yield [15]. When alkyne **5A** was reacted directly with 2-bromo-6-methylpyridine (**4**) under Sonogashira cross-coupling conditions at ambient temperature, MMPEP (**2**) was isolated in 93% yield (Scheme 2). This demonstrated that Stille coupling was not required and that **2** can be prepared in excellent yield of 62% over only three reaction steps and on 1 g scale.

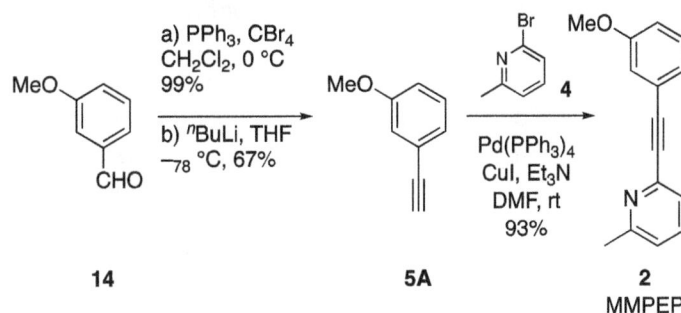

Scheme 2. Improved three step synthesis of MMPEP (**2**) with 1-ethynyl-3-methoxybenzene (**5A**).

We next sought to explore an analogous synthetic strategy for the construction of MTEP (**3**). Our recent report on the synthesis and properties of novel ABP688 derivative (**16**, ThioABP) [24] established the successful application of Sonogashira cross-coupling between 4-bromo-2-methylthiazole (**8**) and alkyne **15** at ambient temperature in moderate 40% yield (Figure 2). The same bromide **8** in reaction with 3-ethynylpyridine (**9**), however, afforded desired product in only 8% conversion, based on the NMR analysis of isolated mixtures (Figure 2, entry 1). Analogue **3** could not be separated from the major product of the reaction, which was presumed to be result of self-coupling of alkyne **9** but remained uncharacterized. When reaction was repeated under the same conditions, it failed to yield any of the desired **3**, thus proving to be non-reproducible and an inefficient way to obtain **3**. At elevated temperature, reaction of bromide **8** with akyne **9** also failed to yield desired **3** (Figure 2, entry 2). Furthermore, the reaction was unsuccessful with silylated alkyne **17**, which was desilylated with TBAF·THF in situ (Figure 2, entry 3) therefore excluding the possibility of effects of presence of TBAF·THF in the reaction mixture on reactivity of coupling partners. The possibility of TBAF·THF effect on the success of Sonogashira cross-coupling was founded based on our previously published observations whereby in situ desilylated α-fluoroalkynes using TBAF·THF were successfully coupled to bromopyridines under analogous reaction conditions (see Figure 3, alkyne **22**) [25].

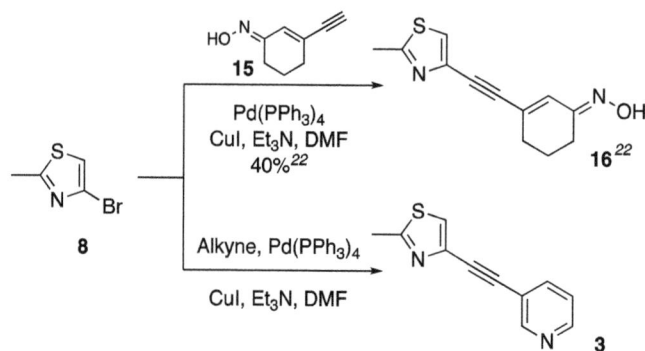

Figure 2. 4-Bromo-2-methylthiazole (**8**) as a reacting partner in Sonogashira coupling *en route* to MTEP (**3**).

Our findings suggested that both reacting partners play a significant role in the cross-coupling and are determinants in the reaction success, which lead us to conduct a comparison with the previously reported synthesis of **3**.

The literature report of the synthesis of MTEP (**3**) is analogous to the one depicted in Scheme 3. Silylated alkyne **20** was prepared in two steps starting from commercially available acid chloride **18** with 76% overall yield. The Sonogashira cross-coupling between **20** and **11** was performed at 60 °C, in the presence of TBAF·THF which was added via syringe pump over several hours [15]. In our hands, this protocol afforded 52% of **3** (entry 1).

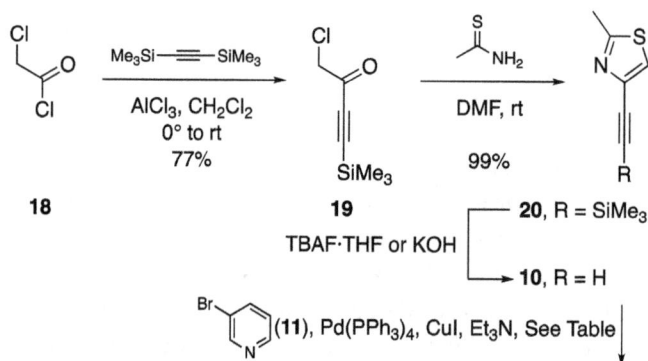

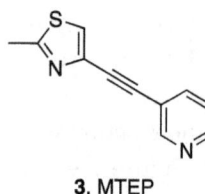

Scheme 3. Synthesis of MTEP (**3**) at elevated reaction temperature with 4-alkynyl-2-methylthiazoles (**10** or **20**) as coupling partners.

Our synthesis thus compared favourably to the one previously published with 39% overall yield vs. 25% reported over the same number of steps. Using the same reacting partners the reaction was then performed at ambient temperature and TBAF·THF was added in one portion (entry 2, an approach previously applied successfully for the series of α-fluorinated oximes with pyridinyl bromides) [25] but this failed to give the desired coupling product in a meaningful amounts. Alkyne **20** was then desilylated to give **10** prior to its addition to the reaction mixture and attempted Sonogashira cross-coupling at ambient temperature gave only trace amounts of desired product (entry 3). To further confirm effects TBAF·THF may have **10** was prepared either as neat material when desilylation was perfomed with KOH as a base, or as a crude mixture containing TBAF·THF when desilylation was done using TBAF solution. Interestingly, either attempt afforded only trace (<1%) amounts of desired product (see Supplementary Materials). With these results in hand we aimed to assess possible reason for different reactivity of the same bromide (e.g., reaction of **8** with **15** and **9** or **17**). Considering the electronegativity of the halides as an important factor [21,22] an explanation was sought through calculation of the respective HOMO energies.

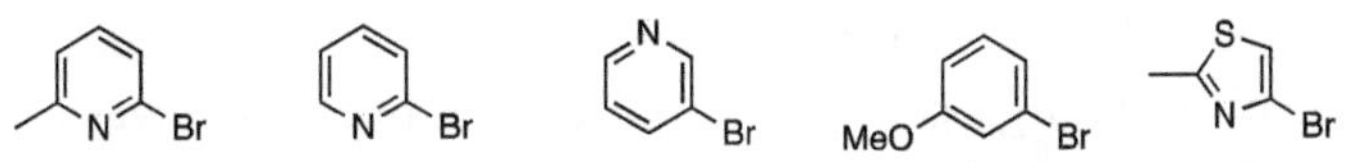

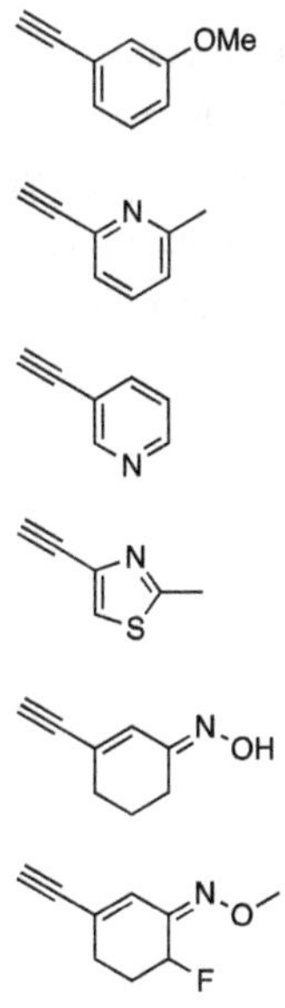

		4 ΔE_{HOMO} / Yield (%)	**21** ΔE_{HOMO} / Yield (%)	**11** ΔE_{HOMO} / Yield (%)	**7A** ΔE_{HOMO} / Yield (%)	**8** ΔE_{HOMO} / Yield (%)
	5A	−0.64 / 93	−0.85 / —	−0.87 / —	−0.13 / —	−0.34 / —
	6	−0.20 / —	−0.41 / —	−0.43 / —	0.31 / 0	0.10 / —
	9	0.01 / —	−0.20 / —	−0.22 / —	0.52 / —	0.31 / 0-8 [a]
	10	−0.48 / —	−0.69 / —	−0.71 / 1 (52) [b]	0.03 / —	−0.18 / —
	15	−0.65 / 70 [30]	−0.86 / 85 [30]	−0.88 / —	−0.14 / —	−0.35 / 41 [24]
	22	−0.57 / 68 [25]	−0.78 / 63 [25]	−0.80 / —	−0.06 / —	−0.27 / —

[a] Conversion of 8% obtained in one instance only.
[b] Reaction of neat **10** afforded 1% (at 23 °C in DMF), while *in situ* formed **10** yielded 52% (at 60 °C in DME)

Figure 3. Difference in values of HOMO energies of reacting partners (ΔE_{HOMO}) calculated using DFT method compared to experimental yields. Note: "—" indicates that reaction was not performed experimentally.

Equilibrium as well as HOMO and LUMO energies were calculated using the DFT method within the Spartan Molecular Modeling kit (the values are provided in the Supplementary Materials). The DFT method as well as the basis set used has previously been applied successfully for other computational studies on the mechanism of Sonogashira coupling [22]. The HOMO energies were calculated for both reacting partners, the halide and the alkyne. As discussed in the Introduction, it has been reported that the lower the HOMO energy of the halide, the more facile oxidative insertion of the palladium into the aryl-halide bond (i.e., more facile interaction between HOMO of the halide and the respective a1 acceptor orbital on the metal). However, our experimental data showed different reactivity of the same aryl halides, thus suggesting that HOMO energy of the aryl halide is not the only determinant of the reaction success. For this reason, HOMO energies of halides and reacting alkynes were compared with respect to the experimentally obtained yields and the difference in HOMO values between the two (ΔE_{HOMO} = E_{HOMO} (halide) − E_{HOMO} (alkyne)) is provided in Figure 3. It was found that product formation was not guaranteed if halide reacted with the alkyne which HOMO energies were of the same value or higher. Meaningful yields of desired products up to 93% were obtained when the HOMO energy of halide was lower than the HOMO energy of the reacting alkyne. In mechanistic terms, oxidative insertion of palladium to halide will proceed at the same rate for halides of equal HOMO energies, and the reaction outcome is further determined by the co-ordination of alkyne to copper(I). While the oxidative insertion of palladium (i.e., first catalytic cycle) is studied and well understood, the subsequent catalytic cycle (i.e., transmetalation) is poorly known and some studies [21] show the possibility of tandem palladium/cooper catalysis. Considering the possibility that both metals can react, and to facilitate oxidative addition, our findings suggest that the product formation is dependent on the HOMO energy of both coupling partners. Although only a subset of reacting possibilities for given halides and alkynes of interest was explored experimentally, in those cases the isolated yields were in agreement with the computationally based hypothesis. Furthermore, results in Figure 3 indicate that cyclic aliphatic alkynes outperform heterocyclic alkynes in terms of reactivity in Sonogashira coupling reactions thus showcasing importance of electronic nature of alkyne coupling partners.

Furthermore, for the explored halides and alkynes HOMOs were different not only in terms of their respective energies, but their nature too. For example for alkynes **5A**, **6** and **9** HOMOs were centered on the aromatic ring unlike **10** in which HOMO was centered on the alkyne. While HOMO of oxime **15** was distributed across the conjugated system of alkyne, cyclic alkene and *N*-oxime (see Supplementary Materials), oxime **22** had HOMO centered on the *N*-oxime functionality only (Figure 4).

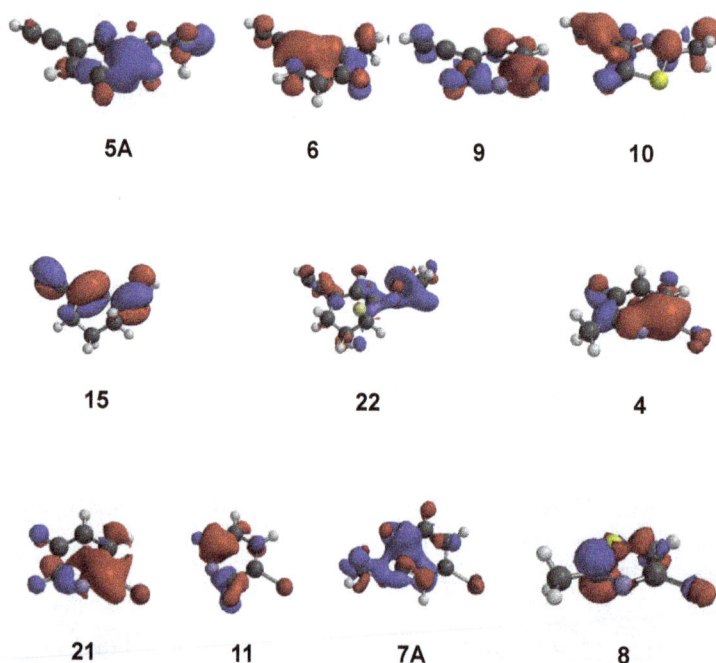

Figure 4. HOMO diagrams for all computationally investigated molecules (alkynes and halides) calculated using DFT method within the Spartan Molecular Modeling kit.

Similarly, for two of the bromides (**4** and **21**) HOMO was centered on the carbon bearing bromide, whereas HOMO was centered in the position *para* to the bromide-bearing carbon for bromides **11**, **7A** and **8**, thus suggesting that the nature of HOMO varied significantly amongst the investigated alkynes/halides. For this reason, HOMO energy alone may not be sufficient indicator of the complex nature of reactive species in the Sonogashira cross-coupling reaction; however our computational findings have allowed explanation for the experimental results observed in the syntheses of MMPEP and MTEP.

3. Materials and Methods

3.1. General Techniques

All reactions requiring anhydrous conditions were conducted in flame-dried glass apparatus under an atmosphere of inert gas. All chemicals and anhydrous solvents were purchased from Aldrich (St. Gallen, Switzerland) or ABCR (Karlsruhe, Germany) and used as received, unless otherwise noted. Reported density values are for ambient temperature. Preparative chromatographic separations were performed on Aldrich Science silica gel 60 (35–75 μm) and reactions followed by TLC analysis using Sigma-Aldrich (St. Gallen, Switzerland) silica gel 60 plates (2–25 μm) with fluorescent indicator (254 nm) and visualized with UV or potassium permanganate. ^{1}H- and ^{13}C-NMR spectra were recorded in Fourier transform mode at the field strength specified on Avance FT-NMR spectrometers (Bruker, Faellanden, Switzerland). Spectra were obtained from the specified deuterated solvents in 5 mm diameter tubes. Chemical shift in ppm is quoted relative to residual solvent signals calibrated as follows: **CDCl$_3$** δ_H (CHCl$_3$) = 7.26 ppm, δ_C = 77.2 ppm. Multiplicities in the ^{1}H-NMR spectra are described as: s = singlet, d = doublet, t = triplet, q = quartet, quint. = quintet, m = multiplet, b = broad; coupling constants are reported in Hz.

3.2. Syntheses

1-Ethynyl-3-methoxybenzene (**5A**). A one-necked round bottom flask was charged with triphenylphosphine (10.5 g, 40 mmol, 4 eq.), then carbon tetrabromide (6.63 g, 20 mmol, 2 eq.) and the yellow solid mixture was carefully dissolved in anhydrous dichloromethane (36 mL; CAUTION: vigorous reaction!) and the resulting orange mixture was allowed to cool to 0 °C (the ice bath). The heterogeneous and red in colour mixture was allowed to stir and then treated with *m*-anisaldehyde (1.2 mL, 1.36 g, 10 mmol, 1 eq., d = 1.119) dropwise over 1 min and the resulting dark orange mixture was allowed to stir at 0 °C for 30 min and then the cooling bath was removed and stirring continued at ambient temperature for 38 min. After this time the crude mixture was quenched with ice cold H$_2$O (40 mL) and diluted with hexanes (25 mL) and the two layers were well shaken and separated. The aqueous phase was extracted with hexanes (5 × 25 mL). The combined organic extracts were concentrated in vacuo and the crude mixture was purified by chromatography on a silica gel column (eluting with 100% hexanes) to afford 1-(2,2-dibromovinyl)-3-methoxybenzene (2.88 g, 9.9 mmol, 99%): ^{1}H-NMR (400 MHz, CDCl$_3$) δ 7.46 (bs, 1H), 7.29 (t, *J* = 8.0 Hz, 1H), 7.12 (tm, *J* = 1.9 Hz, 1H), 7.09 (ddt, *J* = 7.7, 1.4, 0.8 Hz, 1H), 6.89 (ddd, *J* = 8.3, 2.6, 0.8 Hz, 1H), 3.82 (s, 3H) ppm. The compound was in complete agreement with previously reported data [26,27].

A one-necked round bottom flask was charged with a solution of 1-(2,2-dibromovinyl)-3-methoxybenzene (2.88 g, 9.9 mmol, 1 eq.) in anhydrous tetrahydrofuran (30 mL) and the resulting pale yellow solution was allowed to cool to −78 °C (dry ice/acetone bath) and the mixture was then treated with *n*-butyllithium (15 mL, 21.9 mmol, 2.2 eq., c = 1.47 M) dropwise over 13 min during which time mixture turned brighter yellow, red and finally purple. The mixture was allowed to further stir at −78 °C over 1.5 h. After this time the cooling bath was removed and mixture allowed to stir at ambient temperature for 1.8 h. After this time brown homogeneous mixture was quenched with saturated aq. NH$_4$Cl (20 mL) and the mixture was further diluted with H$_2$O (20 mL) and Et$_2$O (50 mL) and the two layers were well shaken and separated. The aqueous phase was extracted with Et$_2$O (2 × 50 mL).

The combined organic extracts were washed with brine (40 mL), dried (Na_2SO_4) and concentrated in vacuo to give dark yellow oily residue. The residue was purified by chromatography on a silica gel column (eluting with 100% hexanes) to afford the title compound (884 mg, 6.7 mmol, 67%): ^{1}H-NMR (400 MHz, $CDCl_3$) δ 7.23 (ddm, J = 7.5 Hz, 1H), 7.09 (ddd, J = 7.6, 1.2 Hz, 1H), 7.02 (dd, J = 2.6, 1.4 Hz, 1H), 6.91 (ddd, J = 8.3, 2.6, 1.0 Hz, 1H), 3.80 (s, 3H), 3.06 (s, 1H) ppm. The compound was in complete agreement with previously reported data [26,28].

2-((3-Methoxyphenyl)ethynyl)-6-methylpyridine (**2**). A two-necked round bottom flask was evacuated, backfilled with an inert atmosphere and then charged with anhydrous *N,N′*-dimethylformamide (7 mL) and 2-bromo-6-methylpyridine (0.66 mL, 998 mg, 5.8 mmol, 1 eq., d = 1.512) was added and colourless solution was treated with tetrakis(triphenylphosphine)palladium(0) (201 mg, 0.174 mmol, 0.3 eq.) in one portion and the resulting yellow heterogeneous mixture was allowed to stir at ambient temperature over 13 min. After this time triethylamine (2.42 mL, 1.76 g, 17.4 mmol, 3 eq., d = 0.726) was added and mixture further allowed to stir for 14 min. During this time mixture became completely homogeneous and pale yellow and it was further treated with copper(I)iodide (110 mg, 0.58 mmol, 0.1 eq.) and then a solution of *m*-ethynylanisole (766 mg, 5.80 mmol, 1 eq.) in anhydrous *N,N′*-dimethylformamide (7 mL) was added and the resulting green-brown mixture was allowed to stir at ambient temperature over 47.5 h. After this time the mixture was quenched with saturated aq NH_4Cl (100 mL) and then diluted with EtOAc (150 mL) and the two layers were well shaken and separated. The aqueous phase was extracted with EtOAc (2 × 150 mL). The combined organic extracts were washed with H_2O (3 × 110 mL), brine (120 mL), dried (Na_2SO_4) and concentrated in vacuo. The crude reaction mixture was purified by chromatography on a silica gel column (eluting with a gradient 10% to 20% EtOAc/pentane) to afford the title compound (1.2 g, 5.4 mmol, 93%): ^{1}H-NMR (400 MHz, $CDCl_3$) δ 7.57 (dd, J = 7.7 Hz, 1H), 7.36 (dm, J = 7.6 Hz, 1H), 7.26 (dd, J = 7.3 Hz, 1H), 7.20 (ddd, J = 7.6, 1.3 Hz, 1H, some roofing observed), 7.14 (dd, J = 2.6, 1.4 Hz, 1H), 7.11 (dm, J = 7.8 Hz, 1H), 6.92 (ddd, J = 8.1, 2.6, 1.1 Hz, 1H), 3.82 (s, 3H), 2.59 (s, 3H) ppm. The compound was in complete agreement with previously published data [14].

2-((3-Methoxyphenyl)ethynyl)-6-methylpyridine hydrochloride salt (**2·HCl**). A one-necked round bottom flask was charged with 2-((3-methoxyphenyl)ethynyl)-6-methylpyridine (108 mg, 0.48 mmol, 1 eq.) and ethanol (1 mL) was added and pale yellow solution was allowed to cool to 0 °C (the ice bath) and it was then treated with ethanolic solution of HCl dopwise over 1 min and the resulting bright yellow solution was allowed to stir at 0 °C for 1 h. After this time the cooling bath was removed and bright yellow mixture was concentrated in vacuo to give crude mixture which was further recrystallized from ^{i}PrOH:EtOH 2:1 to afford the title compound (110 mg, 0.42 mmol, 87%): ^{1}H-NMR (400 MHz, $CDCl_3$) δ 8.12 (dd, J = 7.9 Hz, 1H), 7.66 (dm, J = 7.85 Hz, 1H), 7.49–7.45 (m, 2H), 7.43 (ddd, J = 7.5, 1.1 Hz, 1H, some roofing observed), 7.31 (ddm, J = 8.2 Hz, 1H), 7.02 (ddd, J = 8.4, 2.6, 1.0 Hz, 1H), 3.87 (s, 3H), 3.05 (s, 3H) ppm. The compound was in complete agreement with previously published data [14].

4-Bromo-2-methylthiazole (**8**). A flame dried flask was charged with 2,4-dibromothiazole (500 mg, 2.1 mmol, 1 eq.) and anhydrous diethyl ether was added (12 mL) and the colourless solution was allowed to cool to −78 °C (dry ice/acetone bath) and it was then treated with *n*-butyl lithium (1.6 mL, 2.3 mmol, 1.1 eq., c = 1.47 M) dropwise over 1 min. The mixture turned pale yellow and it was allowed to stir at −78 °C over 79 min. After this time the mixture a solution of dimethyl sulfate (0.6 mL, 779 mg, 6.2 mmol, 3 eq., d = 1.33) in anhydrous diethyl ether (0.5 mL) was added dropwise over 4 min and the resulting mixture allowed to stir at −78 °C over 4 h and then warm to ambient temperature and stir under N_2 over 15 h. After this time the crude mixture (red in colour) was quenched with saturated $NaHCO_3$ (5 mL) and then diluted with H_2O (8 mL) and EtOAc (20 mL). The two layers were well shaken and separated and the aqueous phase was extracted with EtOAc (2 × 20 mL). The combined organic extracts were washed brine (20 mL), dried (Na_2SO_4) and concentrated in vacuo to give crude mixture. The crude mixture was purified by chromatography on a silica gel column (eluting with 10% EtOAc/pentane) to give the title compound (194.3 mg, 1.09 mmol, 53%): ^{1}H NMR (400 MHz, $CDCl_3$) δ

7.06 (s, 1H), 2.73 (s, 3H) ppm. The compound was in complete agreement with previously published data [29].

3-((Trimethylsilyl)ethynyl)pyridine (**17**).   A one-necked round bottom flask was charged with 3-ethynyl-pyridine (150 mg, 1.46 mmol, 1 eq.), anhydrous tetrahydrofuran (4.8 mL) was added and pale brown solution was allowed to cool to −78 °C (dry ice/acetone bath) and it was then treated with a solution of lithium hexamethyldisilazide (2 mL, 1.9 mmol, 1.3 eq., c = 1 M) dropwise over 2 min during which time the mixture turned orange and it was allowed to stir at −78 °C for 1 h. After this time orange mixture was treated with trimethylchlorosilane (0.27 mL, 238 mg, 2.19 mmol, 1.5 eq., d = 0.856) and the mixture was allowed to slowly warm to ambient temperature and further stir over 17.5 h. After this time the crude mixture was quenched with H_2O (10 mL) and then diluted with Et_2O (10 mL) and the two layers were well shaken and separated. The aqueous phase was further extracted with Et_2O (2 × 10 mL). The combined organic extracts were washed with brine (10 mL), dried (Na_2SO_4) and concentrated in vacuo. The crude mixture was purified by chromatography on a silica gel column (eluting with 5% EtOAc/pentane) to afford the title compound (56.1 mg, 0.32 mmol, 22%): ^{1}H-NMR (400 MHz, CDCl$_3$) δ 8.69 (dd, J = 2.0, 0.7 Hz, 1H), 8.52 (dd, J = 4.9, 1.7 Hz, 1H), 7.74 (ddd, J = 7.8, 1.9 Hz, 1H), 7.23 (ddd, J = 7.9, 4.9, 0.9 Hz, 1H), 0.26 (s, 9H) ppm. The compound was also available from commercial sources and the spectral data were in complete agreement.

1-Chloro-4-(trimethylsilyl)but-3-yn-2-one (**19**).   A one-necked round bottom flask was charged with aluminium trichloride (5.5 g, 42 mmol, 1.3 eq.) and anhydrous dichloromethane (63 mL) was added and the resulting yellow suspension was allowed to cool to 0 °C (the ice bath). The mixture was then treated with a solution of chloroacetyl chloride (2.6 mL, 3.65 g, 32.3 mmol, 1 eq., d = 1.417) and bis(trimethylsilyl)acetylene (6.6 mL, 5 g, 29.34 mmol, 0.9 eq., d = 0.752) in anhydrous dichloromethane (38 mL) dropwise over 50 min during which time mixture turned darker yellow and finally brown and it was allowed to stir at 0 °C over 1 h. The cooling bath was then removed and the stirring continued at ambient temperature over 65 min. After this time the mixture was allowed to cool to 0 °C (the ice bath) and it was carefully quenched with 1 M aq. HCl (65 mL). The two layers were well shaken and separated. The aqueous phase was further extracted with CH_2Cl_2 (2 × 125 mL). The combined organic extracts were washed with H_2O (125 mL), saturated aq. $NaHCO_3$ (125 mL), brine (125 mL), dried (Na_2SO_4) and concentrated in vacuo to give brown reside. The crude mixture was purified via Kugelrorh distillation (temperature: 75 °C) at 2×10^{-2} kPa to afford the title compound (4.33 g, 24.8 mmol, 77%): ^{1}H-NMR (400 MHz, CDCl$_3$) δ 4.23 (s, 2H), 0.26 (s, 9H) ppm. The compound was in complete agreement with previously published data [15].

2-Methyl-4-((trimethylsilyl)ethynyl)thiazole (**20**).   A one-necked round bottom flask was charged with 1-chloro-4-(trimethylsilyl)-3-butyn-2-one (4.3 g, 24.6 mmol, 1 eq.)   and anhydrous *N,N′*-dimethylformamide (43 mL) was added and the clear yellow solution was treated with thioacetamide (2.4 g, 31.8 mmol, 1.3 eq.) in one portion and the resulting yellow homogeneous mixture was allowed to stir at ambient temperature over 17 h. After this time the crude mixture was diluted with EtOAc (200 mL) and the organic phase was washed with H_2O (3 × 150 mL), brine (150 mL), dried (Na_2SO_4) and concentrated in vacuo to give brown oily residue. The crude mixture was purified by chromatography on a silica gel column (eluting with gradient 2% to 4% EtOAc/hexanes) to afford the title compound (4.75 g, 24.3 mmol, 99%): ^{1}H-NMR (400 MHz, CDCl$_3$) δ 7.32 (s, 1H), 2.70 (s, 3H), 0.24 (s, 9H) ppm. The compound was in complete agreement with previously published data [15].

4-Ethynyl-2-methylthiazole (**10**).   A one-necked round bottom flask was charged with 2-methyl-4-((trimethylsilyl)ethynyl)thiazole (400 mg, 2.05 mmol, 1 eq.) and methanol (0.5 mL) was added and the red mixture was further treated with a solution of potassium hydroxide (230 mg, 4.1 mmol, 2 eq.) in methanol (4.8 mL) in one portion and the resulting dark brown mixture was allowed to stir over 3.5 h. After this time the mixture was quenched with H_2O (10 mL) and diluted with EtOAc

(10 mL) and the two layers were well shaken and separated. The aqueous phase was extracted with EtOAc (3 × 8 mL). The combined organic extracts were washed with brine (8 mL), dried (Na_2SO_4) and concentrated in vacuo to give crude mixture. The crude mixture was purified by chromatography on a silica gel column (eluting with gradient 5% to 10% EtOAc/pentane) to afford the title compound (172.6 mg, 1.40 mmol, 68%): ^{1}H-NMR (400 MHz, $CDCl_3$) δ 7.37 (s, 1H), 3.09 (s, 1H), 2.71 (s, 3H) ppm. The compound was also available from commercial sources and the spectral data were in complete agreement.

2-Methyl-4-(pyridin-3-ylethynyl)thiazole (**3**). A one-necked round bottom flask was charged with 2-methyl-4-[(trimethylsilyl)ethynyl]-1,3-thiazole (3.84 g, 19.7 mmol, 1 eq.) and 3-bromopyridine (2.1 mL, 3.42 g, 21.6 mmol, 1.1 eq., d = 1.64) was added in one portion and then 1,2-dimethoxyethane (50 mL) was added and the resulting brown heterogeneous mixture was treated with triethylamine (5.5 mL, 3.98 g, 39.4 mmol, 2 eq.) in one portion and the mixture was sparged with N_2 and the flask was allowed to heat (temperature of preheated oil bath: 70 °C). Immediately upon heating tetrakis(triphenylphosphine)palladium (0) (446 mg, 0.39 mmol, 0.02 eq.) was added and sparging continued for another 14 min. After this time sparging was discontinued and the mixture treated with a solution of tetrabutylammonium fluoride (25 mL, 25.4 mmol, 1.3 eq., c = 1 M) in tetrahydrofuran was added via syringe pump (5 mL/h in 20 mL syringe) whilst the mixture was heated over 20 h. The crude mixture was concentrated in vacuo and the residue dissolved in EtOAc (400 mL) and the organic phase washed with H_2O (200 mL). The organic layer was dried (Na_2SO_4) and concentrated in vacuo to give brown oily residue. The crude reaction mixture was purified by chromatography on a silica gel column (eluting with gradient 30% to 50% EtOAc/hexanes) to give the title compound (2.06 g, 10.3 mmol, 52%). The material was then recrystallized from hot EtOAc layered with cold hexanes to afford yellow needles (1.32 g, 6.6 mmol, 33%): ^{1}H-NMR (400 MHz, $CDCl_3$) δ 8.79 (bd, J = 1.3 Hz, 1H), 8.57 (dd, J = 4.8, 1.4 Hz, 1H), 7.83 (ddd, J = 7.9, 1.9 Hz, 1H), 7.43 (s, 1H), 7.29 (ddd, J = 7.8, 4.9, 0.8 Hz, 1H), 2.75 (s, 3H) ppm. The compound was in complete agreement with previously published data [15,17].

2-Methyl-4-(pyridin-3-ylethynyl)thiazole hydrochloride salt (**3·HCl**). A one-necked round bottom flask was charged with 2-methyl-4-(pyridin-3-ylethynyl)thiazole (214 mg, 1.07 mmol, 1 eq.) and ethanolic solution of hydrochloric acid (1.1 mL, 1.07 mmol, 1 eq., c = 1 M) was added but material did not completely dissolve and additional EtOH (1 mL) was added and the resulting heterogeneous mixture allowed to stir at ambient temperature over 30 min. After this time the mixture was concentrated in vacuo and the residue recrystallized from ^{i}PrOH to yield the title compound (168.3 mg, 0.71 mmol, 66%): ^{1}H-NMR (400 MHz, $CDCl_3$) δ 8.87 (bs, 1H), 8.74 (bd, J = 5.4 Hz, 1H), 8.46 (bddd, J = 8.1, 1.6 Hz, 1H), 7.92 (bdd, J = 8.0, 1.6 Hz, 1H), 7.63 (s, 1H), 2.77 (s, 3H) ppm. The compound was also available from commercial sources and the spectral data were in complete agreement.

2-Ethynyl-6-methylpyridine (**6**). A solution of 2-bromo-6-methylpyridine (700 mg, 4.06 mmol, 1 eq.) in triethylamine (degassed, 11.7 mL) was at ambient temperature treated with trimethylsilylacetylene (0.63 mL, 438 mg, 4.47 mmol, 1.1 eq., d = 0.709), copper(I)iodide (76 mg, 0.4 mmol, 0.1 eq.) and *trans*-dichlorobis(triphenylphospine)palladium (280 mg, 0.4 mmol, 0.1 eq.). The resulting solution was allowed to stir at ambient temperature over 17 h. After this time the crude mixture was quenched with H_2O (8 mL) and further extracted with EtOAc (3 × 10 mL). The combined organic extracts were dried (Na_2SO_4) and concentrated in vacuo and the crude mixture was purified by chromatography on a silica gel column (eluting with 5% Et_2O/pentane) to afford 2-methyl-6-((trimethylsilyl)-ethynyl)pyridine (537 mg, 2.84 mmol, 70%): ^{1}H-NMR (400 MHz, $CDCl_3$) δ 7.52 (dd, J = 7.7 Hz, 1H), 7.28 (dm, J = 7.9 Hz, 1H), 7.09 (dm, J = 7.6 Hz, 1H), 2.55 (s, 3H), 0.26 (s, 9H) ppm. The compound was in complete agreement with previously published data [14].

A yellow solution of 2-methyl-6-((trimethylsilyl)ethynyl)pyridine (226 mg, 1.19 mmol, 1 eq.) in methanol (0.3 mL) was treated with the solution of potassium hydroxide (134 mg, 2.39 mmol, 2 eq.) in methanol (2.5 mL) and the resulting colourless solution was allowed to stir at ambient temperature over 2.5 h. After this time the crude mixture was quenched with H_2O (6 mL) and diluted with EtOAc (5 mL) and the two layers were well shaken and separated. The aqueous phase was extracted with EtOAc (3 × 5 mL). The combined organic extracts were washed with brine (3 mL), dried (Na_2SO_4) and concentrated in vacuo. The crude reaction mixture was purified by chromatography on a silica gel column (eluting with gradient 5% to 10% EtOAc/pentane) to afford the title compound (84 mg, 0.72 mmol, 60%): ^{1}H-NMR (400 MHz, $CDCl_3$) δ 7.54 (dd, J = 7.8 Hz, 1H), 7.29 (dm, J = 7.8 Hz, 1H), 7.13 (dm, J = 7.8 Hz, 1H), 3.12 (s, 1H), 2.55 (s, 3H) ppm. The compound was in complete agreement with previously published data [14].

4. Conclusions

In conclusion, employing Sonogashira cross-coupling reaction, two mGlu5 antagonists MMPEP (**2**) and MTEP (**3**) were prepared by an improved synthetic method in 62% and 40% overall yields, respectively. Computationally calculated HOMO energies for the reacting partners suggested that product formation is controlled by both reacting partners, the halide and the alkyne. Our findings revealed that synthetically meaningful yields were achieved when HOMO energy of the halide was lower than that of the alkyne. Furthermore, our results point to possibility of other high-lying molecular orbitals which may be more critical predictors of reactivity. While not all halide-alkyne combinations were attempted, the experimental data of our study support the computationally obtained conclusions, thus furthering our understanding of the requirements for the successful Sonogashira cross-coupling.

Acknowledgments: Bernhard Pfeiffer (Altman group) is acknowledged for technical assistance with the NMR analysis. Mark A. Sephton (ZHAW) is acknowledged for proof-reading the manuscript and useful suggestions. A. Pius Schubiger is acknowledged for many fruitful discussions.

Author Contributions: B.M. performed the experiments, L.M., R.S. and S.M.A. contributed to the design of the study, discussion of the results, and reviewed the manuscript, and S.M.S. performed the experiments and computational study, designed the study and wrote the paper.

Conflicts of Interest: The authors declare no conflict of interest.

References

1. Rouse, S.T.; Marino, M.J.; Bradley, S.R.; Awad, H.; Wittmann, M.; Conn, P.J. Distribution and Roles of Metabotropic Glutamate Receptors in the Basal Ganglia Motor Circuit: Implications for Treatment of Parkinson's Disease and Related Disorders. *Pharmacol. Ther.* **2000**, *88*, 427–435. [CrossRef]

2. Daggett, L.P.; Sacaan, A.I.; Akong, M.; Rao, S.P.; Hess, S.D.; Liaw, C.; Urrutia, A.; Jachec, C.; Ellis, S.B.; Dreessen, J.; et al. Molecular and Functional Characterization of Recombinant Human Metabotropic Glutamate Receptor Subtype 5. *Neuropharmacology* **1995**, *34*, 871–886. [CrossRef]

3. Tanabe, Y.; Masu, M.; Ishii, T.; Shigemoto, R.; Nakanishi, S. A Family of Metabotropic Glutamate Receptors. *Neuron* **1992**, *8*, 169–179. [CrossRef]

4. Ossowska, K.; Konieczny, J.; Wardas, J.; Pietraszek, M.; Kuter, K.; Wolfarth, S.; Pilc, A. An Influence of Ligands of Metabotropic Glutamate Receptor Subtypes on Parkinsonian-like Symptoms and the Striatopallidal Pathway in Rats. *Amino Acids* **2007**, *32*, 179–188. [CrossRef] [PubMed]

5. Bruno, V.; Ksiazek, I.; Battaglia, G.; Lukic, S.; Leonhardt, T.; Sauer, D.; Gasparini, F.; Kuhn, R.; Nicoletti, F.; Flor, P. Selective Blockade of Metabotropic Glutamate Receptor Subtype 5 Is Neuroprotective. *Neuropharmacology* **2000**, *39*, 2223–2230. [CrossRef]

6. Wang, Q.; Walsh, D.M.; Rowan, M.J.; Selkoe, D.J.; Anwyl, R. Block of Long-Term Potentiation by Naturally Secreted and Synthetic Amyloid Beta-Peptide in Hippocampal Slices Is Mediated via Activation of the Kinases c-Jun N-Terminal Kinase, Cyclin-Dependent Kinase 5, and p38 Mitogen-Activated Protein Kinase as Well as metabotropic glutamate receptor type 5. *J. Neurosci.* **2004**, *24*, 3370–3378. [CrossRef] [PubMed]

7.   Ritzén, A.; Mathiesen, J.M.; Thomsen, C. Molecular Pharmacology and Therapeutic Prospects of Metabotropic Glutamate Receptor Allosteric Modulators. *Basic Clin. Pharmacol. Toxicol.* **2005**, *97*, 202–213. [CrossRef] [PubMed]

8.   Gasparini, F.; Lingenhöhl, K.; Stoehr, N.; Flor, P.J.; Heinrich, M.; Vranesic, I.; Biollaz, M.; Allgeier, H.; Heckendorn, R.; Urwyler, S.; et al. 2-Methyl-6-(Phenylethynyl)-Pyridine (MPEP), a Potent, Selective and Systemically Active mGlu5 Receptor Antagonist. *Neuropharmacology* **1999**, *38*, 1493–1503. [CrossRef]

9.   Pilc, A.; Kłodzińska, A.; Brański, P.; Nowak, G.; Pałucha, A.; Szewczyk, B.; Tatarczyńska, E.; Chojnacka-Wójcik, E.; Wierońska, J. Multiple MPEP Administrations Evoke Anxiolytic- and Antidepressant-like Effects in Rats. *Neuropharmacology* **2002**, *43*, 181–187. [CrossRef]

10.   Ametamey, S.M.; Honer, M.; Schubiger, P.A. Molecular Imaging with PET. *Chem. Rev.* **2008**, *108*, 1501–1516. [CrossRef] [PubMed]

11.   Mu, L.; Shubiger, P.A.; Ametamey, S.M. Radioligands for the PET Imaging of Metabotropic Glutamate Receptor Subtype 5 (mGluR5). *Curr. Top. Med. Chem.* **2010**, *10*, 1558–1568. [CrossRef] [PubMed]

12.   Ametamey, S.M.; Kessler, L.J.; Honer, M.; Wyss, M.T.; Buck, A.; Hintermann, S.; Auberson, Y.P.; Gasparini, F.; Schubiger, P.A. Radiosynthesis and Preclinical Evaluation of 11C-ABP688 as a Probe for Imaging the Metabotropic Glutamate Receptor Subtype 5. *J. Nucl. Med.* **2006**, *47*, 698–705. [PubMed]

13.   Ametamey, S.M.; Treyer, V.; Streffer, J.; Wyss, M.T.; Schmidt, M.; Blagoev, M.; Hintermann, S.; Auberson, Y.; Gasparini, F.; Fischer, U.C.; et al. Human PET Studies of Metabotropic Glutamate Receptor Subtype 5 with 11C-ABP688. *J. Nucl. Med.* **2007**, *48*, 247–252. [PubMed]

14.   Alagille, D.; Baldwin, R.M.; Roth, B.L.; Wroblewski, J.T.; Grajkowska, E.; Tamagnan, G.D. Synthesis and Receptor Assay of Aromatic-Ethynyl-Aromatic Derivatives with Potent mGluR5 Antagonist Activity. *Bioorg. Med. Chem.* **2005**, *13*, 197–209. [CrossRef] [PubMed]

15.   Cosford, N.D.P.; Tehrani, L.; Roppe, J.; Schweiger, E.; Smith, N.D.; Anderson, J.; Bristow, L.; Brodkin, J.; Jiang, X.; McDonald, I.; et al. 3-[(2-Methyl-1,3-Thiazol-4-Yl)ethynyl]-Pyridine: A Potent and Highly Selective Metabotropic Glutamate Subtype 5 Receptor Antagonist with Anxiolytic Activity. *J. Med. Chem.* **2003**, *46*, 204–206. [CrossRef] [PubMed]

16.   McIldowie, M.J.; Gandy, M.N.; Skelton, B.W.; Brotchie, J.M.; Koutsantonis, G.A.; Spackman, M.A.; Piggott, M.J. Physical and Crystallographic Characterisation of the mGlu5 Antagonist MTEP and Its Monohydrochloride. *J. Pharm. Sci.* **2010**, *99*, 234–245. [CrossRef] [PubMed]

17.   Iso, Y.; Grajkowska, E.; Wroblewski, J.T.; Davis, J.; Goeders, N.E.; Johnson, K.M.; Sanker, S.; Roth, B.L.; Tueckmantel, W.; Kozikowski, A.P. Synthesis and Structure-Activity Relationships of 3-[(2-Methyl-1,3-Thiazol-4-Yl)ethynyl]pyridine Analogues as Potent, Noncompetitive Metabotropic Glutamate Receptor Subtype 5 Antagonists; Search for Cocaine Medications. *J. Med. Chem.* **2006**, *49*, 1080–1100. [CrossRef] [PubMed]

18.   Sonogashira, K.; Tohda, Y.; Hagihara, N. A Convenient Synthesis of Acetylenes: Catalytic Substitutions of Acetylenic Hydrogen with Bromoalkenes, Iodoarenes and Bromopyridines. *Tetrahedron Lett.* **1975**, *16*, 4467–4470. [CrossRef]

19.   Peixoto, D.; Begouin, A.; Queiroz, M.J.R.P. Synthesis of 2-(Hetero)arylthieno[2,3-b] or [3,2-b]Pyridines from 2,3-Dihalopyridines, (Hetero)arylalkynes, and Na_2S. Further Functionalizations. *Tetrahedron* **2012**, *68*, 7082–7094. [CrossRef]

20.   Khairnar, B.J.; Dey, S.; Jain, V.K.; Bhanage, B.M. Dimethylaminoalkyl Chalcogenolate Palladium(II) Complexes as an Efficient Copper- and Phospine-free Catalyst for Sonogashira Reaction. *Tetrahedron Lett.* **2014**, *55*, 716–719. [CrossRef]

21.   Chinchilla, R.; Nájera, C. Recent Advances in Sonogashira Reactions. *Chem. Soc. Rev.* **2011**, *40*, 5084–5121. [CrossRef] [PubMed]

22.   An der Heiden, M.R.; Plenio, H.; Immel, S.; Burello, E.; Rothenberg, G.; Hoefsloot, H.C.J. Insights into Sonogashira Cross-Coupling by High-Throughput Kinetics and Descriptor Modeling. *Chemistry* **2008**, *14*, 2857–2866. [CrossRef] [PubMed]

23.   Kessler, L.J. Development of Novel Ligands for PET Imaging of the Metabotropic Glutamate Receptor Subtype 5 (mGluR5). Ph.D. Thesis, ETH Zürich, Zürich, Switzerland, 2004. [CrossRef]

24.   Sephton, S.M.; Mu, L.; Müller, A.; Wanger-Baumann, C.A.; Schibli, R.; Krämer, S.D.; Ametamey, S.M. Synthesis and in Vitro/in Vivo Pharmacological Evaluation of [11C]-ThioABP, a Novel Radiotracer for Imaging mGluR5 with PET. *Medchemcomm* **2013**, *4*, 520–526. [CrossRef]

25. Milicevic Sephton, S.; Mu, L.; Schweizer, W.B.; Schibli, R.; Krämer, S.D.; Ametamey, S.M. Synthesis and Evaluation of Novel α-Fluorinated (E)-3-((6-Methylpyridin-2-Yl)ethynyl)cyclohex-2-Enone-O-Methyl Oxime (ABP688) Derivatives as Metabotropic Glutamate Receptor Subtype 5 PET Radiotracers. *J. Med. Chem.* **2012**, *55*, 7154–7162. [CrossRef] [PubMed]

26. Khan, Z.A.; Wirth, T. Synthesis of Indene Derivatives via Electrophilic Cyclization. *Org. Lett.* **2009**, *11*, 229–231. [CrossRef] [PubMed]

27. Ding, Y.; Green, J.R. Benzocycloheptynedicobalt Complexes by Intramolecular Nicholas Reactions. *Synlett* **2005**, *2005*, 271–274. [CrossRef]

28. Ding, C.; Babu, G.; Orita, A.; Hirate, T.; Otera, J. Synthesis and Photoluminescence Studies of Siloles with Arylene Ethynylene Strands. *Synlett* **2007**, *2007*, 2559–2563. [CrossRef]

29. Karama, U.; Höfle, G. Synthesis of Epothilone 16,17-Alkyne Analogs by Replacement of the C13−C15(O)-Ring Segment of Natural Epothilone C. *Eur. J. Org. Chem.* **2003**, *2003*, 1042–1049. [CrossRef]

30. Baumann, C.; Mu, L.; Johannsen, S.; Honer, M.; Schubiger, P.A.; Ametamey, S.M. Structure-Activity Relationships of Fluorinated (*E*)-3-((6-Methylpyridin-2-yl)ethynyl)cyclohex-2-enone-*O*-methyloxime (ABP688(=) Derivatives and the Discovery of a High Affinity Analogue as a Potential Candidate for Imaging Metabotropic Glutamate Receptors Subtype 5 (mGluR5) with Positron Emission Tomography (PET). *J. Med. Chem.* **2010**, *53*, 4009–4017. [CrossRef] [PubMed]

11

Self-Assembled Supramolecular Nanoparticles Improve the Cytotoxic Efficacy of CK2 Inhibitor THN7

Abdelhamid Nacereddine [1,2], Andre Bollacke [2], Eszter Róka [3,4], Christelle Marminon [1] (ID), Zouhair Bouaziz [1] (ID), Ferenc Fenyvesi [3], Ildikó Katalin Bácskay [3], Joachim Jose [2] (ID), Florent Perret [4,*] (ID) and Marc Le Borgne [2,*] (ID)

[1] Faculté de Pharmacie—ISPB, EA 4446 Bioactive Molecules and Medicinal Chemistry, SFR Santé Lyon-Est CNRS UMS3453—INSERM US7, Université de Lyon, Université Claude Bernard Lyon 1, 8 Avenue Rockefeller, F-69373 Lyon CEDEX 8, France; a.nacereddine@gmail.com (A.N.); christelle.marminon-davoust@univ-lyon1.fr (C.M.); zouhair.bouaziz@univ-lyon1.fr (Z.B.)
[2] Institute of Pharmaceutical and Medicinal Chemistry, PharmaCampus, Westfälische Wilhelms-Universität Münster, Corrensstr. 48, 48149 Münster, Germany; andre.bollacke@uni-muenster.de (A.B.); joachim.jose@uni-muenster.de (J.J.)
[3] Department of Pharmaceutical Technology, Faculty of Pharmacy, University of Debrecen, Nagyerdei körút 98, H-4032 Debrecen, Hungary; eszter.roka@gmail.com (E.R.); fenyvesi.ferenc@pharm.unideb.hu (F.F.); bacskay.ildiko@pharm.unideb.hu (I.K.B.)
[4] CSAp, Institut de Chimie et Biochimie Moléculaires et Supramoléculaires, Bâtiment Raulin, Université de Lyon, Université Lyon 1, 43 Bd du 11 novembre 1918, 69622 Villeurbanne CEDEX, France
* Correspondence: florent.perret@univ-lyon1.fr (F.P.); marc.le-borgne@univ-lyon1.fr (M.L.B.)

Abstract: Since the approval of imatinib in 2001, kinase inhibitors have revolutionized cancer therapies. Inside this family of phosphotransferases, casein kinase 2 (CK2) is of great interest and numerous scaffolds have been investigated to design CK2 inhibitors. Recently, functionalized indeno[1,2-b]indoles have been revealed to have high potency against human cancer cell lines such as MCF-7 breast carcinoma and A-427 lung carcinoma. 4-Methoxy-5-isopropyl-5,6,7,8-tetrahydroindeno[1,2-b]indole-9,10-dione (THN7), identified as a potent inhibitor of CK2 (IC_{50} = 71 nM), was selected for an encapsulation study in order to evaluate its antiproliferative activity as THN7-loaded cyclodextrin nanoparticles. Four α-cyclodextrins (α-CDs) were selected to encapsulate THN7 and all experiments indicated that the nanoencapsulation of this CK2 inhibitor in α-CDs was successful. No additional surface-active agent was used during the nanoformulation process. Nanoparticles formed between THN7 and α-C_6H_{13} amphiphilic derivative gave the best results in terms of encapsulation rate (% of associated drug = 35%), with a stability constant (K_{11}) of 298 mol·L^{-1} and a size of 132 nm. Hemolytic activity of the four α-CDs was determined before the in cellulo evaluation and the α-C_6H_{13} derivative gave the lowest value of hemolytic potency (HC_{50} = 1.93 mol·L^{-1}). Only the THN7-loaded cyclodextrin nanoparticles showing less toxicity on human erythrocytes (α-C_6H_{13}, α-C_8H_{17} and α-C_4H_9) were tested against A-427 cells. All drug-loaded nanoparticles caused more cytotoxicity against A-427 cells than THN7 alone. Based on these results, the use of amphiphilic CD nanoparticles could be considered as a drug delivery system for indeno[1,2-b]indoles, allowing an optimized bioavailability and offering perspectives for the in vivo development of CK2 inhibitors.

Keywords: indeno[1,2-b]indole; CK2 inhibitor; cyclodextrin; nanoparticles; in cellulo; human erythrocytes; A427 cells

1. Introduction

The protein kinase CK2 is an ubiquitous and pleiotropic serine/threonine kinase with hundreds of endogenous substrates that are implicated in a wide variety of cellular functions (e.g., growth, proliferation, differentiation, apoptosis) [1]. CK2 is generally described as a tetrameric structure composed of two catalytic (α or α') and two regulatory (β) subunits. CK2 is involved in several pathological processes [2] and it is especially linked to cancer such as leukemia [3,4], glioblastoma [5], and hepatocellular carcinoma [6].

Researchers are currently exploring a wide range of scaffolds to design small molecule inhibitors of CK2 [7]. Among these inhibitors, indeno[1,2-*b*]indole derivatives have been identified as ATP-competitive inhibitors of CK2 [8,9]. Structure-Activity Relationship (SAR) studies through the systematic modification of the four rings A-D brought to light the main positions that identified potent inhibitors of CK2. In fact, the introduction of an alkoxy group in position 4 (ring A) [10] or an alkyl group in position 7 [11] was associated with the most favorable inhibitory effects on CK2. The 4-methoxy-5-isopropyl-5,6,7,8-tetrahydroindeno[1,2-*b*]indole-9,10-dione (THN7, Figure 1) was identified as a potent inhibitor of CK2 (IC_{50} = 71 nM, unpublished data) and then selected for new encapsulation in a set of amphiphilic cyclodextrins (CDs). A "proof of concept" study was previously carried out and validated the use of these macrocyclic oligosaccharides as nanocarriers [12]. The investigation of drug formulations remains a key point in the use of bioactive molecules, especially for indenoindoles used as CK2 inhibitors.

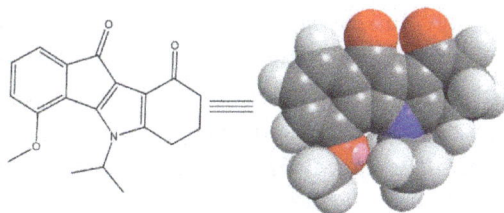

Figure 1. Structure of THN7 derivative.

Over the years, cyclodextrins became efficient vehicles to solubilize drugs and then to optimize diverse biological parameters (e.g., potency, absorption, distribution, metabolism, excretion, and toxicity (ADMET) properties) [13,14]. Moreover, amphiphilic cyclodextrin derivatives have been developed [15–17] in order to favor the interaction of CDs with cell membranes, to form self-assembled nanoparticles for drug encapsulation, enhancing interaction with hydrophobic drugs [18]. For example, amphiphilic cyclodextrins are useful to formulate stable nanoparticles of acyclovir, without the use of any surfactant [19].

Hydrocarbonated and fluorinated amphiphilic α- and β-CDs derivatives were well studied by our group, and it has been shown that these molecules could form very stable nanoparticles that could entrap hydrophilic and hydrophobic drugs [20–22]. As demonstrated previously for an indeno[1,2-*b*]indole analog [12], nanoparticles made from these derivatives can not only encapsulate this CK2 inhibitor, but they can also release it in a controlled manner. We also demonstrated that nanoparticles made from α-CDs derivatives (Figure 2) are more resistant than those made from β-CDs derivatives, even if the complexations are weaker.

In this study, we investigated a new formulation study in which compound THN7 (cLogP 3.326, www.molinspiration.com/cgi-bin/properties, accession date: 16 September 2017) is directly loaded into α-cyclodextrin nanoparticles. Our works were for the first time completed by cell-based assays to demonstrate (i) the safety profile of the four α-cyclodextrins used as nanocarriers and (ii) the improved in cellulo activity of CK2 inhibitor THN7. Red blood cells (RBCs) and A-427 cell line were selected to achieve our goal.

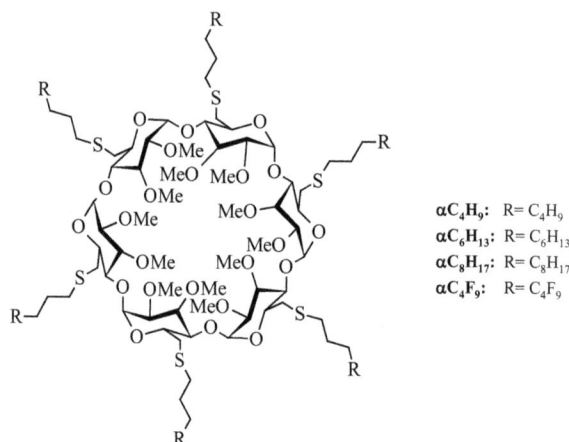

αC$_4$H$_9$: R= C$_4$H$_9$
αC$_6$H$_{13}$: R= C$_6$H$_{13}$
αC$_8$H$_{17}$: R= C$_8$H$_{17}$
αC$_4$F$_9$: R= C$_4$F$_9$

Figure 2. Fluorinated and hydrocarbonated amphiphilic α-cyclodextrins used in this study.

2. Results

2.1. Characterization of THN7:Amphiphilic Cyclodextrin Inclusion Complexes

Due to its very simple utilization, UV/Vis spectroscopy is the method of choice for studying the complexation between amphiphilic α-cyclodextrin derivatives and UV-visible THN7 molecules in ethanol. It has also been chosen for comparison with previously obtained constants determined by the same technique [12]. By using Job and Benesi-Hildebrand plots, stoichiometry and stability constants (K_{11}), respectively, can be easily and rapidly determined. All amphiphilic CD derivatives form 1:1 complexes with THN7 (maximum at 0.5 ratio) (Supplementary Information (SI) Figures S1–S4) and Benesi-Hildebrand plots are linear (SI Figure S5). The results obtained from these plots are given in Table 1.

Table 1. Stoichiometry and stability constants (K_{11}) of complexes in ethanol.

α-Cyclodextrin	Stoichiometry	K_{11} (mol·L^{-1})
C$_4$H$_9$	1:1	057
C$_6$H$_{13}$	1:1	298
C$_8$H$_{17}$	1:1	417
C$_4$F$_9$	1:1	828

The chain lengths and nature on the α-cyclodextrin derivatives seem to have an impact on the association at the molecular scale. Indeed, the K_{11} values increased with the chain length and were higher in the fluorinated derivative. For α-C$_4$H$_9$ the complexation was weak (57 mol·L^{-1}), meaning that at the molecular level, it had no affinity for THN7. Nevertheless, by increasing the length of the hydrocarbonated chain, the affinity also increased (298 mol·L^{-1} and 417 mol·L^{-1} for α-C$_6$H$_{13}$ and α-C$_8$H$_{17}$, respectively), with the higher association constant being observed with the fluorinated analog α-C$_4$F$_9$ (828 mol·L^{-1}). We also noticed that these values are in the same range as those observed previously by our group for another CK2 inhibitor. The differences in the behavior were quite similar: a higher association constant was observed with the fluorinated derivative [12]. All these observations also indicate that the THN7 molecule should be located between the hydrophobic chains rather than in the cyclodextrin cavity, as the molecule is too bulky to fit into the cavity.

2.2. THN7 Loading of Nanoparticles Based on Amphiphilic α-Cyclodextrins

The loading of THN7 compound into α-CDs nanoparticles was achieved as previously described [12,20]. Ethanol was used as an organic solvent because it has been shown that, among other solvents, for nanoparticle formation, ethanol gave the smallest particle size and better polydispersity [23]. At the end of the process, for each amphiphilic α-cyclodextrin used, a 20-mL stock solution of nanoparticles containing 600 μM THN7 was obtained and then stored before use.

Dynamic Light Scattering was employed for measuring sizes of the nanoparticles (SI Figures S6–S9) and the percentage of associated drug was determined after two days. The results are given in Table 2.

As seen in Table 2, the mean particle sizes varies from 66 to 132 nm. Unlike our previous observations of another CK2 inhibitor [12], for the same chain length, fluorinated nanoparticles are bigger (104 vs. 82 nm for α-C_4F_9 and α-C_4H_9, respectively). This may be due to the THN7 molecule's better affinity for these fluorinated derivatives at the molecular scale, implying either more molecules inside the particles, or THN7 coating on the surface. Nevertheless, all of the particle size distributions are monodisperse, with a low polydispersity index (<0.2).

Table 2. Mean diameter (nm) and polydispersity index (PdI) of nanospheres based on different amphiphilic α-cyclodextrins and % of associated THN7.

α-Cyclodextrin	Nanosphere Size (nm)	PdI	Associated THN7 (%)
C_4H_9	82.2 ± 0.2	0.07 ± 0.01	24 ± 3
C_6H_{13}	131.9 ± 0.4	0.07 ± 0.03	35 ± 2
C_8H_{17}	65.8 ± 3.0	0.18 ± 0.02	14 ± 5
C_4F_9	104.3 ± 1.0	0.09 ± 0.02	19 ± 3

The loading capacities ranged from 14 to 35% (for α-C_8H_{17} and α-C_6H_{13}, respectively). This is relatively low compared to the previous ones observed with another indenoindole derivative [12]. Nevertheless, it is worth noting that these encapsulation rates are still in the same range as those observed for other systems. No correlation between the loading capacities and the association constant determined at the molecular level was observed.

2.3. Controlled Release Studies

The in vitro release experiments were performed in order to confirm what has previously been observed in similar systems: the benefit of nanoparticle encapsulation. Figure 3 displays the release profile of THN7 from loaded nanoparticles based on four α-CDs amphiphilic derivatives.

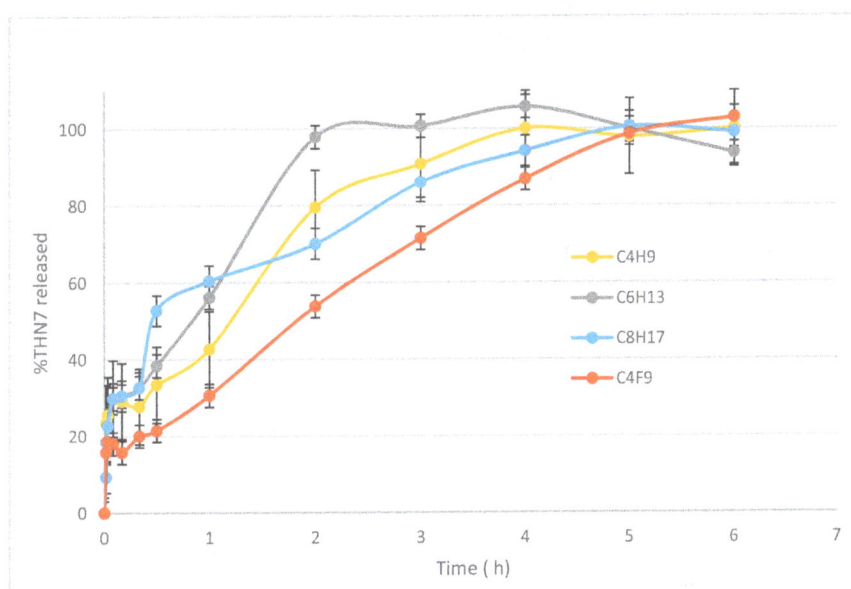

Figure 3. Release profiles of THN7 from loaded nanospheres. The data are the average of three experiments and the error bars indicate the three experiments.

In all cases, a fast release of up to 30% THN7 was observed within the first 30 min, followed by a much more controlled delivery of THN7, meaning that some of the THN7 molecules were probably coated on the surface of the nanospheres as expected before, and the remainder was solubilized inside the hydrophobic core of the nanoparticles. Complete drug release was reached in 1 to 5 h, the longer release being observed for the fluorinated derivative nanoparticles. This confirms the observations made by Krafft et al. [24] on the better resistance and low permeability of fluorinated colloidal systems.

2.4. Hemolytic Activity of α-CD Nanoparticles

C_4F_9 showed a relatively high hemolytic effect as its HC_{50} value was 3.04 ± 0.22 mmol·L^{-1} compared to the other derivatives. The ranking of the hemolytic effect in the case of other α-CD nanoparticles was classified as follows (smallest to largest): $C_6H_{13} > C_4H_9 > C_8H_{17}$ (Figure 4).

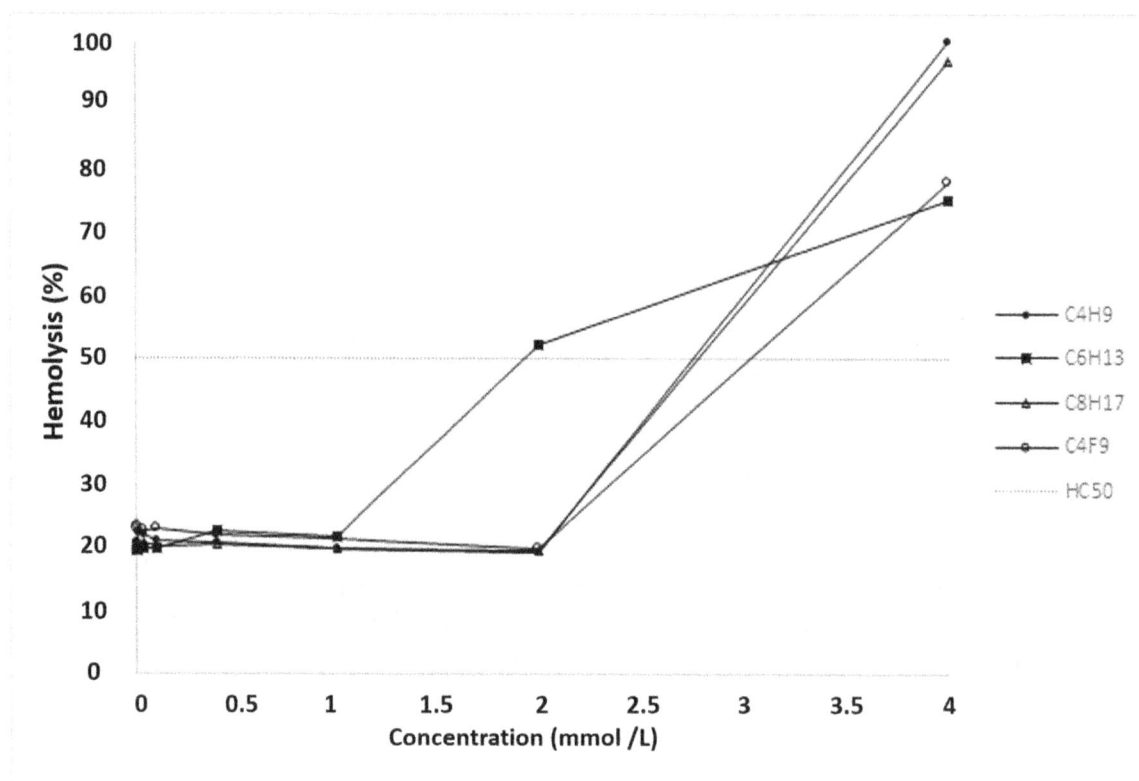

Figure 4. Hemolytic effect of different α-CD nanoparticles on human red blood cells (RBCs). Hemolysis was expressed as the percentage of the untreated control in the function of α-CD nanoparticle concentration. The positive control was purified water and the negative control was phosphate-buffered saline (PBS). Values presented are means $\pm$ SD. All data were obtained from three independent replicates, and in the same experiment, two to four parallel concentrations were measured. HC_{50} values were calculated as follows: $C_6H_{13} = 1.93 \pm 0.11$ mmol·L^{-1}, $C_4H_9 = 2.59 \pm 0.8$ mmol·L^{-1}, $C_8H_{17} = 2.79 \pm 0.75$ mmol·L^{-1} and $C_4F_9 = 3.04 \pm 0.22$ mmol·L^{-1}.

2.5. Improved Cytotoxic Activity of THN7-Loaded α-Cyclodextrin Nanoparticles on A-427 Lung Cancer Cells

To evaluate the cytotoxic effect of THN7-loaded α-cyclodextrin nanoparticles, we treated human lung cancer cells A427 with THN7 alone and each solution of THN7-loaded nanoparticles. In all experiments THN7 was used at a final concentration of 6 μM. A427 cells were selected as a model because they have been reported to overexpress CK2α, the target of kinase inhibitors from the class of indeno[1,2-b]indoles [25,26]. Moreover, other indenoindoles known to be potent CK2 inhibitors were described to have a significant antiproliferative effect on human A427 cells [8]. Cell viability of A427 cells was determined using an MTT assay, and the results are depicted in Figure 5.

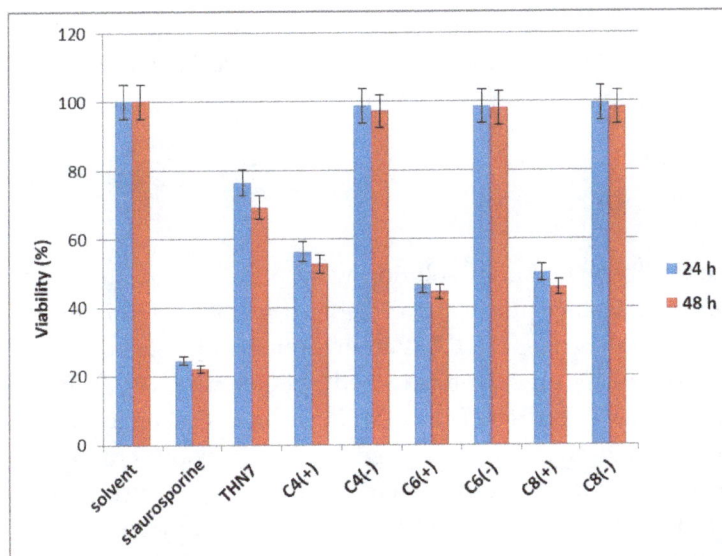

Figure 5. Cytotoxic activity of THN7-loaded α-cyclodextrin nanoparticles on A-427 lung cancer cells. C4: C_4H_9; C6: C_6H_{13}; C8: C_8H_{17}. (+) loaded cyclodextrins; (−) empty cyclodextrins. Viability of A427 cells were determined using an MTT assay. The viability of cells treated with 1% of the appropriate solvent was set 100%. Staurosporine served as a control for the correctly performance of the MTT assay using A427 cells. In all experiments THN7 was used at a final concentration of 6 μM.

The viability of A427 cells was decreased to 75% after treatment with 6 μM THN7 for 24 h. This effect is enhanced by an additional 20% in the case where cells were treated with α-cyclodextrin nanoparticles loaded with THN7. Empty nanoparticles had no effect on cell viability. An additional increase after 48 h incubation with or without nanoparticles was not observed.

After treatment with staurosporine at a concentration of 20 μM, cell viability was reduced to a residual 20%. This demonstrated that the MTT assay worked properly for the determination of cell viability of A427 cells. The cytotoxic effect of staurosporine on different cancer cell lines is well documented by many investigations [27,28].

3. Discussion

Amphiphilic α-cyclodextrin derivatives spontaneously formed nanoparticles in water and efficiently enclosed CK2 inhibitors. Unloaded cyclodextrin nanoparticles had no cytotoxic effect on A-427 lung cancer cells, while THN7-loaded α-cyclodextrin nanoparticles had a more pronounced cytotoxic effect after 24 and 48 h of exposure compared to THN7 alone. This phenomenon can be explained by several mechanisms. First of all, the solubilization of THN7 by amphiphilic cyclodextrins plays an important role in the improvement of its efficacy. The interaction of THN7 with cyclodextrin nanoparticles can prevent its aggregation in water, thus the CK2 inhibitor will penetrate freely through the cell membrane. On the other hand, it has also recently been revealed that both cyclodextrins [29,30] and poly-cationic amphiphilic cyclodextrin complexes [31] are able to enter the cells by endocytosis. Cellular internalization of loaded nanoparticles is a key step for their action and can highly increase the intracellular CK2 inhibitor concentration. To test and visualize the cellular internalization of amphiphilic α-cyclodextrin nanoparticles, the labeling of cyclodextrins with fluorophore is needed. Using fluorescent techniques, the interactions of nanoparticles with cells can be revealed. Our further aim is to functionalize the amphiphilic cyclodextrins by fluorophores and targeting moieties such as folates [32] or specific binding proteins. Targeting receptors or membrane proteins can improve the internalization efficiency, while by the fluorophores the intracellular distribution and fate of nanoparticles can be visualized and determined. A novel, multi-functional nanoscale drug delivery system, based on the nanoparticle formation of functionalized amphiphilic α-cyclodextrins, is under construction and will be tested on cancer cell lines. With a suitable targeting moiety, the in vivo efficacy, distribution, and toxicity of this carrier system can be characterized and used to improve the CK2 inhibitory effect on animal tumor models.

4. Materials and Methods

4.1. Materials

All chemicals and phosphate buffer solution were purchased from Acros Organics or Sigma Aldrich and used without further purification. Other solvents were of chemical grade and were used as received. 4-methoxy-5-isopropyl-5,6,7,8-tetrahydroindeno[1,2-*b*]indole-9,10-dione (THN7) was synthetized according to the same procedure described by References [10,33]. The α-cyclodextrins were purchased from Roquette Frères (Lestrem, France) and their modification to amphiphilic CDs (Figure 2) was conducted according to the syntheses described previously by our group [34]. The structures and the purities of these amphiphilic derivatives were confirmed by spectral experiments according to techniques such as ^{1}H and ^{13}C NMR at 300 and 125 MHz, respectively, and MALDI mass spectroscopy. In order to simplify the name of each compound, shorter names have been assigned. For example, α-C_4F_9 refers to hexakis[6-deoxy-6-(3-perfluorobutylpropanethio)-2,3-di-*O*-methyl]-α-cyclodextrin.

4.2. Cell Culture

The nanoparticles were tested on the human lung cancer cell line A427, which was obtained from the German Collection of Microorganisms and Cell Culture (DSMZ, Braunschweig, Germany). A427 cells were grown at 37 °C in a humidified atmosphere of 5% CO_2 in RPMI-1640 medium supplemented with 10% fetal calf serum (FCS).

4.3. Characterization of Inclusion Complexes Using the UV/Vis Spectroscopy

The continuous variation method was used to determine the stoichiometry of the fluorinated and hydrocarbonated amphiphilic cyclodextrin:THN7 complexes. Two solutions of equal concentration (4×10^{-4} M) of amphiphilic α-CDs and THN7 were prepared in ethanol. These solutions were mixed in different portions without variation of the final volume, and stirred for seven days. The absorbency (Aread) of each solution was measured at 460 nm. The absorbency change (ΔA) was then calculated (ΔA = Aread-AT). The Job plots showed a maximum at a specific molar ratio indicating the stoichiometry of the complexes (see supporting information). For the determination of the equilibrium constant (K), the double-reciprocal (Benesi/Hildebrand) plot was used as previously described [22].

4.4. Preparation of Nanoparticles

These results being the continuity of those published previously [20], we used the same highly loaded method: the THN7 loaded nanoparticles based on amphiphilic α-cyclodextrin derivatives were prepared by the nanoprecipitation technique, using 10 mL of a 4×10^{-4} M solution of preformed 1:1 THN7:CD complexes overloaded with an additional 20 mL of a 4×10^{-4} M THN7 solution in ethanol phase. This ethanolic solution (30 mL) was poured dropwise into deionized water (2×30 mL) and stirred at 400 rpm. Solvent and a part of water were evaporated under reduced pressure, and the total volume was adjusted to 20 mL with deionized water. The final concentration of THN7 in each nanoparticle stock solution was 600 μM. In addition, a DMSO stock solution of THN7 was prepared (also with a concentration of 600 μM).

4.5. Particle Size Measurements

The mean particle size (diameter, nm) and the polydispersity index (PDI) of nanospheres were measured by dynamic light scattering using a NanoZS instrument (Malvern Instruments,

Malvern, UK) [22]. The measurements were carried out at 25 °C. Each value was the average of three measurements.

4.6. Determination of the Encapsulation Efficiency

For measuring the loading efficiency [12], after the formation of nanoparticle suspensions, unbound THN7 molecules in the nanoparticle dispersions were separated by centrifugation at 50,000 rpm for 1 h at +4 °C by an Optima™ MAX-E centrifuge (Beckman-Coulter), in order to settle down the loaded nanoparticles. The supernatant was removed. The precipitate was then dried overnight and the resulting powder containing the loaded nanoparticles was dissolved in ethanol to obtain a clear solution, the absorbance of which was analyzed using a spectrophotometer at a wavelength of 460 nm for the calculation of the encapsulated drug quantity. Experiments were conducted in triplicate. Loading capacity was expressed in terms of associated drug percentage:

Associated drug % = [determined drug quantity (μmol)]/[initial drug quantity (μmol)] × 100.

4.7. In Vitro-Controlled Release Profile

The suspensions of nanoparticles charged in THN7 (1 mL) were introduced into a dialysis tube (Sigma, Pur-A-Lyzer Mega 1000 Dialysis Kit, MWCO: 1 kDa). This tube was then placed in PBS (pH 7.4 with a volume of 10 mL), at room temperature, for a period of time. Aliquots of 1 mL of the buffered solution were taken from the media at specific time intervals and replaced by fresh PBS. The proportion of released and encapsulated THN7 molecules were measured by UV spectrometry at 460 nm [12]. Experiments were conducted three times.

4.8. Hemolysis Test

A hemolysis test was performed on fresh human blood, collected from healthy donors [35]. Erythrocytes were separated from citrated blood by centrifugation at $2500 \times g$ for 10 min, washed three times with PBS, and resuspended in the same solution. Aliquots of the cell suspension with the respective RBC number of 5×10^7 were added to the PBS solution (pH 7.2) containing increasing concentrations of the samples investigated in the study. After mixing them gently, each solution was incubated at 37 °C for 10 min and then centrifuged at $5000 \times g$. Finally, the absorbance of the hemoglobin released into the supernatant was measured at 540 nm with a FLUOstar OPTIMA Microplate Reader. The percentage of hemolysis was expressed as the ratio of hemoglobin in the supernatant of the sample solutions related to the hemoglobin concentration after the complete hemolysis of erythrocytes in water. The dose-response curve was determined, and the concentration inducing hemolysis in 50% of the erythrocyte population (HC_{50}) was subsequently calculated [36].

4.9. Cell Viability Assay

For the determination of cell viability of A427 cells, an MTT assay was performed. A427 cells were seeded at a density of 10^4 cells per well into 96-well plates in 100 μL of growth medium. After 24 h, the medium was replaced by fresh medium containing either a working solution containing THN7 alone (1 μL of THN7 stock solution added to 99 μL medium) or a working solution of THN7-loaded nanoparticles (1 μL of stock solution of THN7-loaded nanoparticles added to 99 μL medium). Then, in each well the final concentration of THN7 (alone or in nanoparticle solution) was 6 μM. Blank experiments were also conducted with empty cyclodextrins. Medium containing 1% of the solvent served as a control. The concentration of staurosporin used in the experiment was 0.5 μM. After 24 h and 48 h, respectively, 10 μL of the MTT solution (5 mg/mL in PBS) were added to each well and the plate was incubated for 2 h at 37 °C. The MTT assay is based on the ability of the mitochondrial succinate-tetrazolium reductase system to convert 3-(4,5-dimethylthiazol-2-yl)-2,5-diphenyltetrazolium bromide (MTT) to the purple-colored formazan. The produced formazan was dissolved by the addition of 100 µL of the MTT stop solution (0.04 M HCl in isopropanol) and the plates were incubated for one additional hour at 37 °C before recording the absorbance at 570 nm.

5. Conclusions

The development of advanced drug delivery systems dedicated to kinase inhibitors is important to investigate for enhancing the uptake of anticancer drugs into tumors. In the present study, four α-CDs were used to encapsulate an indenoindole-type CK2 inhibitor, THN7. All experiments indicated that the nanoencapsulation of THN7 in α-CDs was successful. In parallel, after testing the hemolytic activity of the four selected α-CDs, only three THN7-loaded cyclodextrin nanoparticles (α-C_6H_{13}, α-C_8H_{17}, and α-C_4H_9) were tested against A-427 cells. It is important to note that all THN7-loaded nanoparticles were more cytotoxic against A-427 cells than THN7 alone.

Further studies should be investigated to optimize the drug-loading capacity of our amphiphilic α-cyclodextrin-based nanoparticles. In the present study, we only obtained an encapsulation rate of 35% with the α-C_6H_{13} amphiphilic derivative. The structural modulation of both amphiphilic α-cyclodextrins and indeno[1,2-*b*]indoles could be rapidly achieved, giving new insight into amphiphilic α-cyclodextrin derivatives for targeted drug delivery to tumors. As suggested in the perspectives, we will examine how amphiphilic α-cyclodextrins could assist the bioactive molecule (in this case, a CK2 inhibitor) to enhance in cellulo activity against cancer cells (e.g., A-427, MCF-7). This is a crucial point to study before undertaking an in vivo development project.

Acknowledgments: This scientific work was made possible by financial support from Rhône-Alpes region through the Cluster 5 Chemistry and the Canceropôle Lyon Auvergne Rhône-Alpes (CLARA). Joachim Jose thanks Dagmar Aichele for her support in cell culture experiments. Florent Perret thanks Julien Leclaire for his financial help. Marc Le Borgne thanks Thi Huong Nguyen for her technical assistance. M. Abdelhamid Nacereddine thanks the Algerian Ministry of Foreign Affairs and the "Institut Français d'Algérie" for his doctoral fellowship. The present work was supported by the "Partenariats Hubert Curien" (PHC) (Campus France, Programme Balaton, Grant Agreement No. 890278K). The work of Ferenc Fenyvesi was supported by the János Bolyai Research Scholarship of the Hungarian Academy of Sciences and FK_17 research grant (FK124634) of the National Research, Development, and Innovation Office. Marc Le Borgne and Florent Perret thank Miklós Vecsernyés for his precious help to establish a partnership between Lyon and Debrecen.

Author Contributions: A.N., A.B., and E.R. performed the experiments; C.M. and Z.B. managed the synthesis of compound THN7; F.F., I.K.B., J.J., and F.P. conceived and designed the experiments; I.K.B., J.J., F.P., and M.L.B. analyzed the data and wrote the paper.

Conflicts of Interest: The authors declare no conflict of interest.

References

1. De Villavicencio-Diaz, T.N.; Rabalski, A.J.; Litchfield, D.W. Protein kinase CK2: Intricate relationships within regulatory cellular networks. *Pharmaceuticals* **2017**, *10*, 27. [CrossRef] [PubMed]

2. Jose, J.; Le Borgne, M.; Pinna, L.A.; Montenarh, M. An updated view on an emerging target: Selected papers from the 8th international conference on protein kinase CK2. *Pharmaceuticals* **2017**, *10*, 33. [CrossRef] [PubMed]

3. Buontempo, F.; McCubrey, J.A.; Orsini, E.; Ruzzene, M.; Cappellini, A.; Lonetti, A.; Evangelisti, C.; Chiarini, F.; Evangelisti, C.; Barata, J.T.; et al. Therapeutic targeting of CK2 in acute and chronic leukemias. *Leukemia* **2018**, *32*, 1–10. [CrossRef] [PubMed]

4. Gowda, C.; Sachdev, M.; Muthusami, S.; Kapadia, M.; Petrovic-Dovat, L.; Hartman, M.; Ding, Y.; Song, C.; Payne, J.L.; Tan, B.H.; et al. Casein kinase II (CK2) as a therapeutic target for hematological malignancies. *Curr. Pharm. Des.* **2017**, *23*, 95–107. [CrossRef] [PubMed]

5. Rowse, A.L.; Gibson, S.A.; Meares, G.P.; Rajbhandari, R.; Nozell, S.E.; Dees, K.J.; Hjelmeland, A.B.; McFarland, B.C.; Benveniste, E.N. Protein kinase CK2 is important for the function of glioblastoma brain tumor initiating cells. *J. Neurooncol.* **2017**, *132*, 219–229. [CrossRef] [PubMed]

6. Zhang, H.X.; Jiang, S.S.; Zhang, X.F.; Zhou, Z.Q.; Pan, Q.Z.; Chen, C.L.; Zhao, J.J.; Tang, Y.; Xia, J.C.; Weng, D.S. Protein kinase CK2α catalytic subunit is overexpressed and serves as an unfavorable prognostic marker in primary hepatocellular carcinoma. *Oncotarget* **2015**, *6*, 34800–34817. [PubMed]

7. Cozza, G. The development of CK2 inhibitors: From traditional pharmacology to in silico rational drug design. *Pharmaceuticals* **2017**, *10*, 26. [CrossRef] [PubMed]

8. Hundsdoerfer, C.; Hemmerling, H.-J.; Hamberger, J.; Le Borgne, M.; Bednarski, P.; Goetz, C.; Totzke, F.; Jose, J. Novel indeno[1,2-*b*]indoloquinones as inhibitors of the human protein kinase CK2 with antiproliferative activity towards a broad panel of cancer cell lines. *Biochem. Biophys. Res. Commun.* **2012**, *424*, 71–75. [CrossRef] [PubMed]

9. Hundsdoerfer, C.; Hemmerling, H.-J.; Goetz, C.; Totzke, F.; Bednarski, P.; Le Borgne, M.; Jose, J. Indeno[1,2-*b*]indole derivatives as a novel class of potent human protein kinase CK2 inhibitors. *Bioorg. Med. Chem.* **2012**, *20*, 2282–2289. [CrossRef] [PubMed]

10. Gozzi, G.J.; Bouaziz, Z.; Winter, E.; Daflon-Yunes, N.; Honorat, M.; Guragossian, N.; Marminon, C.; Valdameri, G.; Bollacke, A.; Guillon, J.; et al. Phenolic indeno[1,2-*b*]indoles as ABCG2-selective potent and non-toxic inhibitors stimulating basal ATPase activity. *Drug Des. Dev. Ther.* **2015**, *9*, 3481–3495.

11. Alchab, F.; Ettouati, L.; Bouaziz, Z.; Bollacke, A.; Delcros, J.-G.; Gertzen, C.G.; Gohlke, H.; Pinaud, N.; Marchivie, M.; Guillon, J.; et al. Synthesis, biological evaluation and molecular modeling of substituted indeno[1,2-*b*]indoles as inhibitors of human protein kinase CK2. *Pharmaceuticals* **2015**, *8*, 279–302. [CrossRef] [PubMed]

12. Perret, F.; Marminon, C.; Zeinyeh, W.; Nebois, P.; Bollacke, A.; Jose, J.; Parrot-Lopez, H.; Le Borgne, M. Preparation and characterization of CK2 inhibitor-loaded cyclodextrin nanoparticles for drug delivery. *Int. J. Pharm.* **2013**, *441*, 491–498. [CrossRef] [PubMed]

13. Gidwani, B.; Vyas, A. A comprehensive review on cyclodextrin-based carriers for delivery of chemotherapeutic cytotoxic anticancer drugs. *BioMed Res. Int.* **2015**, *2015*. [CrossRef] [PubMed]

14. Muankaew, C.; Loftsson, T. Cyclodextrins-based formulations: A non-invasive platform for targeted drug delivery. *Basic Clin. Pharmacol. Toxicol.* **2018**, *122*, 46–55. [CrossRef] [PubMed]

15. Bilensoy, E. Amphiphilic cyclodextrin nanoparticles for effective and safe delivery of anticancer drugs. *Adv. Exp. Med. Biol.* **2015**, *822*, 201. [PubMed]

16. Sallas, F.; Darcy, R. Amphiphilic cyclodextrins—Advances in synthesis and supramolecular chemistry. *Eur. J. Org. Chem.* **2008**, *2008*, 957–969. [CrossRef]

17. Varan, G.; Varan, C.; Erdogar, N.; Hincal, A.A.; Bilensoy, E. Amphiphilic cyclodextrin nanoparticles. *Int. J. Pharm.* **2017**, *531*, 457–469. [CrossRef] [PubMed]

18. Erdogar, N.; Bilensoy, E. *Cyclodextrins in Drug Delivery*; CRC Press: Boca Raton, FL, USA, 2015; pp. 178–209.

19. Parrot-Lopez, H.; Perret, F.; Bertino-Ghera, B. Les cyclodextrines amphiphiles et leurs applications: Élaboration de nanoparticules de cyclodextrines amphiphiles pour des applications biomédicales. *Ann. Pharm.* **2010**, *68*, 12–26. [CrossRef] [PubMed]

20. Bertino-Ghera, B.; Perret, F.; Chevalier, Y.; Parrot-Lopez, H. Novel nanoparticles made from amphiphilic perfluoroalkyl α-cyclodextrin derivatives: Preparation, characterization and application to the transport of acyclovir. *Int. J. Pharm.* **2009**, *375*, 155–162. [CrossRef] [PubMed]

21. Bertino-Ghera, B.; Perret, F.; Fenet, B.; Parrot-Lopez, H. Control of the regioselectivity for new fluorinated amphiphilic cyclodextrins: Synthesis of di- and tetra(6-deoxy-6-alkylthio)- and 6-(perfluoroalkylpropanethio)-α-cyclodextrin derivatives. *J. Org. Chem.* **2008**, *73*, 7317–7326. [CrossRef] [PubMed]

22. Perret, F.; Duffour, M.; Chevalier, Y.; Parrot-Lopez, H. Design, synthesis, and in vitro evaluation of new amphiphilic cyclodextrin-based nanoparticles for the incorporation and controlled release of acyclovir. *Eur. J. Pharm. Biopharm.* **2013**, *83*, 25–32. [CrossRef] [PubMed]

23. Galindo-Rodriguez, S.; Allemann, E.; Fessi, H.; Doelker, E. Physicochemical parameters associated with nanoparticle formation in the salting-out, emulsification-diffusion, and nanoprecipitation methods. *Pharm. Res.* **2004**, *21*, 1428–1439. [CrossRef] [PubMed]

24. Krafft, M.P. Fluorocarbons and fluorinated amphiphiles in drug delivery and biomedical research. *Adv. Drug Deliv. Rev.* **2001**, *47*, 209–228. [CrossRef]

25. Hung, M.S.; Xu, Z.; Chen, Y.; Smith, E.; Mao, J.H.; Hsieh, D.; Lin, Y.C.; Yang, C.T.; Jablons, D.M.; You, L. Hematein, a casein kinase II inhibitor, inhibits lung cancer tumor growth in a murine xenograft model. *Int. J. Oncol.* **2013**, *43*, 1517–1522. [CrossRef] [PubMed]

26. Zhang, S.; Wang, Y.; Mao, J.H.; Hsieh, D.; Kim, I.J.; Hu, L.M.; Xu, Z.; Long, H.; Jablons, D.M.; You, L. Inhibition of ck2α down-regulates hedgehog/gli signaling leading to a reduction of a stem-like side population in human lung cancer cells. *PLoS ONE* **2012**, *7*, e38996. [CrossRef] [PubMed]

27. Ding, Y.; Wang, B.; Chen, X.; Zhou, Y.; Ge, J. Staurosporine suppresses survival of hepg2 cancer cells through omi/htra2-mediated inhibition of pi3k/akt signaling pathway. *Tumor Biol.* **2017**, *39*. [CrossRef] [PubMed]

28. Zhang, Y.; Yu, S.; Ou-Yang, J.; Dong, X.; Wang, M.; Li, J. Effect of protein kinase c alpha, caspase-3 and survivin on apoptosis of oral cancer cells induced by staurosporine. *Acta Pharmacol. Sin.* **2005**, *26*, 1365–1372. [CrossRef] [PubMed]

29. Fenyvesi, F.; Reti-Nagy, K.; Bacso, Z.; Gutay-Toth, Z.; Malanga, M.; Fenyvesi, E.; Szente, L.; Varadi, J.; Ujhelyi, Z.; Feher, P.; et al. Fluorescently labeled methyl-beta-cyclodextrin enters intestinal epithelial caco-2 cells by fluid-phase endocytosis. *PLoS ONE* **2014**, *9*, e84856. [CrossRef] [PubMed]

30. Reti-Nagy, K.; Malanga, M.; Fenyvesi, E.; Szente, L.; Vamosi, G.; Varadi, J.; Bacskay, I.; Feher, P.; Ujhelyi, Z.; Roka, E.; et al. Endocytosis of fluorescent cyclodextrins by intestinal caco-2 cells and its role in paclitaxel drug delivery. *Int. J. Pharm.* **2015**, *496*, 509–517. [CrossRef] [PubMed]

31. O'Neill, M.J.; Guo, J.; Byrne, C.; Darcy, R.; O'Driscoll, C.M. Mechanistic studies on the uptake and intracellular trafficking of novel cyclodextrin transfection complexes by intestinal epithelial cells. *Int. J. Pharm.* **2011**, *413*, 174–183. [CrossRef] [PubMed]

32. Evans, J.C.; Malhotra, M.; Sweeney, K.; Darcy, R.; Nelson, C.C.; Hollier, B.G.; O'Driscoll, C.M. Folate targeted amphiphilic cyclodextrin nanoparticles incorporating a fusogenic peptide deliver therapeutic sirna and inhibit the invasive capacity of 3d prostate cancer tumours. *Int. J. Pharm.* **2017**, *532*, 511–518. [CrossRef] [PubMed]

33. Marminon, C.; Nacereddine, A.; Bouaziz, Z.; Nebois, P.; Jose, J.; Le Borgne, M. Microwave-assisted oxidation of indan-1-ones into ninhydrins. *Tetrahedron Lett.* **2015**, *56*, 1840–1842. [CrossRef]

34. Bertino-Ghera, B.; Perret, F.; Baudouin, A.; Coleman, A.W.; Parrot-Lopez, H. Synthesis and characterization of *O*-6-alkylthio- and perfluoroalkylpropanethio-α-cyclodextrins and their *O*-2-, *O*-3-methylated analogues. *New J. Chem.* **2007**, *31*, 1899–1906. [CrossRef]

35. Roka, E.; Ujhelyi, Z.; Deli, M.; Bocsik, A.; Fenyvesi, E.; Szente, L.; Fenyvesi, F.; Vecsernyes, M.; Varadi, J.; Feher, P.; et al. Evaluation of the cytotoxicity of α-cyclodextrin derivatives on the caco-2 cell line and human erythrocytes. *Molecules* **2015**, *20*, 20269–20285. [CrossRef] [PubMed]

36. Nornoo, A.O.; Osborne, D.W.; Chow, D.S.L. Cremophor-free intravenous microemulsions for paclitaxel: Formulation, cytotoxicity and hemolysis. *Int. J. Pharm.* **2008**, *349*, 108–116. [CrossRef] [PubMed]

12

Iron in Friedreich Ataxia: A Central Role in the Pathophysiology or an Epiphenomenon?

David Alsina, Rosa Purroy⬛, Joaquim Ros and Jordi Tamarit *⬛

Departament de Ciències Mèdiques Bàsiques, IRBLleida, Universitat de Lleida, 25198 Lleida, Spain; david.alsina@cmb.udl.cat (D.A.); rosa.purroy@irblleida.udl.cat (R.P.); joaquim.ros@cmb.udl.cat (J.R.)
* Correspondence: jordi.tamarit@cmb.udl.cat

Abstract: Friedreich ataxia is a neurodegenerative disease with an autosomal recessive inheritance. In most patients, the disease is caused by the presence of trinucleotide GAA expansions in the first intron of the frataxin gene. These expansions cause the decreased expression of this mitochondrial protein. Many evidences indicate that frataxin deficiency causes the deregulation of cellular iron homeostasis. In this review, we will discuss several hypotheses proposed for frataxin function, their caveats, and how they could provide an explanation for the deregulation of iron homeostasis found in frataxin-deficient cells. We will also focus on the potential mechanisms causing cellular dysfunction in Friedreich Ataxia and on the potential use of the iron chelator deferiprone as a therapeutic agent for this disease.

Keywords: Iron-sulfur; Friedreich Ataxia; Oxidative stress; Iron chelators

---

1. The Disease

Friedreich's Ataxia (FRDA) is a neurodegenerative disease described at the end of the 19th century by the German physician Nikolaus Friedreich from whom acquired the name. Friedreich observed in a group of patients that during the puberty a characteristic symptomatology began to manifest, specifically: ataxia, dysarthria, loss of sensitivity, muscle weakness, scoliosis, pes cavus, and heart symptoms. Later, a greater incidence of diabetes mellitus in patients than in the rest of the population was also reported [1]. It is considered a rare disease that follows a pattern of autosomal recessive inheritance. The frequency of carriers oscillates, depending on the area, between 1:50 and 1:100, while those affected by the disease are approximately 1:50,000, which makes this disease the most common form of hereditary ataxia [2].

The mutation responsible for the disease is an expansion of GAA trinucleotides in the first intron of the FXNor X25 gene (located in chromosome 9), which codes for the mitochondrial protein frataxin [3]. This expansion of triplets, which in patients can reach up to more than 1000 copies, results in a marked decrease in protein frataxin levels (below 5%–30% of normal levels) [4]. The number of GAA expansions has an inversely proportional relation to the age at which the first symptoms of the disease begin to manifest and it also determines their severity [5–7]. Besides GAA expansions, epigenetic modifications might also contribute to the variability in the onset and disease progression. Sarsero and collaborators reported differences in DNA methylation patterns between patients upstream and downstream the GAA expansion. Such differences caused variations in frataxin gene expression [8]. Finally, a small percentage of patients, around 4%, are compound heterozygous for a GAA expansion and a frataxin (FXN) point mutation or deletion [9].

2. Frataxin, an Ancestral Conserved Protein

Frataxin is a highly conserved protein throughout evolution and homologues can be found in most species. Its structure is formed by two helix alpha joined by a series of antiparallel beta sheets and is highly conserved (Figure 1). Despite the high degree of conservation in the three-dimensional structure, the stability of this protein varies significantly between species. One of the factors that are responsible for the differences in the stability of the protein is the C-terminal endpoint. While in Yfh1 (the yeast's homologue), this region is virtually nonexistent, in the human protein this fragment is found inserted between the two alpha helixes. This protects the hydrophobic nucleus of the protein and increases its stability [10].

hFxn   **Yfh1**

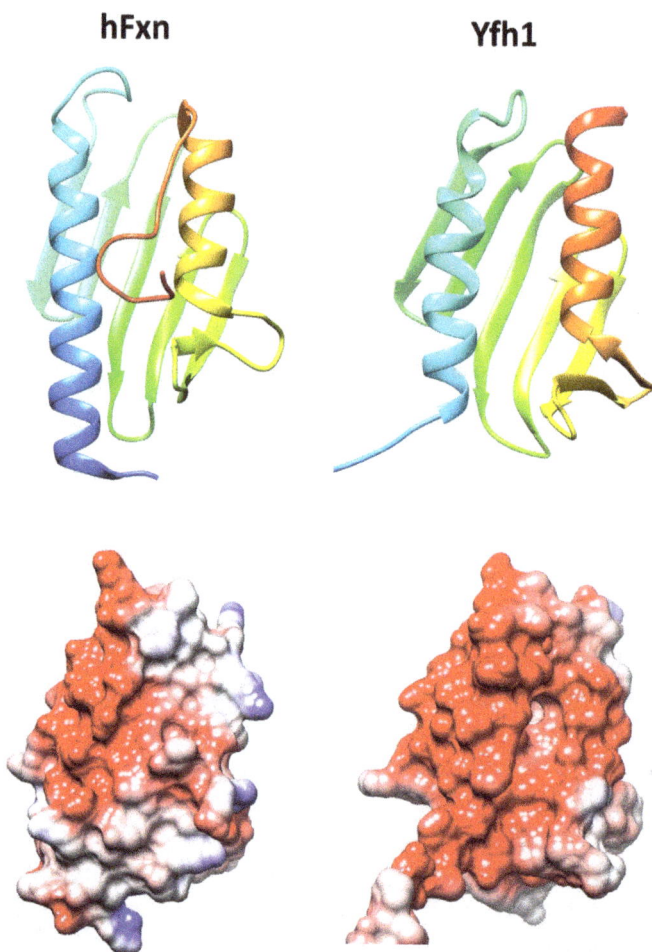

Figure 1. Structures of human frataxin (hFxn, pdb code 3s4m) and Yeast Frataxin Homologue 1 (Yfh1, pdb code 2fql). Top, ribbons representations showing the conserved alpha-beta-alpha structure. Structures are colored according to sequence, from dark blue (N-terminal) to red (C-terminal). In human frataxin the C-terminal region folds over the hydrophobic cavity formed between both alpha helices. Below, coulumbic surface coloring of the same structures. The red color indicates the presence of a marked acidic ridge, which may be involved in iron binding. Molecular graphics and analyses were performed with the UCSF Chimera package [11].

Frataxin is a mitochondrial protein, and as such, it has a signal peptide at its N-terminal end. It was soon identified, both for Yfh1 and for mouse frataxin, that Mitochondrial Processing Peptidase interacted with frataxin and was responsible for its processing [12,13]. This processing involves two sequential cleavages, which first produce an intermediate form of frataxin and subsequently the mature form. For human frataxin, the cleavage positions described are between amino acids 41–42 (intermediate form) and between amino acids 80–81 (mature form), although other less abundant forms that correspond to alternative cleavage sites (for instance, positions 55–56) have also been identified [14,15]. In these works, it was shown that the mature form of frataxin corresponds to FXN^{81-210}. This form is fully active and capable of improving the survival and phenotypes of frataxin deficient cells. Despite the demonstration that the FXN^{81-210} form is the dominant form and that it is active, there is some debate over the role that could be developed by the intermediate forms, as these forms can also be detected in certain tissues (although at low levels) [16]. It was shown that processing of the intermediate form was slower than that of the precursor form, which suggested that this could be a mechanism for controlling the levels of the different frataxin forms [17]. More recently, it has been suggested that the different forms of frataxin might play different roles. This point will be discussed in the next section. In addition to post-translational processing, alternative splicing mechanisms have also been observed that may generate different isoforms of frataxin. Work by Xia and collaborators suggested that these alternative forms could be tissue-specific and could have different functions and locations [18]. However, there are not additional evidences about the nature and relevance of these alternative forms.

3. Frataxin Function

Although very early after the discovery of frataxin as the gene that was responsible for Friedreich's Ataxia, it was established that iron homeostasis was altered by frataxin deficiency, the specific function of this protein remains controversial. Over the years, different functions have been proposed for frataxin, most of them related to iron metabolism and the control of oxidative stress in mitochondria.

3.1. Frataxin, an Iron Binding and Storage Protein

It has been proposed that frataxin could work like a metalochaperone and iron storage protein. In several studies with purified protein, it has been observed that frataxin has the ability to interact with metal ions, but the coordination environment of these metal binding sites has not been properly defined. There is also uncertainty on the number of metal ions that are bound per frataxin monomer. It has been described that frataxin can bind divalent metal ions using a group of exposed acidic residues. These amino acids are located in a specific area of the protein forming an acidic ridge, quite conserved, different from the canonical iron binding motifs where cysteine and/or histidine amino acids are usually found. This acidic zone results in a weak and non-specific electrostatic bonding of iron, which also allows the coordination of other divalent metals [19]. The estimated Kd for Fe^{2+} and Fe^{3+} of this region was calculated on the micromolar range [20]. Gentry and collaborators reported the potential presence of a high affinity iron binding site. They showed that three metal ions could be bound by each frataxin monomer, and that His86 was required for one of these binding sites. This residue is located in the disordered N-terminal tail and had not been previously reported to be involved in metal coordination. They calculated that this site would have an affinity for Fe^{2+} higher than the iron chelator ferrozine, while the remaining two sites would have lower affinities [21]. His86 is not included in most of the frataxin structures that are found in the protein data bank nor is conserved in yeast and bacterial homologues. More recently, while using NMR to investigate iron binding, it was also proposed that frataxin tightly binds a single Fe^{2+} but not Fe^{3+} [22].

Isaya and collaborators noticed that iron binding to yeast and bacterial frataxin promoted its oligomerization to complexes of high molecular weight (850–1100 kDa) [23–25]. These oligomeric forms resembled those that were formed by ferritin, the main protein responsible for iron storage in eukaryotes. Indeed, oligomeric frataxin was shown to use a ferrooxidation reaction to build a ferrihydrite mineral core inside the particles. Therefore it was proposed that frataxin could act as a mitochondrial ferritin. Although this function would be redundant in higher eukaryotes due to the presence of a mitochondrial ferritin, this hypothesis acquired some strength when subsequent studies demonstrated that the expression of mitochondrial ferritin in frataxin deficient yeast was able to partially recover some of the observed phenotypes. Specifically, the heterologous expression of mitochondrial ferritin partially prevented the accumulation of iron, the cells were more resistant to oxidizing agents and they partially recovered the activities of enzymes with iron-sulfur centers (which is a common described consequence of frataxin deficiency) [26]. Regarding human frataxin, it has been claimed that the mature form (FXN^{81-210}) does not form aggregates [27] and that only the intermediate forms FXN^{42-210} and FXN^{56-210} would be assembled into larger structures. Based on this observation, it has been suggested that different frataxin proteoforms would perform different functions. The mature form would be monomeric and involved in iron binding and delivery to biochemical pathways requiring this metal, while FXN^{56-210} and FXN^{42-210} would be able to oligomerize and store iron. A caveat to these hypotheses is that the long frataxin isoforms are not observed in most tissues by western blot. Mass spectrometry data also suggests that these long frataxin isoforms may be present at very low concentrations: data collected in the PeptideAtlas repository indicates that the theoretically likely frataxin peptides between positions 42 and 81 have never been observed, while those from the FXN^{81-210} have been observed at least 400 times. (PeptideAtlas is a publicly accessible compendium of peptides identified in mass spectrometry proteomics experiments) [28]. Recently, it has been shown that FXN^{81-210} can also undergo oligomerization under certain conditions, although the stability of these oligomers would be lower than that of bacterial frataxin [29].

Nevertheless, there are other caveats on the ferritin-like hypothesis. It has been argued that physiological conditions of calcium and magnesium stabilize the monomeric frataxin form and consequently frataxin would not oligomerize in vivo [27]. It has also been shown that mitochondrial iron in yeast strains expressing different Yfh1 concentrations, presented nearly identical chemical and biochemical characteristics [30]. Another point to take into account is which could be the contribution of frataxin to mitochondrial iron storage or trafficking from a quantitative point of view. Most iron that is present in mitochondria is found at the active sites of proteins. Despite that, non-proteinaceous labile metal iron pools have also been detected within cells. These pools are thought to be involved in cellular trafficking, regulation, signaling, and/or storage of metal ions. Due to their lability (and their presence at low concentrations), their structure and functions are not completely understood. For instance, mitochondria contain 0.7–2 mM Fe, but the proportion of labile iron is not completely known, with estimates ranging from 1 to 100 µM [31,32]. These differences in the estimates may be due to real differences between the models or experimental conditions used, but also on the methodological approaches used to analyze this elusive iron pool. Also, the nature of these nonproteinaceous metal complexes is not known. Based on the abundance of GSH within the mitochondria it has been hypothesized that could be an FeII (GSH) adduct. Citrate, which is also present in the mitochondrial matrix at high concentrations, has also been considered as a potential ligand for non-proteinaceous iron complexes (reviewed in [32]). In yeast, by using Mössbauer spectroscopy, it has been shown that the proportion and nature of these labile iron pools may vary depending on the metabolic state of the cell. Respiring mitochondria where estimated to contain ~15 µM labile non-heme high spin Fe^{2+}, while this pool in fermenting mitochondria increased to ~150 µM. The concentration of yeast frataxin in mitochondria has been estimated to be three orders of magnitude lower, around 35 nM [33]. Therefore, as monomeric frataxin has been claimed to bind three iron atoms, it cannot contribute significantly to store iron in a non-reactive easy deliverable form. However, it could play a role in iron trafficking as a temporary carrier or catalyzing its speciation between different forms. For instance, it could bind Fe^{2+} and promote its controlled oxidation to Fe^{3+}, which would be then stored in the form of Fe^{3+}-phosphate nanoparticles. Regarding oligomeric frataxin, the mineralization process would allow for this protein to bind much more iron atoms per subunit. The yeast 48 subunit oligomer can store ~50–75 iron atoms per subunit in 1–2 nm cores [34]. This raises the iron potentially bound by frataxin up to the µM range, but still this amount may not be a significant contribution to the whole mitochondrial iron pool. In comparison, around 35% of mitochondrial iron in fermenting mitochondria may be stored in the form of Fe^{3+} nanoparticles [33]. That said, the contribution of mitochondrial ferritin to iron storage in mitochondria is also intriguing, as the concentration of this protein according to the PaxDb database is much lower than that of frataxin (PaxDB is a database that contains protein abundance information across organisms and tissues) [35].

3.2. Frataxin in the Biosynthesis of Iron Containing Proteins

It has also been proposed that frataxin could participate in the biosynthesis of both heme groups and of iron-sulfur centers. This hypothesis has several fundamentals: (a) frataxin deficiency leads to a loss in proteins which contain iron-sulfur centers or heme groups; (b) frataxin has the ability to bind iron atoms; and, (c) several studies have shown the ability of frataxin to interact with proteins that areinvolved in heme or iron-sulfur biosynthesis.

3.2.1. Biosynthesis of Heme Groups

The incorporation of the iron atom into protoporphyrin IX is the last step in the biosynthesis of heme groups. This step is catalyzed by ferrochelatase, but it is not known how iron is provided to this enzyme. In in vitro studies, it was shown that there was a physical interaction between frataxin and ferrochelatase with a 1 to 2 stoichiometry, which seems logical, since ferrochelatase functions as a dimer. In addition, this interaction resulted in the formation of heme groups [36]. A study in which NMR spectroscopy was used to analyze the binding between both of the proteins suggested that ferrochelatase interacted with frataxin in a manner that included its iron-binding interface [37]. More recently, Söderberg and collaborators presented a model of the interaction of trimeric Yfh1 (yeast frataxin) and ferrochelatase in which one of the subunits of the Yfh1 trimer interacted with one subunit of the ferrochelatase dimer, whereas another trimer subunit was positioned for iron delivery [38]. These results support the hypothesis of frataxin acting as an iron donor in the biosynthesis of heme groups. However, heme deficiency is not always observed in frataxin-deficient cells and anemia has not been shown to be a symptom of FRDA. Indeed, no alterations where observed in heme synthesis in erythroid progenitor stem cells that were obtained from FRDA patients [39]. Moreover, experiments using either conditional frataxin-deficient T-Rex-293 cells or yeasts have shown that heme deficiency is a late consequence of frataxin deficiency [40,41]. These observations suggest that heme deficiency may be an epiphenomenon observed in certain frataxin-deficient cells which could be caused by poor iron availability or by metabolic remodeling. In this regard, we have shown in frataxin-deficient yeast that heme deficiency could be caused by the induction of Cth2, a protein induced in response to iron limitation, which promotes the degradation of mRNAs from iron-containing proteins [42].

3.2.2. Biosynthesis of Iron-Sulfur Centers

In addition to interacting with ferrochelatase, frataxin also interacts with the proteins that form the central biosynthesis machinery of iron-sulfur centers: IscU (Isu1 in yeast), Nfs1, and Isd11 [43,44]. Several authors have shown that this interaction facilitates the formation of an iron-sulfur center into IscU, the scaffold protein where these cofactors are first assembled. It was initially suggested that frataxin would act as an iron donor in the biosynthesis of these centers [45]. More recently, it has been suggested that frataxin would participate in the biosynthesis of iron-sulfur centers as an allosteric regulator and not as an iron donor. In works that were carried out in vitro with the CyaY protein (bacterial homologue of frataxin), it was shown that this protein had an inhibitory effect on the production of iron-sulfur centers. As this effect was increased in response to iron concentration, the authors suggested that frataxin could adapt the production of iron-sulfur to the number of final acceptor proteins [46]. Surprisingly, studies with human proteins demonstrated that eukaryotic frataxins would have a contrary effect. In this case, they stimulated the production of iron-sulfur centers by favoring the desulfurase activity of Nfs1 [47–49].

Today, despite the intense debate that is generated around the function or functions of frataxin, this non-essential activity in the metabolism of iron as an allosteric regulator of the biosynthesis of iron-sulfur centers has strong support from in vitro biochemical data and is the most accepted hypothesis. A detailed explanation of this complex biochemical process can be found in recent reviews [50,51]. However, this hypothesis also presents caveats when exposed to in vivo biological data. Remarkably, iron-sulfur cluster deficiency is not observed in several models of frataxin deficiency, such as flies [52], patient fibroblasts [53], or rat cardiac myocytes [54]. Moreover, detailed analysis of the cellular events that are caused by frataxin deficiency in yeast, have shown that iron-sulfur deficiency is an epiphenomenon that is caused by a metabolic remodeling program activated in response to disrupted iron homeostasis [41,55]. These observations question the role of frataxin in iron-sulfur biogenesis or at least suggest the possibility of additional functions for frataxin beyond iron-sulfur biogenesis. From these observations, it also becomes obvious that frataxin is not essential for iron-sulfur biogenesis.

3.3. Control of Oxidative Stress and the Generation of Ros

One of the phenotypes most consistently observed in frataxin-deficient cells is sensitivity to oxidizing agents [56,57]. Some authors have linked such sensitivity to oxidative stress to impaired biosynthesis of iron-sulfur centers. This hypothesis suggests that a vicious cycle would be created in which the deficient formation of iron-sulfur clusters would increase mitochondrial free iron that would increase the production of reactive oxygen species (ROS) through Fenton reaction. Then, ROS would further damage iron-sulfur clusters and promote the formation of more free iron. In fact, increased presence of labile iron has been reported in frataxin deficient yeast [58], T-Rex-293 cells [40] and in a mouse model of hepatic FXN deficiency [59]. However, no differences where observed between the mitochondrial iron pools from human lymphoblasts and fibroblasts that were obtained from either controls or FRDA patients [31]. Nevertheless, some observations suggest that oxidative stress could be the cause (and not the consequence) of iron-sulfur deficiency. For instance, in fibroblasts or lymphocytes from patients [53], or in frataxin-deficient cardiac myocytes [54], oxidative stress could be observed while the activities of iron-sulfur proteins remained unaltered. Moreover, there are evidences that iron-sulfur deficiency can be modulated by oxygen concentration or antioxidant treatment. In this regard, frataxin is not required for iron-sulfur biogenesis in yeasts grown at low oxygen tensions [60,61]. In some fly models, iron-sulfur deficiency is only observed under hyperoxic conditions [52], while in other models it can be prevented by antioxidants [62].

Which could be the origin of oxidative stress? Since frataxin has the ability to bind iron, a redox active metal, and oxidize it to Fe^{3+}, it has been proposed that frataxin could prevent oxidative stress by limiting the presence of free Fe^{2+} through its binding and the subsequent controlled oxidation to Fe^{3+}. This reaction would prevent the formation of reactive oxygen species through the reaction of Fe^{2+} with oxygen [63,64]. Therefore, the vicious cycle would have its origin in free iron than would then generate oxidative stress that would damage iron-sulfur clusters and generate more free iron. Another potential source of reactive oxygen species in frataxin-deficient cells could be the OXPHOS system. In this regard, an interaction was described between frataxin and mitochondrial electron transport chain proteins [65]. Also, decreased activity of the mitochondrial electron transport chain has been observed in several biological models of frataxin deficiency [53,66,67]. Any alteration in the OXPHOS system that was caused by frataxin deficiency could increase electron leakage and thus generate ROS [68].

Rustin and collaborators observed that frataxin-deficient cells could not properly activate the NRF2 signaling pathway in response to oxidative damage and in consequence they had a deficient response to oxidative insults and hypersensitivity to oxidative stress. They hypothesized that this impairment was related to actin remodeling [69]. This phenomenon has also been described in frataxin-deficient motor neurons [70], and in the frataxin-deficient YG8R mouse model where transcriptomic analysis showed a downregulation of NRF2-dependent antioxidant enzymes [71].

4. Evidences of Iron Accumulation and Its Relation to Pathophysiology in FRDA

Iron accumulation in a frataxin deficient cell model was first described in yeast *yfh1* mutants [72]. This early observation has been subsequently confirmed by several other researchers. Using Mössbauer spectroscopic analysis, Dancis and collaborators showed that in *Dyfh1* mitochondria iron was present as amorphous nano-particles of ferric phosphate [73]. Iron accumulation is caused by increased iron uptake due to activation of the iron sensor Aft1 [58], but the mechanisms leading to such activation are not completely understood. It has been assumed that it would be caused by iron-sulfur cluster loss, as Aft1 is known to be regulated by the presence of these cofactors. However, previous research from our group using conditional Yfh1 mutants provided two observations that challenged this hypothesis: (i) activation of Aft1 was observed earlier than iron-sulfur loss [41]; and, (ii) loss of iron-sulfur containing proteins in Yfh1 deficient yeasts was not observed in *cth2* cells. Therefore iron-sulfur loss was an epiphenomenon mainly caused by Cth2, which is an Aft1 target that binds to mRNAs from iron-containing proteins and promotes its degradation [42]. Moreover, we have also observed that nitric oxide can prevent Aft1 activation in Yfh1-deficient cells, but not in cells that are deficient in iron-sulfur biogenesis [74]. This observation also indicates that in Yfh1 deficient yeast Aft1 may be activated by a mechanism different than iron-sulfur cluster deficiency. Besides yeast, iron deposits or accumulation have also been clearly observed in frataxin deficient flies [75,76] and in cardiac muscles from frataxin deficient mice [77] and FRDA patients [78]. Iron in the heart from cardiac KO conditional mouse (the MCK mutant) was found in mitochondrial aggregates 100–400 nm in diameter, markedly different from those observed for mammalian ferritin. Energy-dispersive X-ray analysis showed that, in addition to iron, phosphorus and sulfur were present in these aggregates. Mössbauer spectra also confirmed that these aggregates where different than mammalian ferritin. The absorption profile observed was consistent with paramagnetic high-spin Fe(III) [79]. These observations are consistent with those that were obtained in frataxin-deficient yeast, and suggest that iron could be in the form of ferric-phosphate nanoparticles in both models. In other tissues or mammalian cell types, iron accumulation is not consistently observed. For instance, in fibroblasts or lymphoblasts from patients, there are no evidences of iron accumulation [31], while some authors have observed it in the nervous system [80]. Changes in the iron-responsive proteins, ferritin, divalent metal transporter 1 (DMT1), transferrin receptor 1 (TfR1), and ferroportin have been reported in the dentate nucleus of affected individuals [81]. Similar to yeast, iron deregulation in mammals might be caused by Iron-responding protein 1 (IRP1) activation [82,83], but the mechanisms causing this activation are not completely understood. It could be caused by deficiencies in iron supply to mitochondrial iron-dependent pathways that would activate the mechanisms of response to iron deficiency [59]. Frataxin has also been shown to interact with IRP1 and modulate the switch between its aconitase and RNA-binding forms. This function would be carried on by a cytosolic form of frataxin [84]. However, some authors are skeptical about the existence of an extra mitochondrial form of frataxin, and therefore question the physiological relevance of the observed interaction between IRP1 and frataxin.

As indicated above, many evidences support that frataxin deficiency causes a dysregulation in iron homeostasis, and it has also been shown in several models that the modulation of iron homeostasis ameliorates several phenotypes caused by frataxin deficiency [74,85]. However, the contribution of iron accumulation to the pathophysiology of FRDA has not been clearly determined. In this regard, several hypotheses have been formulated. It has been proposed that iron accumulation would be toxic and could be contributing to the formation of reactive oxygen species through the Fenton reaction. Iron overload could be also inducing the synthesis of sphingolipids, which, through the Pdk1/Mef2 pathway, would trigger neurodegeneration [76,80]. Iron toxicity could be also related to the formation of iron-phosphate aggregates that would compromise phosphate availability [86]. Nevertheless, it has also been suggested that iron accumulation would not be toxic per se, and that pathological consequences of frataxin deficiency would be mostly related to deficient iron supply to iron-dependent proteins. In this regard, it has been shown that IRP1 activation has a protective effect in a mouse model of hepatic FXN deficiency, as it contributes to sustain mitochondrial iron needs and mitochondrial function in these mice [59]. It has also been observed that dietary iron supplementation limits cardiac hypertrophy in MCK mutant mice [79].

These contradictory observations suggest that the pathological mechanisms could be more complex and specific for different models and tissues. For instance, in yeast, we have observed that activation of Aft1 causes the overexpression of Cth2, an mRNA binding protein that downregulates the expression of most iron-binding proteins that are required for aerobic growth. Thus, the activation of such pathway has a strong contribution to the alterations observed in yeast [42]. Beyond yeast, there are several evidences that frataxin deficiency may be causing perturbations in signaling pathways that could contribute to pathology. For instance, as mentioned before, neurodegeneration has been linked to the activation of the Pdk1/Mef2 pathway [76,80]. Cardiac hypertrophy could be related to the activation of the NFAT/calcineurin pathway, which has been observed in rat frataxin deficient cardiac myocytes [87]. Therefore, pathophysiology could be related to the pathways activated in different cells and tissues in response to the perturbations caused by frataxin deficiency.

Besides iron, some authors have reported deregulation of the homeostasis of other metals as a consequence of frataxin deficiency. In frataxin deficient yeast, we observed a decrease in manganese content and limited copper availability [58,88]. Subsequent studies using a conditional frataxin mutant indicated that manganese deficiency was caused by downregulation of Smf2, a Mn transporter that was degraded in response to iron accumulation [41]. In frataxin deficient flies it was found that the levels of zinc, copper, and manganese were increased, and that copper and zinc chelation improved the impaired motor performance of these flies [89]. In Dorsal Root Ganglia from FRDA patients, zinc and iron related proteins displayed major shifts in their cellular localization [90]. Alterations in calcium homeostasis have also been reported in several models of FRDA [87,91]. These alterations are mostly considered to be consequences of the deregulation of iron homeostasis, which may impact other metals. Nevertheless, frataxin is known to have also the capacity to chelate metals that are different than iron, such as manganese or copper [92]. The biological significance of these interactions has not been explored yet.

5. Targeting Iron as a Therapeutic Approach in FRDA

There is currently no cure for FRDA but several therapeutic approaches are being investigated. Some drugs have already entered clinical trials. Briefly, therapeutic approaches can be divided into compounds that improve mitochondrial function and reduce oxidative stress, drugs that modulate the altered metabolic pathways, and strategies to increase the expression or content of frataxin, either by promoting its expression, by supplying it through gene therapy (reviewed in [93]) or by protein replacement strategies [94].

Due to the alterations that were observed in iron homeostasis in different models and patients of FRDA, the use of iron chelators as a treatment to eliminate the excess iron accumulating in mitochondria was proposed many years ago. Deferoxamine was not considered to be a suitable iron chelator for depleting the intracellular iron deposits found in FRDA, as it does not cross the blood brain barrier and poorly penetrates biological membranes. It also has a high affinity for iron, which could compromise iron availability. The proposed alternative was deferiprone, an orally administered, lipidsoluble iron chelator that had been previously used to treat iron overload in polytransfused individuals with hemoglobinopathies. This compound can easily cross the blood–brain barrier and cellular membranes and therefore reach intracellular (or mitochondrial) iron deposits. In addition, since its affinity for iron is lower than that of transferrin, it has been shown that it can redistribute iron from intracellular iron deposits to this protein [95]. Indeed, the cellular properties that are affected by frataxin deficiency in HEK-293 cells were corrected by deferiprone treatment [96].

Several clinical trials have been performed with deferiprone in FRDA patients. In summary, these studies suggested that low doses of deferiprone would be beneficial on cardiac parameters. Higher doses of the drug worsened the condition and could result in agranulocytosis (reviewed in [97]). We can speculate that this dose dependent effect could be a consequence of different pathological mechanisms that are exerted by frataxin deficiency. Some of them would be caused by iron accumulation, while others would be caused by deficient iron availability. Therefore, low doses of the chelator would partially prevent the toxic effects that are caused by iron accumulation, while higher doses of deferiprone would compromise iron availability, and therefore worsen those pathological conditions caused by inefficient iron availability. Nevertheless, it has been proposed that deferiprone at low doses could be combined with other drugs. A pilot study with five FRDA patients suggested that combined therapy of deferiprone and idebenone (a Q10 analogue) was relatively safe and it could provide some benefits on neurological function and heart hypertrophy [98].

6. Concluding Remarks

Many evidences indicate that the lack of frataxin leads to alterations in iron cellular homeostasis. However, the precise mechanism(s) causing iron deregulation in frataxin-deficient cells are not completely understood. Several hypotheses have been formulated, but although most of them are well supported by in vitro data, all of them present caveats when exposed to biological data. In Figure 2, we have summarized two potential mechanisms which in our opinion could explain iron accumulation and oxidative stress: (1) the iron-sulfur hypothesis proposes that frataxin contributes to iron-sulfur biogenesis and its deficiency activates cellular iron sensors that would promote iron uptake; and, (2) the iron toxicity hypothesis assumes that frataxin would be involved in controlled iron ferrooxidation, and its deficiency would lead to ROS generation and the increased formation of ferric-phosphate nanoparticles. The iron-sulfur hypothesis is well supported by in vitro data, but its major caveat is the absence of iron-sulfur deficiency in many models of frataxin deficiency. On the other hand, the iron toxicity hypothesis does not provide a clear explanation for the activation of iron sensors.

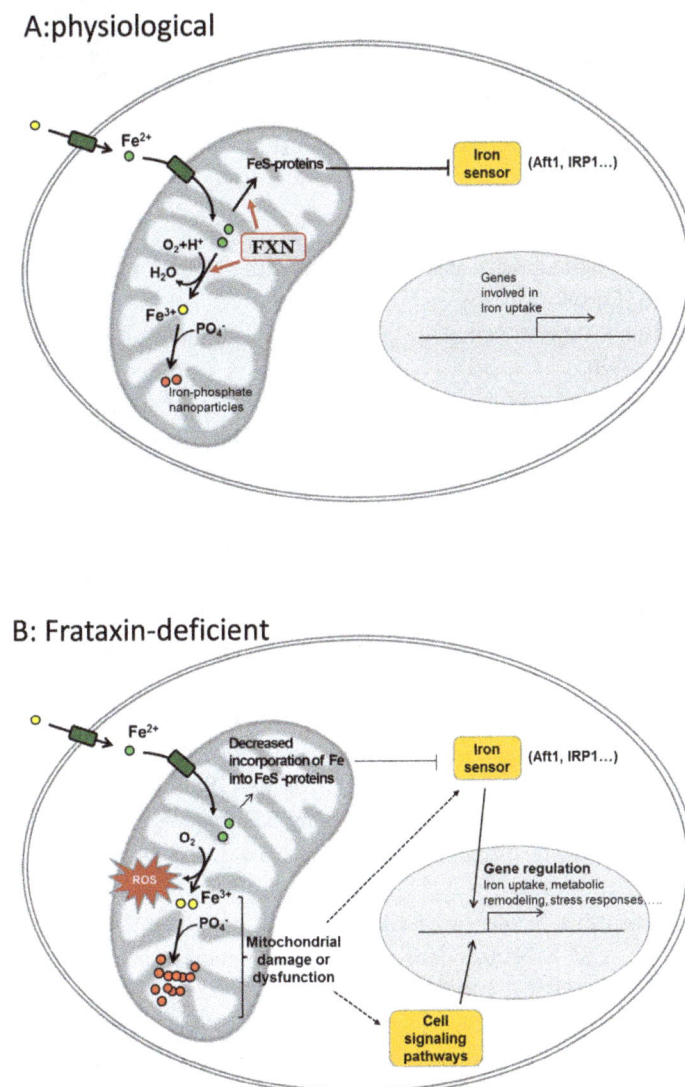

Figure 2. Potential contribution of frataxin to iron homeostasis and cellular consequences of its deficiency. (**A**), physiological: frataxin (FXN) binds Fe^{2+} and contributes to its controlled oxidation to

Fe^{3+} and/or to incorporate it into Fe-containing proteins. These Fe-containing proteins (notably FeS proteins) keep the iron sensor inactive and genes involved in iron uptake are not expressed. Oxidized iron (Fe^{3+}) is stored in the form of ferric-phosphate nanoparticles. (**B**), frataxin-deficient: loss of frataxin leads to decreased incorporation of iron into Fe-proteins and/or uncontrolled oxidation of Fe^{2+} by O_2. Such events lead to reactive oxygen species (ROS) generation, decreased phosphate availability, and mitochondrial dysfunction. Iron sensors and other cell signaling pathways are activated and regulate the expression of genes involved in iron uptake and/or other cell-specific pathways involved on metabolic remodeling, hypertrophy or neurodegeneration.

Also, it is not clear the contribution of iron to FRDA pathology, which could be related either to iron accumulation or to limited iron availability. Indeed, iron homeostasis deregulation could be an epiphenomenon that is not linked to pathology. In fact, many evidences suggest that the mechanisms causing cellular dysfunction could be tissue or model specific. They could also be related to the signaling pathways activated in response to the alterations that are caused by frataxin deficiency. This complexity may explain the limited effects of iron chelators on clinical trials, as these compounds would only prevent certain pathological mechanisms in a limited number of tissues.

Funding: This work has been supported by grant SAF2017-83883-R from Ministerio de Economia Industria y Competitividad (Spain).

Acknowledgments: Molecular graphics and analyses were performed with the UCSF Chimera package. Chimera is developed by the Resource for Biocomputing, Visualization, and Informatics at the University of California, San Francisco (supported by NIGMS P41-GM103311).

Conflicts of Interest: The authors declare no conflict of interest.

References

1. Ashby, D.W.; Tweedy, P.S. Friedreich's ataxia combined with diabetes mellitus in sisters. *Br. Med. J.* **1953**, *1*, 1418–1421. [CrossRef] [PubMed]

2. Koeppen, A.H. Friedreich's ataxia: Pathology, pathogenesis, and molecular genetics. *J. Neurol. Sci.* **2011**, *303*, 1–12. [CrossRef] [PubMed]

3. Campuzano, V.; Montermini, L.; Molto, M.D.; Pianese, L.; Cossee, M.; Cavalcanti, F.; Monros, E.; Rodius, F.; Duclos, F.; Monticelli, A.; et al. Friedreich's ataxia: Autosomal recessive disease caused by an intronic GAA triplet repeat expansion. *Science* **1996**, *271*, 1423–1427. [CrossRef] [PubMed]

4. Campuzano, V.; Montermini, L.; Lutz, Y.; Cova, L.; Hindelang, C.; Jiralerspong, S.; Trottier, Y.; Kish, S.J.; Faucheux, B.; Trouillas, P.; et al. Frataxin is Reduced in Friedreich Ataxia Patients and is Associated with Mitochondrial Membranes. *Hum. Mol. Genet.* **1997**, *6*, 1771–1780. [CrossRef] [PubMed]

5. Filla, A.; De Michele, G.; Cavalcanti, F.; Pianese, L.; Monticelli, A.; Campanella, G.; Cocozza, S. The relationship between trinucleotide (GAA) repeat length and clinical features in Friedreich ataxia. *Am. J. Hum. Genet.* **1996**, *59*, 554–560. [PubMed]

6. Isnard, R.; Kalotka, H.; Dürr, A.; Cossée, M.; Schmitt, M.; Pousset, F.; Thomas, D.; Brice, A.; Koenig, M.; Komajda, M. Correlation between left ventricular hypertrophy and GAA trinucleotide repeat length in Friedreich's ataxia. *Circulation* **1997**, *95*, 2247–2249. [CrossRef] [PubMed]

7. McDaniel, D.O.; Keats, B.; Vedanarayanan, V.; Subramony, S.H. Sequence variation in GAA repeat expansions may cause differential phenotype display in Friedreich's ataxia. *Mov. Disord.* **2001**, *16*, 1153–1158. [CrossRef] [PubMed]

8. Evans-Galea, M.V.; Carrodus, N.; Rowley, S.M.; Corben, L.A.; Tai, G.; Saffery, R.; Galati, J.C.; Wong, N.C.; Craig, J.M.; Lynch, D.R.; et al. FXN methylation predicts expression and clinical outcome in Friedreich ataxia. *Ann. Neurol.* **2012**, *71*, 487–497. [CrossRef] [PubMed]

9. Galea, C.A.; Huq, A.; Lockhart, P.J.; Tai, G.; Corben, L.A.; Yiu, E.M.; Gurrin, L.C.; Lynch, D.R.; Gelbard, S.; Durr, A.; et al. Compound heterozygous *FXN* mutations and clinical outcome in friedreich ataxia. *Ann. Neurol.* **2016**, *79*, 485–495. [CrossRef] [PubMed]

10. Adinolfi, S.; Nair, M.; Politou, A.; Bayer, E.; Martin, S.; Temussi, P.; Pastore, A. The factors governing the thermal stability of frataxin orthologues: How to increase a protein's stability. *Biochemistry* **2004**, *43*, 6511–6518. [CrossRef] [PubMed]

11. Pettersen, E.F.; Goddard, T.D.; Huang, C.C.; Couch, G.S.; Greenblatt, D.M.; Meng, E.C.; Ferrin, T.E. UCSF Chimera—A visualization system for exploratory research and analysis. *J. Comput. Chem.* **2004**, *25*, 1605–1612. [CrossRef] [PubMed]

12. Koutnikova, H.; Campuzano, V.; Koenig, M. Maturation of wild-type and mutated frataxin by the mitochondrial processing peptidase. *Hum. Mol. Genet.* **1998**, *7*, 1485–1489. [CrossRef] [PubMed]

13. Branda, S.S.; Cavadini, P.; Adamec, J.; Kalousek, F.; Taroni, F.; Isaya, G. Yeast and human frataxin are processed to mature form in two sequential steps by the mitochondrial processing peptidase. *J. Biol. Chem.* **1999**, *274*, 22763–22769. [CrossRef] [PubMed]

14. Condò, I.; Ventura, N.; Malisan, F.; Rufini, A.; Tomassini, B.; Testi, R. In vivo maturation of human frataxin. *Hum. Mol. Genet.* **2007**, *16*, 1534–1540. [CrossRef] [PubMed]

15. Schmucker, S.; Argentini, M.; Carelle-Calmels, N.; Martelli, A.; Puccio, H. The in vivo mitochondrial two-step maturation of human frataxin. *Hum. Mol. Genet.* **2008**, *17*, 3521–3531. [CrossRef] [PubMed]

16. Gakh, O.; Bedekovics, T.; Duncan, S.F.; Smith, D.Y.; Berkholz, D.S.; Isaya, G. Normal and Friedreich ataxia cells express different isoforms of frataxin with complementary roles in iron-sulfur cluster assembly. *J. Biol. Chem.* **2010**, *285*, 38486–38501. [CrossRef] [PubMed]

17. Cavadini, P.; Adamec, J.; Taroni, F.; Gakh, O.; Isaya, G. Two-step Processing of Human Frataxin by Mitochondrial Processing Peptidase. *J. Biol. Chem.* **2000**, *275*, 41469–41475. [CrossRef] [PubMed]

18. Xia, H.; Cao, Y.; Dai, X.; Marelja, Z.; Zhou, D.; Mo, R.; Al-Mahdawi, S.; Pook, M.A.; Leimkühler, S.; Rouault, T.A.; et al. Novel frataxin isoforms may contribute to the pathological mechanism of Friedreich ataxia. *PLoS ONE* **2012**, *7*, e47847. [CrossRef] [PubMed]

19. Pastore, A.; Puccio, H. Frataxin: A protein in search for a function. *J. Neurochem.* **2013**, *126*, 43–52. [CrossRef] [PubMed]

20. Yoon, T.; Cowan, J.A. Iron−Sulfur Cluster Biosynthesis. Characterization of Frataxin as an Iron Donor for Assembly of [2Fe−2S] Clusters in ISU-Type Proteins. *J. Am. Chem. Soc.* **2003**, *125*, 6078–6084. [CrossRef] [PubMed]

21. Gentry, L.E.; Thacker, M.A.; Doughty, R.; Timkovich, R.; Busenlehner, L.S. His86 from the N-Terminus of Frataxin Coordinates Iron and Is Required for Fe-S Cluster Synthesis. *Biochemistry* **2013**, *52*, 6085–6096. [CrossRef] [PubMed]

22. Cai, K.; Frederick, R.O.; Tonelli, M.; Markley, J.L. Interactions of iron-bound frataxin with ISCU and ferredoxin on the cysteine desulfurase complex leading to Fe-S cluster assembly. *J. Inorg. Biochem.* **2018**, *183*, 107–116. [CrossRef] [PubMed]

23. Adamec, J.; Rusnak, F.; Owen, W.G.; Naylor, S.; Benson, L.M.; Gacy, M.; Isaya, G. Iron-dependent self-assembly of recombinant yeast frataxin: Implications for Friedreich ataxia. *Am. J. Hum. Genet.* **2000**, *67*, 549–562. [CrossRef] [PubMed]

24. Cavadini, P.; O'Neill, H.A.; Benada, O.; Isaya, G. Assembly and iron-binding properties of human frataxin, the protein deficient in Friedreich ataxia. *Hum. Mol. Genet.* **2002**, *11*, 217–227. [CrossRef] [PubMed]

25. Schagerlof, U.; Elmlund, H.; Gakh, O.; Nordlund, G.; Hebert, H.; Lindahl, M.; Isaya, G.; Al-Karadaghi, S. Structural basis of the iron storage function of frataxin from single-particle reconstruction of the iron-loaded oligomer. *Biochemistry* **2008**, *47*, 4948–4954. [CrossRef] [PubMed]

26. Campanella, A.; Isaya, G.; O'Neill, H.A.; Santambrogio, P.; Cozzi, A.; Arosio, P.; Levi, S. The expression of human mitochondrial ferritin rescues respiratory function in frataxin-deficient yeast. *Hum. Mol. Genet.* **2004**, *13*, 2279–2288. [CrossRef] [PubMed]

27. Adinolfi, S.; Trifuoggi, M.; Politou, A.S.; Martin, S.; Pastore, A. A structural approach to understanding the iron-binding properties of phylogenetically different frataxins. *Hum. Mol. Genet.* **2002**, *11*, 1865–1877. [CrossRef] [PubMed]

28. Desiere, F.; Deutsch, E.W.; King, N.L.; Nesvizhskii, A.I.; Mallick, P.; Eng, J.; Chen, S.; Eddes, J.; Loevenich, S.N.; Aebersold, R. The PeptideAtlas project. *Nucleic Acids Res.* **2006**, *34*, D655–D658. [CrossRef] [PubMed]

29. Ahlgren, E.C.; Fekry, M.; Wiemann, M.; Söderberg, C.A.; Bernfur, K.; Gakh, O.; Rasmussen, M.; Højrup, P.; Emanuelsson, C.; Isaya, G.; et al. Iron-induced oligomerization of human FXN81-210 and bacterial CyaY frataxin and the effect of iron chelators. *PLoS ONE* **2017**, *12*, e0188937. [CrossRef] [PubMed]

30. Seguin, A.; Sutak, R.; Bulteau, A.L.; Garcia-Serres, R.; Oddou, J.L.; Lefevre, S.; Santos, R.; Dancis, A.; Camadro, J.; Latour, J.; et al. Evidence that yeast frataxin is not an iron storage protein in vivo. *Biochim. Biophys. Acta-Mol. Basis Dis.* **2010**, *1802*, 531–538. [CrossRef] [PubMed]

31. Sturm, B.; Bistrich, U.; Schranzhofer, M.; Sarsero, J.P.; Rauen, U.; Scheiber-mojdehkar, B.; de Groot, H.; Ioannou, P.; Petrat, F. Friedreich's Ataxia, No Changes in Mitochondrial Labile Iron in Human Lymphoblasts and Fibroblasts A Decrease in Antioxidative Capacity? *J. Biol. Chem.* **2004**, *280*, 6701–6708. [CrossRef] [PubMed]

32. Lindahl, P.A.; Moore, M.J. Labile Low-Molecular-Mass Metal Complexes in Mitochondria: Trials and Tribulations of a Burgeoning Field. *Biochemistry* **2016**, *55*, 4140–4153. [CrossRef] [PubMed]

33. Garber-Morales, J.; Holmes-Hampton, G.P.; Miao, R.; Guo, Y.; Münck, E.; Lindahl, P.A. Biophysical characterization of iron in mitochondria isolated from respiring and fermenting yeast. *Biochemistry* **2010**, *49*, 5436–5444. [CrossRef] [PubMed]

34. Park, S.; Gakh, O.; O'Neill, H.; Mangravita, A.; Nichol, H.; Ferreira, G.C.; Isaya, G. Yeast frataxin sequentially chaperones and stores iron by coupling protein assembly with iron oxidation. *J. Biol. Chem.* **2003**, *278*, 31340–31351. [CrossRef] [PubMed]

35. Wang, M.; Herrmann, C.J.; Simonovic, M.; Szklarczyk, D.; von Mering, C. Version 4.0 of PaxDb: Protein abundance data, integrated across model organisms, tissues, and cell-lines. *Proteomics* **2015**, *15*, 3163–3168. [CrossRef] [PubMed]

36. Yoon, T.; Cowan, J.A. Frataxin-mediated iron delivery to ferrochelatase in the final step of heme biosynthesis. *J. Biol. Chem.* **2004**, *279*, 25943–25946. [CrossRef] [PubMed]

37. He, Y.; Alam, S.L.; Proteasa, S.V.; Zhang, Y.; Lesuisse, E.; Dancis, A.; Stemmler, T.L. Yeast frataxin solution structure, iron binding, and ferrochelatase interaction. *Biochemistry* **2004**, *43*, 16254–16262. [CrossRef] [PubMed]

38. Soderberg, C.G.; Gillam, M.E.; Ahlgren, E.C.; Hunter, G.A.; Gakh, O.; Isaya, G.; Ferreira, G.C.; Al-Karadaghi, S. The Structure of the Complex between Yeast Frataxin and Ferrochelatase: Characterization and pre-Steady State Reaction of Ferrous Iron Delivery and Heme Synthesis. *J. Biol. Chem.* **2016**, *291*, 11887–11898. [CrossRef] [PubMed]

39. Steinkellner, H.; Singh, H.N.; Muckenthaler, M.U.; Goldenberg, H.; Moganty, R.R.; Scheiber-Mojdehkar, B.; Sturm, B. No changes in heme synthesis in human Friedreich's ataxia erythroid progenitor cells. *Gene* **2017**, *621*, 5–11. [CrossRef] [PubMed]

40. Lu, C.; Cortopassi, G. Frataxin knockdown causes loss of cytoplasmic iron-sulfur cluster functions, redox alterations and induction of heme transcripts. *Arch. Biochem. Biophys.* **2007**, *457*, 111–122. [CrossRef] [PubMed]

41. Moreno-Cermeno, A.; Obis, E.; Belli, G.; Cabiscol, E.; Ros, J.; Tamarit, J. Frataxin Depletion in Yeast Triggers Up-regulation of Iron Transport Systems before Affecting Iron-Sulfur Enzyme Activities. *J. Biol. Chem.* **2010**, *285*, 41653–41664. [CrossRef] [PubMed]

42. Moreno-Cermeno, A.; Alsina, D.; Cabiscol, E.; Tamarit, J.; Ros, J. Metabolic remodeling in frataxin-deficient yeast is mediated by Cth2 and Adr1. *Biochim. Biophys. Acta* **2013**, *1833*, 3326–3337. [CrossRef] [PubMed]

43. Schmucker, S.; Martelli, A.; Colin, F.; Page, A.; Wattenhofer-Donze, M.; Reutenauer, L.; Puccio, H. Mammalian Frataxin: An Essential Function for Cellular Viability through an Interaction with a Preformed ISCU/NFS1/ISD11 Iron-Sulfur Assembly Complex. *PLoS ONE* **2011**, *6*, e16199. [CrossRef] [PubMed]

44. Wang, T.; Craig, E.A. Binding of yeast frataxin to the scaffold for Fe-S cluster biogenesis. *J. Biol. Chem.* **2008**, *283*, 12674–12679. [CrossRef] [PubMed]

45. Gerber, J.; Muhlenhoff, U.; Lill, R. An interaction between frataxin and Isu1/Nfs1 that is crucial for Fe/S cluster synthesis on Isu1. *EMBO Rep.* **2003**, *4*, 906–911. [CrossRef] [PubMed]

46. Adinolfi, S.; Iannuzzi, C.; Prischi, F.; Pastore, C.; Iametti, S.; Martin, S.R.; Bonomi, F.; Pastore, A. Bacterial frataxin CyaY is the gatekeeper of iron-sulfur cluster formation catalyzed by IscS. *Nat. Struct. Mol. Biol.* **2009**, *16*, 390–396. [CrossRef] [PubMed]

47. Bridwell-Rabb, J.; Fox, N.G.; Tsai, C.L.; Winn, A.M.; Barondeau, D.P. Human frataxin activates Fe-S cluster biosynthesis by facilitating sulfur transfer chemistry. *Biochemistry* **2014**, *53*, 4904–4913. [CrossRef] [PubMed]

48. Tsai, C.L.; Barondeau, D.P. Human frataxin is an allosteric switch that activates the Fe-S cluster biosynthetic complex. *Biochemistry* **2010**, *49*, 9132–9139. [CrossRef] [PubMed]

49. Parent, A.; Elduque, X.; Cornu, D.; Belot, L.; Le Caer, J.P.; Grandas, A.; Toledano, M.B.; D'Autréaux, B. Mammalian frataxin directly enhances sulfur transfer of NFS1 persulfide to both ISCU and free thiols. *Nat. Commun.* **2015**, *6*, 5686. [CrossRef] [PubMed]

50. Rouault, T.A.; Maio, N. Biogenesis and functions of mammalian iron-sulfur proteins in the regulation of iron homeostasis and pivotal metabolic pathways. *J. Biol. Chem.* **2017**, *292*, 12744–12753. [CrossRef] [PubMed]

51. Braymer, J.J.; Lill, R. Iron-sulfur cluster biogenesis and trafficking in mitochondria. *J. Biol. Chem.* **2017**, *292*, 12754–12763. [CrossRef] [PubMed]

52. Llorens, J.; Navarro, J.; Martínez-Sebastián, M.J.; Baylies, M.K.; Schneuwly, S.; Botella, J.; Moltó, M.D. Causative role of oxidative stress in a Drosophila model of Friedreich ataxia. *FASEB J.* **2007**, *21*, 333–344. [CrossRef] [PubMed]

53. Rötig, A.; de Lonlay, P.; Chretien, D.; Foury, F.; Koenig, M.; Sidi, D.; Munnich, A.; Rustin, P. Aconitase and mitochondrial iron-sulphur protein deficiency in Friedreich ataxia. *Nat. Genet.* **1997**, *17*, 215–217. [CrossRef] [PubMed]

54. Obis, È.; Irazusta, V.; Sanchís, D.; Ros, J.; Tamarit, J. Frataxin deficiency in neonatal rat ventricular myocytes targets mitochondria and lipid metabolism. *Free Radic. Biol. Med.* **2014**, *73*, 21–33. [CrossRef] [PubMed]

55. Gabrielli, N.; Ayte, J.; Hidalgo, E. Cells lacking pfh1, a fission yeast homolog of Mammalian frataxin protein, display constitutive activation of the iron starvation response. *J. Biol. Chem.* **2012**, *287*, 43042–43051. [CrossRef] [PubMed]

56. Tamarit, J.; Obis, È.; Ros, J. Oxidative stress and altered lipid metabolism in Friedreich ataxia. *Free Radic. Biol. Med.* **2016**, *100*, 138–146. [CrossRef] [PubMed]

57. Bayot, A.; Santos, R.; Camadro, J.M.; Rustin, P. Friedreich's ataxia: The vicious circle hypothesis revisited. *BMC Med.* **2011**, *9*, 112–119. [CrossRef] [PubMed]

58. Irazusta, V.; Obis, E.; Moreno-Cermeño, A.; Cabiscol, E.; Ros, J.; Tamarit, J. Yeast frataxin mutants display decreased superoxide dismutase activity crucial to promote protein oxidative damage. *Free Radic. Biol. Med.* **2010**, *48*, 411–420. [CrossRef] [PubMed]

59. Martelli, A.; Schmucker, S.; Reutenauer, L.; Mathieu, J.R.R.; Peyssonnaux, C.; Karim, Z.; Puy, H.; Galy, B.; Hentze, M.W.; Puccio, H. Iron Regulatory Protein 1 Sustains Mitochondrial Iron Loading and Function in Frataxin Deficiency. *Cell Metab.* **2015**, *21*, 311–322. [CrossRef] [PubMed]

60. Bulteau, A.L.; Dancis, A.; Gareil, M.; Montagne, J.J.; Camadro, J.M.; Lesuisse, E. Oxidative stress and protease dysfunction in the yeast model of Friedreich ataxia. *Free Radic. Biol. Med.* **2007**, *42*, 1561–1570. [CrossRef] [PubMed]

61. Gibson, T.J.; Koonin, E.; Musco, G.; Pastore, A.; Bork, P. Friedreich's ataxia protein: Phylogenetic evidence for mitochondrial dysfunction. *Trends Neurosci.* **1996**, *19*, 465–468. [CrossRef]

62. Anderson, P.R.; Kirby, K.; Orr, W.C.; Hilliker, A.J.; Phillips, J.P. Hydrogen peroxide scavenging rescues frataxin deficiency in a Drosophila model of Friedreich's ataxia. *Proc. Natl. Acad. Sci. USA* **2008**, *105*, 611–616. [CrossRef] [PubMed]

63. O'Neill, H.A.; Gakh, O.; Park, S.; Cui, J.; Mooney, S.M.; Sampson, M.; Ferreira, G.C.; Isaya, G. Assembly of human frataxin is a mechanism for detoxifying redox-active iron. *Biochemistry* **2005**, *44*, 537–545. [CrossRef] [PubMed]

64. Gakh, O.; Park, S.; Liu, G.; Macomber, L.; Imlay, J.A.; Ferreira, G.C.; Isaya, G. Mitochondrial iron detoxification is a primary function of frataxin that limits oxidative damage and preserves cell longevity. *Hum. Mol. Genet.* **2006**, *15*, 467–479. [CrossRef] [PubMed]

65. Gonzalez-Cabo, P.; Vazquez-Manrique, R.P.; Garcia-Gimeno, M.A.; Sanz, P.; Palau, F. Frataxin interacts functionally with mitochondrial electron transport chain proteins. *Hum. Mol. Genet.* **2005**, *14*, 2091–2098. [CrossRef] [PubMed]

66. Koutnikova, H.; Campuzano, V.; Foury, F.; Dolle, P.; Cazzalini, O.; Koenig, M. Studies of human, mouse and yeast homologues indicate a mitochondrial function for frataxin. *Nat. Genet.* **1997**, *16*, 345–351. [CrossRef] [PubMed]

67. Lodi, R.; Rajagopalan, B.; Blamire, A.M.; Cooper, J.M.; Davies, C.H.; Bradley, J.L.; Styles, P.; Schapira, A. Cardiac energetics are abnormal in Friedreich ataxia patients in the absence of cardiac dysfunction and hypertrophy: An in vivo 31P magnetic resonance spectroscopy study. *Cardiovasc. Res.* **2001**, *52*, 111–119. [CrossRef]

68. Armstrong, J.S.; Khdour, O.; Hecht, S.M. Does oxidative stress contribute to the pathology of Friedreich's ataxia? A radical question. *FASEB J.* **2010**, *24*, 2152–2163. [CrossRef] [PubMed]

69. Paupe, V.; Dassa, E.P.; Goncalves, S.; Auchere, F.; Lonn, M.; Holmgren, A.; Rustin, P. Impaired nuclear Nrf2 translocation undermines the oxidative stress response in Friedreich ataxia. *PLoS ONE* **2009**, *4*, e4253. [CrossRef] [PubMed]

70. D'Oria, V.; Petrini, S.; Travaglini, L.; Priori, C.; Piermarini, E.; Petrillo, S.; Carletti, B.; Bertini, E.; Piemonte, F. Frataxin deficiency leads to reduced expression and impaired translocation of NF-E2-related factor (Nrf2) in cultured motor neurons. *Int. J. Mol. Sci.* **2013**, *14*, 7853–7865. [CrossRef] [PubMed]

71. Shan, Y.; Schoenfeld, R.A.; Hayashi, G.; Napoli, E.; Akiyama, T.; Carstens, M.; Carstens, E.E.; Pook, M.A.; Cortopassi, G.A. Frataxin deficiency leads to defects in expression of antioxidants and Nrf2 expression in dorsal root ganglia of the Friedreich's ataxia YG8R mouse model. *Antioxid. Redox Signal.* **2013**, *19*, 1481–1493. [CrossRef] [PubMed]

72. Babcock, M.; de Silva, D.; Oaks, R.; Davis-Kaplan, S.; Jiralerspong, S.; Montermini, L.; Pandolfo, M.; Kaplan, J. Regulation of mitochondrial iron accumulation by Yfh1p, a putative homolog of frataxin. *Science* **1997**, *276*, 1709–1712. [CrossRef] [PubMed]

73. Lesuisse, E.; Santos, R.; Matzanke, B.F.; Knight, S.A.B.; Camadro, J.M.; Dancis, A. Iron use for haeme synthesis is under control of the yeast frataxin homologue (Yfh1). *Hum. Mol. Genet.* **2003**, *12*, 879–889. [CrossRef] [PubMed]

74. Alsina, D.; Ros, J.; Tamarit, J. Nitric oxide prevents Aft1 activation and metabolic remodeling in frataxin-deficient yeast. *Redox Biol.* **2018**, *14*, 131–141. [CrossRef] [PubMed]

75. Soriano, S.; Llorens, J.V.; Blanco-Sobero, L.; Gutiérrez, L.; Calap-Quintana, P.; Morales, M.P.; Moltó, M.D.; Martínez-Sebastián, M.J. Deferiprone and idebenone rescue frataxin depletion phenotypes in a Drosophila model of Friedreich's ataxia. *Gene* **2013**, *521*, 274–281. [CrossRef] [PubMed]

76. Chen, K.; Lin, G.; Haelterman, N.A.; Ho, T.S.Y.; Li, T.; Li, Z.; Duraine, L.; Graham, B.H.; Jaiswal, M.; Yamamoto, S.; et al. Loss of Frataxin induces iron toxicity, sphingolipid synthesis, and Pdk1/Mef2 activation, leading to neurodegeneration. *Elife* **2016**, *5*, e16043. [CrossRef] [PubMed]

77. Whitnall, M.; Rahmanto, Y.S.; Sutak, R.; Xu, X.; Becker, E.M.; Mikhael, M.R.; Ponka, P.; Richardson, D.R. The MCK mouse heart model of Friedreich's ataxia: Alterations in iron-regulated proteins and cardiac hypertrophy are limited by iron chelation. *Proc. Natl. Acad. Sci. USA* **2008**, *105*, 9757–9762. [CrossRef] [PubMed]

78. Ramirez, R.L.; Qian, J.; Santambrogio, P.; Levi, S.; Koeppen, A.H. Relation of Cytosolic Iron Excess to Cardiomyopathy of Friedreich's Ataxia. *Am. J. Cardiol.* **2012**, *110*, 1820–1827. [CrossRef] [PubMed]

79. Whitnall, M.; Rahmanto, Y.S.; Huang, M.L.H.; Saletta, F.; Lok, H.C.; Gutierrez, L.; Lázaro, F.J.; Fleming, A.J.; St. Pierre, T.G.; Mikhael, M.R.; et al. Identification of nonferritin mitochondrial iron deposits in a mouse model of Friedreich ataxia. *Proc. Natl. Acad. Sci. USA* **2012**, *109*, 20590–20595. [CrossRef] [PubMed]

80. Chen, K.; Ho, T.S.Y.; Lin, G.; Tan, K.L.; Rasband, M.N.; Bellen, H.J. Loss of Frataxin activates the iron/sphingolipid/PDK1/Mef2 pathway in mammals. *Elife* **2016**, *5*, e20732. [CrossRef] [PubMed]

81. Koeppen, A.H.; Michael, S.C.; Knutson, M.D.; Haile, D.J.; Qian, J.; Levi, S.; Santambrogio, P.; Garrick, M.D.; Lamarche, J.B. The dentate nucleus in Friedreich's ataxia: The role of iron-responsive proteins. *Acta Neuropathol.* **2007**, *114*, 163–173. [CrossRef] [PubMed]

82. Seznec, H.; Simon, D.; Monassier, L.; Criqui-Filipe, P.; Gansmuller, A.; Rustin, P.; Koenig, M.; Puccio, H. Idebenone delays the onset of cardiac functional alteration without correction of Fe-S enzymes deficit in a mouse model for Friedreich ataxia. *Hum. Mol. Genet.* **2004**, *13*, 1017–1024. [CrossRef] [PubMed]

83. Stehling, O.; Elsässer, H.P.; Brückel, B.; Mühlenhoff, U.; Lill, R. Iron-sulfur protein maturation in human cells: Evidence for a function of frataxin. *Hum. Mol. Genet.* **2004**, *13*, 3007–3015. [CrossRef] [PubMed]

84. Condò, I.; Malisan, F.; Guccini, I.; Serio, D.; Rufini, A.; Testi, R. Molecular control of the cytosolic aconitase/IRP1 switch by extramitochondrial frataxin. *Hum. Mol. Genet.* **2010**, *19*, 1221–1229. [CrossRef] [PubMed]

85. Navarro, J.A.; Botella, J.A.; Metzendorf, C.; Lind, M.I.; Schneuwly, S. Mitoferrin modulates iron toxicity in a Drosophila model of Friedreich's ataxia. *Free Radic. Biol. Med.* **2015**, *85*, 71–82. [CrossRef] [PubMed]

86. Seguin, A.; Santos, R.; Pain, D.; Dancis, A.; Camadro, J.M.; Lesuisse, E. Co-precipitation of phosphate and iron limits mitochondrial phosphate availability in Saccharomyces cerevisiae lacking the yeast frataxin homologue (YFH1). *J. Biol. Chem.* **2011**, *286*, 6071–6079. [CrossRef] [PubMed]

87. Purroy, R.; Britti, E.; Delaspre, F.; Tamarit, J.; Ros, J. Mitochondrial pore opening and loss of Ca^{2+} exchanger NCLX levels occur after frataxin depletion. *Biochim. Biophys. Acta-Mol. Basis Dis.* **2018**, *1864*, 618–631. [CrossRef] [PubMed]

88. Irazusta, V.; Cabiscol, E.; Reverter-Branchat, G.; Ros, J.; Tamarit, J. Manganese is the link between frataxin and iron-sulfur deficiency in the yeast model of Friedreich ataxia. *J. Biol. Chem.* **2006**, *281*, 12227–12232. [CrossRef] [PubMed]

89. Soriano, S.; Calap-Quintana, P.; Llorens, J.V.; Al-Ramahi, I.; Gutiérrez, L.; Martínez-Sebastián, M.J.; Botas, J.; Moltó, M.D. Metal Homeostasis Regulators Suppress FRDA Phenotypes in a Drosophila Model of the Disease. *PLoS ONE* **2016**, *11*, e0159209. [CrossRef] [PubMed]

90. Koeppen, A.H.; Kuntzsch, E.C.; Bjork, S.T.; Ramirez, R.; Mazurkiewicz, J.E.; Feustel, P.J. Friedreich ataxia: Metal dysmetabolism in dorsal root ganglia. *Acta Neuropathol. Commun.* **2013**, *1*, 26. [CrossRef] [PubMed]

91. Mincheva-Tasheva, S.; Obis, E.; Tamarit, J.; Ros, J. Apoptotic cell death and altered calcium homeostasis caused by frataxin depletion in dorsal root ganglia neurons can be prevented by BH4 domain of Bcl-xL protein. *Hum. Mol. Genet.* **2013**, *23*, 1829–1841. [CrossRef] [PubMed]

92. Han, T.H.L.; Camadro, J.M.; Santos, R.; Lesuisse, E.; Chahine, J.M.; Ha-Duong, N.T. Mechanisms of iron and copper-frataxin interactions. *Metallomics* **2017**, *9*, 1073–1085. [CrossRef] [PubMed]

93. Tai, G.; Corben, L.A.; Yiu, E.M.; Milne, S.C.; Delatycki, M.B. Progress in the treatment of Friedreich ataxia. *Neurol. Neurochir. Pol.* **2018**, *52*, 129–139. [CrossRef] [PubMed]

94. Britti, E.; Delaspre, F.; Feldman, A.; Osborne, M.; Greif, H.; Tamarit, J.; Ros Salvador, J. Frataxin-deficient neurons and mice models of Friedreich ataxia are improved by TAT-MTScs-FXN treatment. *J. Cell. Mol. Med.* **2017**, *22*, 834–848. [CrossRef] [PubMed]

95. Sohn, Y.S.; Breuer, W.; Munnich, A.; Cabantchik, Z.I. Redistribution of accumulated cell iron: A modality of chelation with therapeutic implications. *Blood* **2008**, *111*, 1690–1699. [CrossRef] [PubMed]

96. Kakhlon, O.; Manning, H.; Breuer, W.; Melamed-Book, N.; Lu, C.; Cortopassi, G.; Munnich, A.; Cabantchik, Z. Cell functions impaired by frataxin deficiency are restored by drug-mediated iron relocation. *Blood* **2008**, *112*, 5219–5227. [CrossRef] [PubMed]

97. Pandolfo, M.; Hausmann, L. Deferiprone for the treatment of Friedreich's ataxia. *J. Neurochem.* **2013**, *126*, 142–146. [CrossRef] [PubMed]

98. Elincx-Benizri, S.; Glik, A.; Merkel, D.; Arad, M.; Freimark, D.; Kozlova, E.; Cabantchik, I.; Hassin-Baer, S. Clinical Experience With Deferiprone Treatment for Friedreich Ataxia. *J. Child Neurol.* **2016**, *31*, 1036–1040. [CrossRef] [PubMed]

13

Research Progress on Rolling Circle Amplification (RCA)-Based Biomedical Sensing

Lide Gu [1] [iD], Wanli Yan [1], Le Liu [1], Shujun Wang [2,3], Xu Zhang [3,4] and Mingsheng Lyu [1,2,3,*]

[1] College of Marine Life and Fisheries, Huaihai Institute of Technology, Lianyungang 222005, China;
     gu_lide@163.com (L.G.); yanwanli003@163.com (W.Y.); liulezz3@163.com (L.L.)
[2] Marine Resources Development Institute of Jiangsu, Lianyungang 222005, China; shujunwang86@163.com
[3] Co-Innovation Center of Jiangsu Marine Bio-industry Technology, Huaihai Institute of Technology,
     Lianyungang 222005, China; xu_zhang@cbu.ca
[4] Verschuren Centre for Sustainability in Energy & the Environment, Cape Breton University,
     Sydney, NS B1P 6L2, Canada
*   Correspondence: mingshenglu@hotmail.com

Abstract: Enhancing the limit of detection (LOD) is significant for crucial diseases. Cancer development could take more than 10 years, from one mutant cell to a visible tumor. Early diagnosis facilitates more effective treatment and leads to higher survival rate for cancer patients. Rolling circle amplification (RCA) is a simple and efficient isothermal enzymatic process that utilizes nuclease to generate long single stranded DNA (ssDNA) or RNA. The functional nucleic acid unit (aptamer, DNAzyme) could be replicated hundreds of times in a short period, and a lower LOD could be achieved if those units are combined with an enzymatic reaction, Surface Plasmon Resonance, electrochemical, or fluorescence detection, and other different kinds of biosensor. Multifarious RCA-based platforms have been developed to detect a variety of targets including DNA, RNA, SNP, proteins, pathogens, cytokines, micromolecules, and diseased cells. In this review, improvements in using the RCA technique for medical biosensors and biomedical applications were summarized and future trends in related research fields described.

Keywords: rolling circle amplification (RCA); biosensor; clinical diagnostics; cancer

1. Introduction

Rolling circle amplification (RCA) is a commonly used research tool in molecular biology, materials science, and medicine [1–3]. Since its discovery at the end of 20th century, the applications of RCA have been increasing consistently with the development of science and technology [4]. RCA is an isothermal enzymatic process that uses DNA or RNA polymerases (e.g., Φ29 DNA polymerase) to produce single stranded DNA (ssDNA) or RNA molecules which are a connection in series of complementary units of a template. The process is simple and efficient [5–10]. An RCA reaction contains four parts: (1) a DNA polymerase and homologous buffer; (2) a relatively short DNA or RNA primer; (3) a circle template; and (4) deoxynucleotide triphosphates (dNTPs). In RCA, nucleotides (nt) were added continuously to a primer annealed to a circular template by polymerase, which produces a long ssDNA with hundreds to thousands of repeat units. It should also be noted that RCA products possess multiple repetitive sequence units, which correspond to the circular DNA template; therefore, they can be processed through modification of the template. By transforming the substrate, the DNA products can be customized to include functional sequences, including DNA aptamers [5,6], spacer domains [6], DNAzymes [7–10], and restriction enzyme sites [11–13]. Furthermore, multifunctional materials with diverse properties can also be made via hybridizing RCA products with complementary oligonucleotides tethered to functional moieties. These include fluorescent dyes, electrochemical tags, biotin, antibodies, enzymes and nanoparticles [14–17], which can then be used for sensitive detection, biorecognition, immunosensing and bioimaging.

Recently, RCA had been utilized to study and develop sensitive detection methods for DNA [9,11,18–24], RNA [25–27], DNA methylation [28,29], single nucleotide polymorphisms (SNP) [30–32], small molecules [7,33,34], target proteins [10,35], and cancer cells [6,36,37]. The circular templates are designed in RCA so that a single binding event can be amplified over a thousand-fold. The signal from a single binding event can be amplified in an exponential manner. RCA is ideal for the required ultrasensitive detection [38]. The feature is especially useful for diagnostics. The isothermal nature of RCA provides new possibilities for targeted therapy compared to other methods, such as polymerase chain reaction (PCR), which uses intricate and expensive apparatus (e.g., temperature gradient). Owing to these inherent excellent properties, multifarious, RCA-based platforms have been applied to test various types of targets, such as DNA, RNA, SNP, proteins, pathogens, cytokines, and tumor cells. In this review, improvements in the use of the RCA technique for medical biosensors and biomedical applications will be summarized and future trends in related research fields will be examined.

2. Enzyme-Aided RCA Biosensor

Organisms contain a variety of enzymes, and changes in these enzymes provide a lot of important information, particularly for medical diagnoses. The study of these enzymes can help not only with the diagnosis, but also with the treatment of various diseases. Because RCA has many advantages (such as simplicity, efficiency, tunability), it thus plays an important role in enzyme research. RCA-mediated enzymatic reaction catalyzed amplification provides dual-amplification for ultrasensitive detection of analytes due to the excellent catalytic nature of some enzymes and efficient amplification of RCA. Some DNAzymes can combine with RCA to detect the sensitivity and specificity of other enzymes, such as DNA ligase and polynucleotide kinase/phosphatase (PNKP). DNA ligase, an extremely important member of the enzyme family, which can connect the 3′-hydroxyl and 5′-phosphoryl termini of fractured DNA to form phosphodiester bonds, and plays indispensable roles in DNA replication, repair, and recombination [39–41]. Recent clinical researches revealed that the activity level of DNA ligase is connected with the pathogenesis of cancer. Inhibiting the activity of DNA ligase can decrease cancer cell proliferation and metastasis, and immensely augment the sensitivity of cancer cells to anticancer drugs [42,43]. Polynucleotide kinase/phosphatase (PNKP) is a bifunctional enzyme with 5′-kinase and 3′-phosphatase activities; once the DNA strand is broken, its end will produce 5′-phosphate and 3′-hydroxyl groups, thus allowing some specific proteins to replace lost nucleotides and regroup broken strands [44]. PNKP also plays an important role in nucleic acid metabolism and DNA repair during strand interruption [45]. Inhibition of PNKP can also promote the sensitivity of human tumors to γ-radiation [46], which could be useful for enhancing the efficacy of existing cancer treatments [45].

In order to ascertain the activity of a DNA ligase, a G-quadruplex DNAzyme-based DNA ligase sensor was developed by Jiang et al. [47]. In their design, the oligonucleotide probes did not need to be labeled due to the use of G-quadruplex DNAzyme; hence, label-free detection was possible. The amplification of RCA will generate multimeric G-quadruplexes containing thousands of G-quadruplex units and revealed highly active hemin-binding sites, resulting in great improvements in sensor sensitivity. This sensor enabled the specific detection of T4 DNA ligase at a level as low as 1.9 U/μL. When the PNKP-triggered 5′-phosphroylation step was added to the substrate DNA, a PNKP sensor was easily designed on the basis of the above sensing strategy (Figure 1), which allowed specific detection of T4 PNKP at a limit of 1.8 U/μL.

This procedure is quite simple. A visual result will be obtained through a colorimetric reaction. It is easy, efficient and accurate. Meantime, the concept is also suitable for analysis of other enzymes.

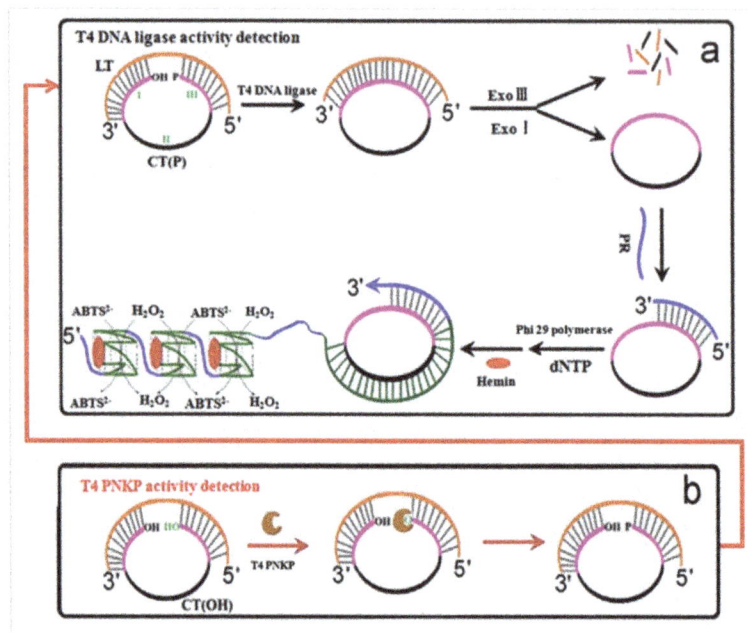

Figure 1. Schematic diagram of G-quadruplex DNAzyme-based DNA ligase sensor. (**a**) The CT composed of three parts. Part I and III could hybridize with LT and form a split ring. Part II was a C-rich area where G-rich sequences are generated to form G-quadruplex structures after RCA. The split was repaired when T4 DNA ligase was introduced; then, LT was excised by Exo I and Exo III After annealing, PR was adhered to the circular template and activated RCA with Phi29 polymerase. Numerous G-rich sequences will be produced to fold into G-quadruplex units and bind hemin to form catalytic G-quadruplex DNAzymes, which can catalyze the oxidation of $ABTS^{2-}$ by H_2O_2 to ABTS, enhancing the absorption signal. (**b**) When the PNKP-triggered 5′-phosphroylation step was added to the substrate DNA, a PNKP sensor was easily designed based on the above sensing strategy. (LT, linear template; CT, circular template; ABTS, 2,2′-azino-bis(3-ethylbenzothiazoline-6-sulfonic acid)) [47].

3. AuNP-RCA Biosensor for Multiple Pathogens Detection

Many diseases are related to the invasion of pathogens. Studying the characteristics of pathogenic bacteria may help in developing treatments for these diseases. A fast and accurate definitive diagnosis of specific pathogenic bacteria is extremely important in clinical diagnostics. There are many effective techniques that are traditionally used to identify pathogens; however, these approaches can only confirm a single pathogen per assay [48–53]. Therefore, developing an all-purpose detection method for concurrent recognition of multiple pathogens is vitally important for improving detection efficacy. SPR biosensors may afford an opportunity to detect diverse pathogens. SPR is an optical detection technology, which utilizes the refraction and reflection of light. In this process, DNA probes are immobilized on the sensor surface and the complex of target molecules are introduced to traverse these clusters continuously [54]. Due to the sensitivity of the optical device, the detection process can be operated and monitored in real-time; therefore, SPR biosensors offer simple, sensitive, and on-site analysis [55]. Shi et al. [56] made a characteristic biosensor for the detection of pathogenic bacteria. In their study, an SPR DNA biosensor with a gold (Au) nanoparticle surface, based on RCA, was developed for isothermal recognition of DNA. The sensor contained a specific padlock probe (PLP) and a capture probe (CP), which were connected by biotin, and an Au nanoparticle-modified probe, the products of RCA were hybridized with them (Figure 2). The CP was fixed on AuNP in order to enhance the binding and hybridizing abilities of the biosensor. The linear PLP was cyclized by ligase after hybridizing with the pathogenic bacteria-specific sequences in 16S rDNA and the circular product was fully complementary with the CP. The corresponding channel on the chip surface distinguished every target gene DNA during the recognition process. The in situ solid-phase RCA reaction was then initiated by the immobilized CPs, which were regarded as primers, and produced long single-stranded DNA. The SPR angle changed with RCA products fixed on the chip surface. Six different bacterial pathogens were simultaneously recognized utilizing this method. At low background signals, the synthetic oligonucleotides and genomic DNA could be detected at 0.5 pM and 0.5 pg/μL, respectively. This study successfully proved that the above method could be used to further establish and refine medical technology and could be used clinically as an additional treatment for human health.

This method affords a very significant platform for the detection of various bacteria pathogens. By taking merit of amplification of AuNP-RCA, the constitutionally high sensitivity of the SPR bio-sensor improved the limit of detection [56]. Successfully it overcame the problem of those single bacteria detection methods which were time-consuming, complex and with low efficiency. Also, more bacteria could be detected at same time.

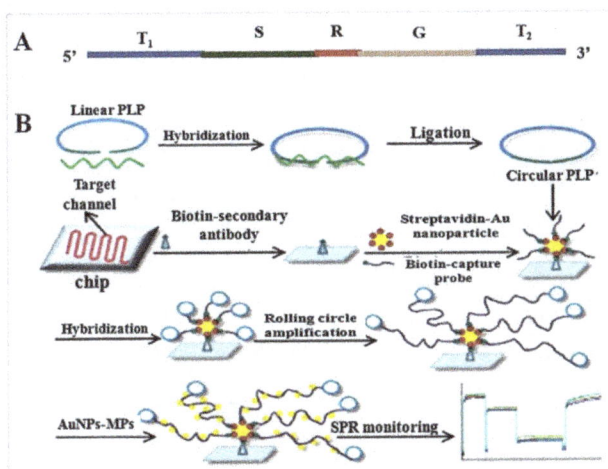

Figure 2. Schematic diagram of AuNP-RCA sensor for multiple pathogens detection. (**A**) The PLP was designed as 5 regions which contain target-complementary sequences at the 5′ and 3′ ends (T1 and T2); the CPs hybridizes with a sequence-specific region (S); a Hpal restriction endonuclease digestion site (R) and the AuNP-MP binding sequences: a general region (G). (**B**) The scheme of detection process. (1) Linear PLP and target sequences were hybridized and linked to form circular template. (2) Immobilizing biotin-secondary antibody on the chip surface and incubated with streptavidin-Au nanoparticles and biotin-capture probe. (3) Circular PLP was added and hybridized with CPs to activate the RCA reaction, which can produce abundant binding sites for AuNP-MP and output signal of SPR [56].

4. Aptamer Biosensor Based on RCA

In clinical medicine, a tumor marker is generally regarded as an indicator of a malignant tumor. Tumor markers are proteins, conjugated proteins, carbohydrates or peptides that are related to tumor formation and are produced by tumor tissues and cells [57,58]. In recent years, the detection of tumor markers has become possible with the continuing development of the aptamer technique. Aptamers are in vitro synthetic single-stranded DNA/RNA oligonucleotides obtained through systematic evolution of ligands by exponential enrichment (SELEX) [59,60]. Aptamers could bind with a great variety of molecules, proteins, nanomaterials, cells, and even chemicals with excellent affinity and specificity because of their three-dimensional structure. Aptamers had been used extensively in drug transfer, protein analysis, immunodiagnosis and treatment, biosensors, due to their many unique properties, such as easy synthesis, excellent affinity, high specificity, nice stability, and simple modification. A variety of novel technologies and programs based aptamers have been studied, including microfluidics [61], fluorescent [62], and electrochemical processes [63].

As a high-efficiency isothermal amplification reaction, RCA is always coupled with biosensing methods for protein analysis. Zhang et al. [64] designed a highly sensitive fluorescent aptasensor for thrombin detection based on competition-triggered RCA All of the reactants were contained in a single reaction. In the lack of target molecule, the ligation-RCA step was inhibited because complementary DNA (cDNA) conjugated with the aptamer probe to generate a double-stranded duplex. Conversely, when the target molecule was introduced, the aptamer probe bonded to the target molecule with high selectivity. As a result, the cDNA hybridized with the PLP rather than with the aptamer probe. The PLP was circularized by DNA T4 ligase and the RCA process was achieved using Phi29 DNA polymerase. The RCA product then hybridized with the loop of molecular beacons, and generated a distinct fluorescence signal (Figure 3). The effects of the length of cDNA and concentration of PLP were studied in this work. After optimizing the operational methods, the target analyte, thrombin, was detected with high sensitivity. This method provided a new possibility for other target analytes.

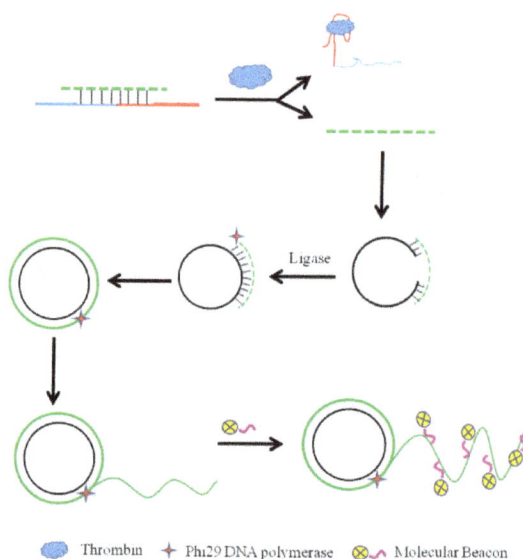

Figure 3. Scheme of the aptasensor design. In the lack of target molecule, the ligation-RCA step was inhibited because complementary DNA (cDNA) was hybridized to the aptamer probe to generate a double-stranded duplex. Conversely, when the target molecule was introduced, the aptamer probe bound to the target molecule with high selectivity. As a result, the cDNA hybridized with the PLP insead of the aptamer probe. The PLP was circularized by DNA T4 ligase for RCA with Phi29 DNA polymerase. The product then hybridized with the loop of molecular beacons and generated a distinct fluorescence signal [64].

Methylene blue, a biological stain, can insert into the double-stranded DNAs from the products of RCA and serves as an electrochemical label [65], allowing for label-free electrochemical sensing. For example, a label-free ultrasensitive electrochemical aptamer sensor, based on hyperbranched rolling circle amplification (HRCA) with the help of DPV, was developed by Wang et al. [66]. In their work, HRCA was coupled to an electrochemical technique to detect platelet-derived growth factor B-chain (PDGF-BB) with high sensitivity and specificity. This combined the excellent sensitivity of HRCA and the inexpensive electrochemical detection. Both the target molecule competitive reaction and the combination of electrochemical technique increased the accuracy of the result; meanwhile, the use of RCA speeded up the process of experiment. Moreover, these strategies are also applicable to other target analytes by tuning the sequence of the aptamer probe.

5. Micromolecular Biosensor Based on Electrochemistry Coupled to RCA

The development of electrochemical technology provides biosensors widely used in disease diagnosis and immunotherapy. RCA could produce a mass of sites on which to fasten DNA recognition probes. Owing to the otherness of binding efficiency between electroactive species and DNA, electroactive species such as tetramethylbenzidine and methylene blue are often used as electrochemical responders to enlarge the electrochemical signal [67]. Therefore, a composite of RCA and electrochemistry could be used to information output for electrochemical study.

Doxorubicin hydrochloride (DOX), a class of important anti-tumor antibiotics, produces a wide range of biochemical effects in organisms. DOX has a strong cytotoxic effect with a main mechanism of action of inhibiting nucleic acid synthesis [68]. Thus, the sensitivity of DNA sensors could be drastically enhanced using DOX as an electroactive indicator. For instance, DOX could be used to establish a high sensitivity DNA sensor [69]. An electrochemical DOX biosensor based on RCA has been established by Lu et al. [70]. In their study, DOX was intercalated into double-stranded GC or CG sequences and the DOX current signal was monitored using differential pulse voltammetry (DPV).

Furthermore, with the help of electrochemical impedance spectroscopy, potassium ferricyanide ($K_3Fe(CN)_6$) and DNA have been used for electrochemical signal output for ultra-sensitive detection of small molecules via ligation-RCA with analyte-mediated sticky ends (Figure 4A). In this method, 2 ss-DNA probes were designed for DNA cyclization. A "hairpin" structure was formed by the left part probe after denaturing, and right part probe also formed a similar "hairpin" structure, based on analyte-activated conformation change. Subsequently, the two probes were ligated via DNA ligase and a circular template for the RCA reaction was formed. When the adenosine was introduced, the RCA products hybridized with the capture probe on the electrode surface, prompting the impedance signal to enhance drastically, because the scheduled kinetics limit between $[Fe(CN)_6]^{3-/4-}$ and the negatively charged phosphate backbone of the DNA (Figure 4B). Using this electrochemical sensing technology, a fairly low detection limit and a wide linear dynamic range were accomplished by Yi et al. [71] with highly specific detection of the target.

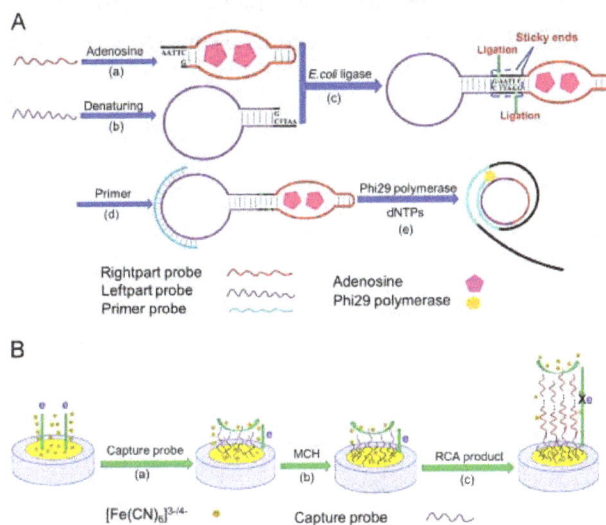

Figure 4. Schematic diagram of micromolecular biosensor based on electrochemistry coupled to RCA. (**A**) Formulation of RCA process based on structure-switching aptamer and sticky ends-based ligation. (a) Right part probe: target-aptamer binding, (b) left part probe: DNA denaturing to form a hairpin structure, (c) double probes were linked by *E. coli* DNA ligase with the same sticky ends, (d) the primer was adhered to the circular template by annealing, (e) RCA was initiated by adding Phi29 DNA polymerase and dNTPs. (**B**) Fabrication of the electrochemical biosensor. (a) Capture probes were anchored to the bare electrode, (b) blocking the electrode with MCH, (c) capture probe–RCA product hybridization for EIS quantitative determination [71].

Although these protocols are complex compared to other designs, the composite of RCA and electrochemical techniques offered a credible method for the detection of numerous small biomolecules.

6. Transcription Factor (TF) Biosensor Based on RCA

A TF is a protein that is capable of binding to a specific nucleotide sequence upstream of a gene. The TF regulates the velocity of transcription of genetic information from DNA to mRNA [72] and may influence multiple transcription-associated cellular processes including cell development, differentiation, and growth [73]. TF plays a vital role in gene transcriptional regulation, and TF proteins have been confirmed to have a variety of unique features closely associated with various human diseases including cancer, abnormal hormone responses, autoimmune disorders, neurological disorders, diabetes, cardiovascular disease [74]. For example, the nuclear factor-kappaB (NF-κB) protein and the TATA-binding protein (TBP) are related to a variety of diseases [75]. Therefore, the quantification of TF proteins is essential for pharmaceutical research and immunodiagnosis.

NF-κB p65 protein, a crucial TF, appears on multiple pathogenesis, such as inflammation, vicious circle, apoptosis, and cancer. Some corresponding measures had been developed to detect TF, such as western blot, electrophoretic mobility shift assay [76], DNase footprinting assay [77], and enzyme-linked immunosorbent assay (ELISA) [78]. However, these processes have some universal drawbacks such as insensitive, high detection limit, etc. Inspired by the advantages of RCA, Deng et al. [33] designed a highly sensitive, reproducible biosensor with good specificity for ultrasensitive TF detection. In their study, a biomedical biosensor was designed to detect TF, based on specific target molecule-DNA adsorption and RCA signal amplification. Here, three ss-DNA probes were designed for the TF biosensor. Probe 1 (P1) was attached to the electrode surface and hybridized with probe 2 (P2) to form a partially complementary dsDNA. The complementary part included a TF binding sites, while the non-complementary part of P2 paired with RCA primer sequence. Probe 3 (P3) was displaced P2 and hybridized with P1 to create a whole complementary dsDNA. In the presence of TF protein, a stable TF-DNA complex formed and initiated the RCA process. Finally, the electrochemical redox probe MB was combined with the RCA product and produced the signal that was detected by DPV (Figure 5). The fabricated biomedical sensor displayed a wide linear range and a low detection limit.

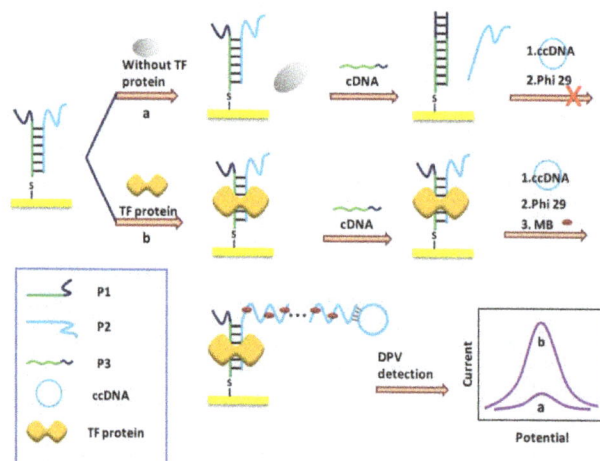

Figure 5. Schematic diagram of TF sensing. Three ss-DNA probes were designed for the TF biosensor. P1 was attached to the electrode surface and hybridized with P2 to form a partially complementary dsDNA. The complementary part included a TF binding sites while the non-complementary part of P2 paired with RCA primer sequence. (a) In the absence of TF protein, P3 was displaced by P2 and hybridized with P1 to form a dsDNA strand, thus stopping RCA. (b) In the presence of TF protein, a stable TF-DNA complex formed and inhibited the displacement of P3, and then, initiated the RCA with ccDNA and Phi29 DNA polymerase. Finally, the electrochemical redox probe MB was combined with the RCA product and produced the signal that was detected by DPV [33].

A mutation in TBP, a kind of TF that could bond with the TATA box specifically, causes a variety of neurodegenerative diseases. Therefore, engineering a high-efficiency immunosensor has become an emerging and powerful strategy for proteome and genomics research, also for clinical diagnosis. An efficient fluorescent-amplification method for fast, quantitative, and low cost detection of TF has been developed by Li et al. [79] utilizing RCA using TBP as a target model. Three components were used in their study: TF binding probe (TFBP), enlargement primer, and dumbbell-probe. When the RCA process was complete, the products were quantized though the signal of SYBR Green I. This strategy had a very low detection limit and a wide linear region. The schematic is similar to that in Figure 5. The above two sensing strategies are simple and accurate, and they can be used for detecting other transcription factors by changing the protein-binding sequence. These protocols have advantage to be a tool for clinic diagnostic applications and high throughput bioanalysis.

7. MiRNAs Biosensor Based on RCA

MicroRNAs (miRNAs) are small (18–25 nt), endogenic, non-coding, single-stranded RNA molecules that could command the expression of messenger RNA in numerous organisms [80]. Since miRNAs were found in eukaryotic cells [81], a mass of studies based on miRNA had verified that disorder in miRNA expression caused many emerging malignancies [82–84]. Therefore, miRNAs as novel biomarkers often be used in the diagnosis and treatment of many types of cancer [85–88], which necessitates simple, fast, reliable, sensitive, and specific tests for miRNA detection.

Traditional techniques for miRNAs detection include Northern blotting [89], RT-PCR [90], and microarrays [91]. Though these methods all have merits, they still have some drawbacks, such as low efficiency, low sensitivity, and being time-consuming. It's necessary to select an effective amplification measure for accurate detection of miRNAs. A number of amplification strategies have been proposed, such as exonuclease (Exo)-assisted signal amplification [92,93], strand displacement amplification (SDA) [94], and RCA [95–98]. Among the many amplification methods, RCA may be the most suitable for miRNA detection because these short RNAs are optimal substrates for the ligation reaction that is needed to launch the process of RCA.

A label-free ultrasensitive colorimetric biosensing scheme for miRNA detection had been reported by Li et al. [99]. To improve the analytical efficiency of RCA-based amplification strategies for miRNA detection, with the mutual assistance of trigger template, C-rich DNA co-modified molecular beacon (MB), G-rich DNA (GDA) probe, MB-mediated SDA, and toehold-initiated rolling circle amplification (TIRCA) to compose into a new-type, functionalized, nucleic acid-based amplification system for miRNAs detection with specificity and sensitivity (Figure 6). The amplification system consists of three parts: MB/GDNA probe, polymerase & nicking enzyme, and a seal prime (dumb-bell-shaped amplification template). MB/GDNA combined with miRNA and promoted the MB-mediated SDA to continuously produce nicking triggers, which then hybridized with the seal probe to launch TIRCA reaction and release a mountain of GDNAs. The connection of GDNAs and hemin to create a G-quadruplex/hemin DNAzyme, a famous horse radish peroxidase mimic, which catalyzed a colorimetric reaction. Notably, the 3'-OH of MB and GDNA could be deactivated by a C6 spacer, which blocked the nonspecific polymerization along with the 5' protruding termini of MB, thus increasing the target molecule identification and decreasing the background signal. The project exhibited high sensitivity and specificity with a wide linear dynamic range, and enabled successful visual analysis the minute amount of miRNA in some real samples via the naked eye. This simple and high-efficiency signal amplification strategy built a fast and sensitive platform for miRNA detection.

Moreover, Deng's group [97] utilized toehold-mediated strand displacement (TMSD) to design a structure-switchable seal probe to activate the RCA reaction of specific RNAs, a proposed that could accomplish the precise recognition and in situ enlargement of the target miRNA. In this miRNA course, the design of a dumbbell-shaped seal probe was the key for TMSD and RCA. The TMSD process was initiated by the target miRNA and caused a structural change in the probe. When miRNA was combined by the toehold domain, spontaneous branch migration prompted the circular form, and started RCA process.

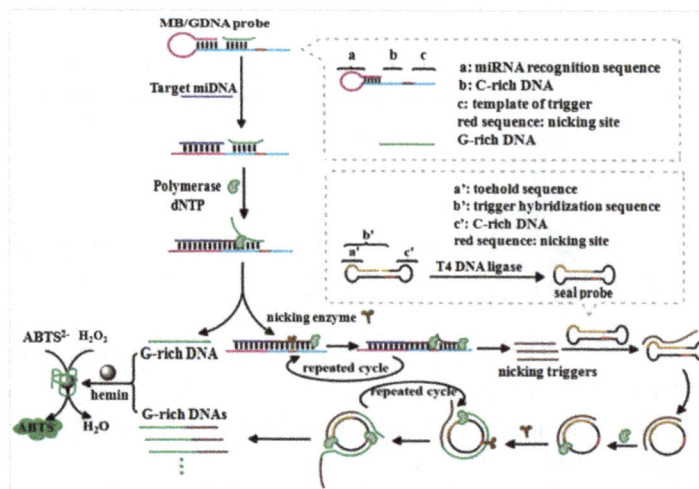

Figure 6. Schematic diagram of the functional nucleic acid-based amplification system for miRNA detection. The MB/ GDNA probe were composed of four domains (see right frame). The hybridization was achieved between target miRNA and domain (a); then, the target miRNA was extended to domain (b) and domain (c) to form a complete duplex by Phi29 DNA polymerase (adhered to the domain b). Then, the duplex nicking site was recognized by the nicking enzyme specifically, and the extended DNA strand was cleaved at domain (c). The TIRCA was triggered when the seal probe was annealed with the primer which were nicking triggers and released by the circulation of the extension and cleavage processes at domain (c). When the toehold domain of seal probe was bound with trigger, the spontaneous branch migration leaded to an activated circular form, and the RCA was initiated. The resultant DNA duplex was cleaved at the nicking site in the circle by nicking enzyme. Hundreds of tandem repeats of GDNA was produced as the primers were extended by Phi29 DNA polymerase. Consequently, once the presence of hemin, the colorimetric detection was amplified by the formation of DNAzyme [99].

Nevertheless, the stabilized dumbbell structure will stop the mismatched miRNA and terminated the amplification. After the seal probe was activated, the target miRNA was enlarged to lots of tandem repeat sequences by RCA and the evident diffraction-limited spot corresponding to a single miRNA will eliminate the FAM-labeled probe interference from background signal. Through this process, both stringent recognition and in situ amplification of the target miRNA can be achieved. The visualization analysis of individual miRNAs in single cells is accomplished.

8. Protein Biosensor Based on RCA

In recent years, with improvements in people's standard of living, a variety of protein-related diseases have appeared. For example, gastric cancer, which was characterized by many oncoprotein biomarkers, such as p21, p27, p53, CyclinE, C-myc, Galectin-3, miR-221, MCM7, Runx3, etc. [100]. Therefore, an accurate and efficient method for protein detection is essential for disease diagnosis and clinical applications. In the traditional method of protein detection, antibodies offered a testing tool for proteins detection [101,102]; however, antibodies are generally from in vivo and cannot be synthesized in vitro. In contrast, aptamers can be synthesized in vitro through the SELEX technique. Aptamers have been widely used to fabricate biosensors in numerous new fields of study [63,103–105].

Optical diffraction biosensors have been widely used to distinguish the binding process of many biomolecules, based on changes in effective height or refractive index on periodically patterned gratings [106]. Utilizing the many advantages of RCA, Lee et al. [107] achieved a diffraction biosensor for proteins using microbead-based RCA. In their work, aptamer and RCA were connected to detect

PDGF-BB, which is related to cancer cell proliferation and transformation [108,109]. In the presence of PDGF-BB, a sandwich complex was formed between two anti-PDGF-BB aptamers (Figure 7). One of the aptamers contained a primer binding site, and the complex of aptamer and primer was used to help the product of RCA to directly localize on PDGF. The RCA reaction was initiated and the primer sequence was extended into a long oligonucleotide with the aid of phi 29 DNA polymerase. The biotinylated aptamers were fixed on the surface where periodic patterns of streptavidin were microcontact printed using a polydimethylsiloxane stamp. After the streptavidin-labeled microbeads were introduced, the diffraction grating was completed and linked with RCA concatemers on the periodic patterns. The number of microbeads on the patterns was the main determinant to generated different intensities diffraction modes with a laser light. In the absence of RCA on periodically patterned gratings, the capacity of the aptamer-based sandwich propose was executed for testing the efficiency of RCA on the periodical patterns as a signal amplification strategy, and the result proved there wasn't any obvious bead-binding was detected, thereby reconfirming the importance of RCA.

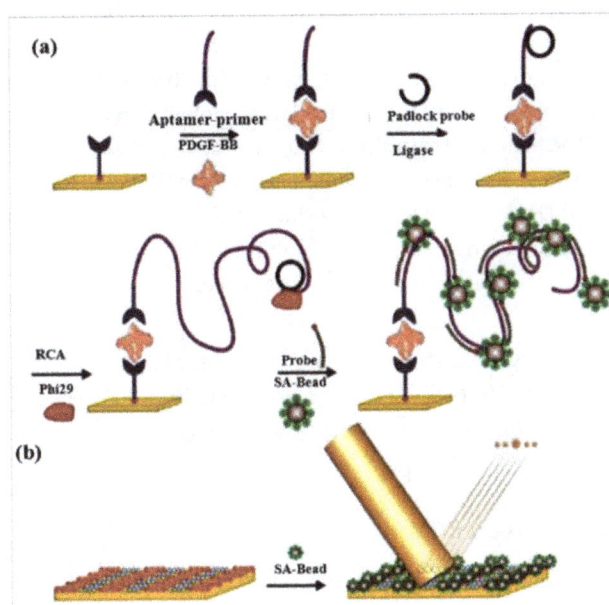

Figure 7. (**a**) Scheme of RCA-based microbead combines with aptamers for detection assay. Streptavidin coated periodic patterns links a biotinylated anti-PDGF-B specific aptamer. PDGF-BB was added and bound by the aptamer. An aptamer-primer complex recognized and bound to the protein. The primer tail of the aptamer was hybridized by a padlock probe, thereby initiating the RCA. The elongated concatemers hybridized with biotinylated probes which bound with streptavidin conjugated beads. (**b**) The diffraction gratings were formed by self-assembled streptavidin (SA)-coated beads on the RCA-based micropattern. The diffraction modes yielded when the illumination with a laser carried out [107].

The same principle, a sensitive protein biosensor, was designed by Guo et al. [110]. They used RCA coupled with thrombin catalysis to design a specific aptamer-based sandwich assay for protein detection on a microplate. This propose makes use of the long-ssDNA, with a series of tandem duplication thrombin-binding sites from RCA and the affinity of aptamer to finish various thrombin labeling and activation for signal producing (Figure 8). First, the target molecule was specifically recognized by an antibody-coated microplate. Then, a familiar sandwich structure is formed by adding aptamer and primer sequence. Following the RCA reaction was initiated to produce the combination sequence for thrombin with the help of primer. More thrombin molecules bound with these combination sequences and catalyzed the chromogenic or fluorogenic peptide substrates transformed to detectable products for final quantification of the target proteins. This protocol was used to identify PDGF-BB. With the help of two systems from RCA and thrombin catalysis, this assay had an extremely low detection limit when a fluorogenic peptide substrate was introduced. This project created a new approach for signal output in RCA relevant studies via direct thrombin labeling and evaded costing too long time on preparation of enzyme-conjugate and affinity probes.

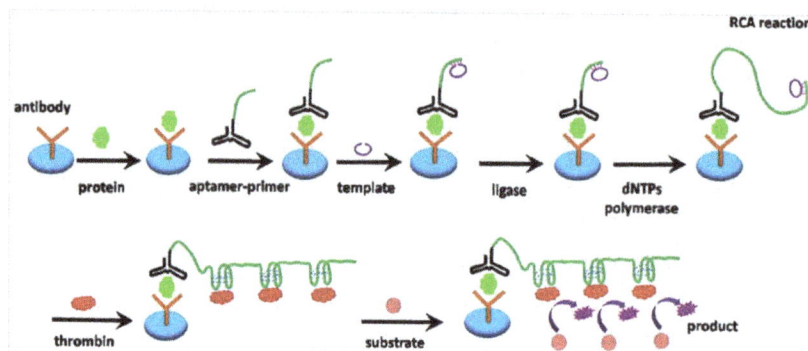

Figure 8. Schematic diagram of using RCA coupled with thrombin catalysis to detect protein. Microplate coated with antibody which captured the target protein. Then, the aptamer-primer complex bound with the protein. The template hybridized with the primer and was circularized by ligase, and it encoded with a complementary sequence of the aptamer for thrombin. Subsequently, the RCA initiated and a long single-stranded DNA sequence was produced for thrombin. The generated ssDNA bound with thrombin molecules, achieving multiple thrombin labeling in sandwich complex. Thrombin catalyzes small peptide substrates into detectable product [110].

By taking advantage of RCA, an antibody coated microplate as a signal enhancement strategy is an excellent biosensing platform. That cleverly avoided the using of complex instruments and offered a visual detection of the molecular binding events under an ordinary experiment conditions. These strategies can be used in analysis of other proteins.

9. Other Novel Biosensors Based on RCA

With the increasing sophistication of experimental techniques, more and more new types of immunosensors have been developed, such as sensors for the capture of oligonucleotides, proteins, cancer cells, and sensors for vitamins [111].

Nucleic acids occupy an extremely significant role in biological inheritance, and variations in them can cause immeasurable damage to an organism. Accordingly, qualitative and quantitative studies of nucleic acids contribute to the development of immunodiagnostics and pharmacogenomics [112]. Abundant methods for the detection of nucleic acids had been reported, such as SPR [113], inductively coupled plasma mass spectrometric (ICPMS) [114], chemiluminescence [115]. Nonetheless, the detection limit for DNA when using these existing scheme is still a major obstacle. Therefore, designing a novel detection method for nucleic acids is imperative. A new style of biosensor, based on RCA and nanoparticle aggregation, for ultrasensitive detection of DNA and tumor cells was developed by Ding et al. [116]. Their work included three primary steps, which are summarized as follows: first, the surface of magnetic beads was immobilized with a "sandwich-type" DNA complex contained target DNA. Then the primer in the "sandwich-type" DNA complex initiated RCA in the system. The new "sandwich-type" DNA complex were formed in the long RCA products for electrochemical detection (Figure 9). With the help of DPV, an extremely low detection limit of target DNA was obtained. Assisted with aptamer technique, this signal output strategy was also used to identify tumor cells, in which an extremely low detection limit was also achieved (Figure 10).

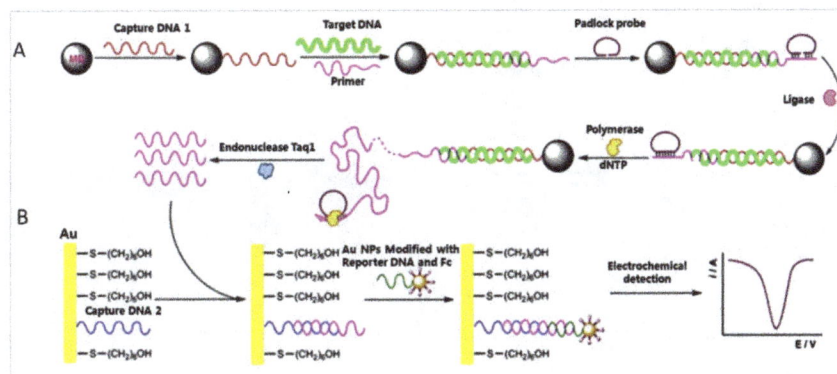

Figure 9. Scheme of RCA and electrochemical detection of DNA. (**A**) MBs connected with capture DNA1, and target DNA was added and tethered with it. Then, the primer DNA connected to the target DNA and the padlock probe after annealing. The RCA process was initiated to yield a long ssDNA after the padlock probe was circularized by ligase. Consequently, the long RCA products was digested to generate a crowd of short single ssDNA with same sequence as transfer DNA (t DNA) after Taq I DNA enzymes were added. (**B**) The surface of the Au electrode was covered by self-assembled DNA 2. And the electrochemical biosensor was formed by t DNA and capture DNA 2. The signal DNA loaded on Au NPs and hybridize with t DNA. The differential pulse voltammetry (DPV) scan monitored the quantity of the t DNA [116].

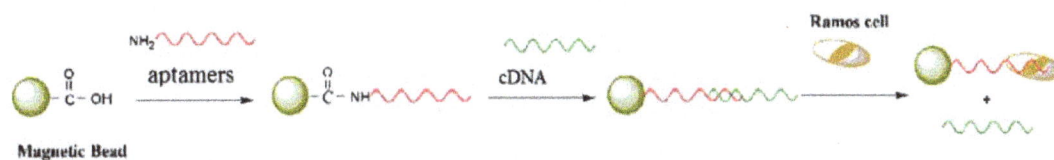

Figure 10. Scheme of the Ramos cells and aptamer reaction. Carboxyl-group-coated MBs connected with amino-modified aptamers of Ramos cells to form MB-DNA bio-complex which hybridized with cDNA. The bio-complex could instead of cDNA because of the stronger affinity between the aptamers and its targets when the presence of Ramos cells [116].

Folic acid (FA), a water-soluble vitamin, promotes the maturation of bone marrow cells in the human. A deficiency in FA can cause megaloblastic anemia and leucopenia, which is particularly important for pregnant women. Therefore, monitoring the FA level is vital for the immunodiagnosis and treatment of cancers and chronic inflammatory diseases [117]. For example, a fluorescence biosensor for folate receptor (FR) in cancer cells based on terminal protection and HRCA was developed by Li et al. [118]. In their work, ssDNA terminally tethered to FA specifically combined with FR and was protected from digestion by exonuclease I (Exo I). The protected ssDNA hybridized with the padlock probe and triggered the HRCA reaction. Conversely, the ssDNA was digested by Exo I and no probe was left to initiate the HRCA reaction without the protection of the target FR. In the presence of SYBR Green I, the HRCA products included a mass of double-stranded DNA and a strong fluorescence signal could be detected (Figure 11). Moreover, the developed biosensor is also used to detect FR in cancer cells (e.g., HeLa cells). The increased fluorescence intensity has shown lower detection limit with a wide linear dynamic range.

This protocol offered a simple, fast and efficient method for the identification of FR. At the same time, it effectively prevented the ssDNA from hydrolysis by Exo I, and made full use of the advantages of HRCA rapid expansion, which not only shortened the working time, but also increased the reliability of the result.

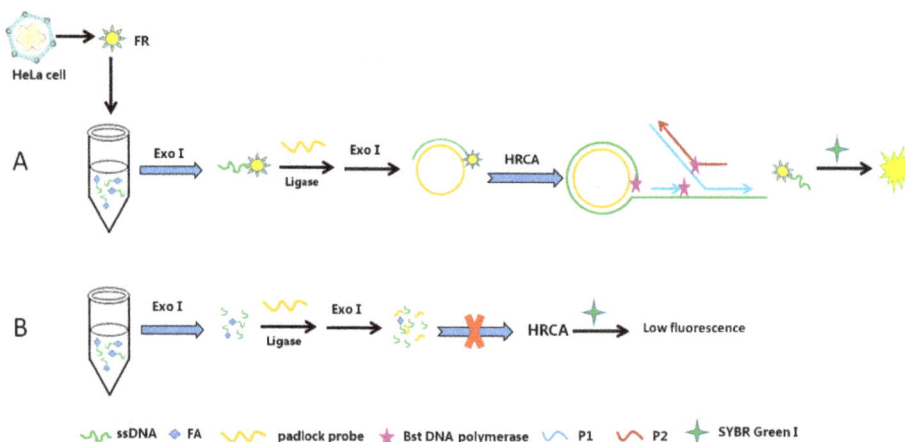

Figure 11. Schematic of a fluorescence biosensor for FR determination, based on HRCA and terminal protection. (**A**) FR connected with FA-ssDNA through FR-FA interaction and prevented the hydrolyzation of Exo I. Then, the compound hybridized with padlock probe, and formed a circular padlock probe with the aid of DNA ligase. Later, the HRCA reaction was activated by Bst DNA polymerase, P1, P2, and dNTPs to launch chain extensions and strand displacements, resulting a mass of long double-strand DNA (dsDNA) and ssDNA yielded. High fluorescence signal was monitored after introducing SYBR Green I. (**B**) In the absence of the target, ssDNA were hydrolyzed by Exo I and the HRCA was inhibited, so only weak fluorescence signal was detected [118].

10. Outlook

RCA is an excellent signal amplification technology. It is a highly versatile DNA amplification tool widely used in many fields where limitations in sensitivity and/or specificity, laborious sample preparation and/or signal amplification procedures had previously hindered the use of other tools. RCA is used for assays and procedures in fields such as immunohistochemistry, immunodiagnostics, nanotechnology, materials science, genomics, proteomics, biosensing, drug discovery, targeted therapy, flow cytometry. Moreover, the combination of RCA with functional nucleic acids, containing aptamers and DNAzymes, and with other assay platforms involve PCR, SELEX, optical diffraction, ELISA, microfluidics, ICPMS, chemiluminescence, SPR, and nanoparticles, presents new opportunities for ultrasensitive detection of a lot of targets, including nucleic acids, proteins, vitamins, small molecules, viruses, hormones, and cells. Particularly, RCA has increased the sensitivity of medical detection and greatly reduced the detection limit. In recent years, the combination of RCA with aptamers and nanomaterials has attracted more attention. Integrating these three technologies will greatly promote human health and medicine. As the standard of living continues to increase, more new diseases will likely emerge, necessitating continued research to ensure human health and social development. The combination of new generations of biosensors with RCA and/or other technologies holds great potential for further applications in biomedical research and early clinical diagnostics.

Acknowledgments: This work was by the National Natural Science Foundation of China (31471719), Jiangsu Science and Technology Development Program (Grant No. BF2016702), and PhD Research Foundation of Huaihai Institute of Technology.

Conflicts of Interest: The authors declare no conflict of interest.

References

1.　Nilsson, M.; Gullberg, M.; Dahl, F.; Szuhai, K.; Raap, A.K. Real-time monitoring of rolling-circle amplification using a modified molecular beacon design. *Nucleic Acids Res.* **2002**, *30*, e66. [CrossRef]

2.　Liu, X.; Xue, Q.; Ding, Y.; Zhu, J.; Wang, L.; Jiang, W. Cascade Signal Amplification Strategy for Sensitive and Label-free DNA Detection Based on Exo III-catalyzed Recycling Coupled with Rolling Circle Amplification. *Analyst* **2014**, *139*, 2884–2889. [CrossRef] [PubMed]

3. Li, Y.; Zeng, Y.; Ji, X.; Li, X.; Ren, R. Cascade signal amplification for sensitive detection of cancer cell based on self-assembly of DNA scaffold and rolling circle amplification. *Sens. Actuators B Chem.* **2012**, *171–172*, 361–366. [CrossRef]

4. Khan, S.A. Plasmid rolling-circle replication: Highlights of two decades of research. *Plasmid* **2005**, *53*, 126–136. [CrossRef] [PubMed]

5. Zhao, W.; Cui, C.H.; Bose, S.; Guo, D.; Shen, C.; Wong, W.P.; Halvorsen, K.; Farokhzad, O.C.; Teo, G.S.L.; Phillips, J.A.; et al. Bioinspired multivalent DNA network for capture and release of cells. *Proc. Natl. Acad. Sci. USA* **2012**, *109*, 19626–19631. [CrossRef] [PubMed]

6. Zhang, Z.; Ali, M.M.; Eckert, M.A.; Kang, D.K.; Chen, Y.Y.; Sender, L.S.; Fruman, D.A.; Zhao, W. A polyvalent aptamer system for targeted drug delivery. *Biomaterials* **2013**, *34*, 9728–9735. [CrossRef] [PubMed]

7. Ali, M.M.; Li, Y. Colorimetric Sensing by Using Allosteric-DNAzyme-Coupled Rolling Circle Amplification and a Peptide Nucleic Acid–Organic Dye Probe. *Angew. Chem.* **2009**, *121*, 3564–3567. [CrossRef]

8. Cheglakov, Z.; Weizmann, Y.; Basnar, B.; Willner, I. Diagnosing viruses by the rolling circle amplified synthesis of DNAzymes. *Org. Biomol. Chem.* **2007**, *5*, 223–225. [CrossRef] [PubMed]

9. Dong, H.; Wang, C.; Xiong, Y.; Lu, H.; Ju, H.; Zhang, X. Highly sensitive and selective chemiluminescent imaging for DNA detection by ligation-mediated rolling circle amplified synthesis of DNAzyme. *Biosens. Bioelectron.* **2013**, *41*, 348–353. [CrossRef] [PubMed]

10. Tang, L.; Liu, Y.; Ali, M.M.; Kang, D.K.; Zhao, W.; Li, J. Colorimetric and ultrasensitive bioassay based on a dual-amplification system using aptamer and DNAzyme. *Anal. Chem.* **2012**, *84*, 4711–4717. [CrossRef] [PubMed]

11. Dahl, F.; Banér, J.; Gullberg, M.; Mendel-Hartvig, M.; Landegren, U.; Nilsson, M. Circle-to-circle amplification for precise and sensitive DNA analysis. *Proc. Natl. Acad. Sci. USA* **2004**, *101*, 4548–4553. [CrossRef] [PubMed]

12. Linck, L.; Reiß, E.; Bier, F.; Resch-Genger, U. Direct labeling rolling circle amplification as a straightforward signal amplification technique for biodetection formats. *Anal. Methods* **2012**, *4*, 1215–1220. [CrossRef]

13. Zhao, W.; Gao, Y.; Kandadai, S.A.; Brook, M.A.; Li, Y. DNA Polymerization on Gold Nanoparticles through Rolling Circle Amplification: Towards Novel Scaffolds for Three-Dimensional Periodic Nanoassemblies. *Angew. Chem. Int. Ed.* **2006**, *45*, 2409–2413. [CrossRef] [PubMed]

14. Ali, M.M.; Aguirre, S.D.; Xu, Y.; Filipe, C.D.M.; Pelton, R.; Li, Y. Detection of DNA using bioactive paper strips. *Chem. Commun.* **2009**, *45*, 6640–6642. [CrossRef] [PubMed]

15. Berr, A.; Schubert, I. Interphase chromosome arrangement in Arabidopsis thaliana is similar in differentiated and meristematic tissues and shows a transient mirror symmetry after nuclear division. *Genetics* **2007**, *176*, 853–863. [CrossRef] [PubMed]

16. Beyer, S.; Nickels, P.; Simmel, F.C. Periodic DNA nanotemplates synthesized by rolling circle amplification. *Nano Lett.* **2005**, *5*, 719–722. [CrossRef] [PubMed]

17. Su, H.; Yuan, R.; Chai, Y.; Mao, L.; Zhuo, Y. Ferrocenemonocarboxylic–HRP@ Pt nanoparticles labeled RCA for multiple amplification of electro-immunosensing. *Biosens. Bioelectron.* **2011**, *26*, 4601–4604. [CrossRef] [PubMed]

18. Thomas, D.; Lizardi, P.; Nardone, G.; Winndeen, E. Cascade rolling circle amplification, a homogeneous fluorescence detection system for DNA diagnostics. *Clin. Chem.* **1997**, *11*, 38.

19. Smolina, I.; Lee, C.; Frank-Kamenetskii, M. Detection of low-copy-number genomic DNA sequences in individual bacterial cells by using peptide nucleic acid-assisted rolling-circle amplification and fluorescence in situ hybridization. *Appl. Environ. Microbiol.* **2007**, *73*, 2324–2328. [CrossRef] [PubMed]

20. Xu, W.; Xie, X.; Li, D.; Yang, Z.; Li, T.; Liu, X. Ultrasensitive Colorimetric DNA Detection using a Combination of Rolling Circle Amplification and Nicking Endonuclease-Assisted Nanoparticle Amplification (NEANA). *Small* **2012**, *8*, 1846–1850. [CrossRef] [PubMed]

21. Johne, R.; Müller, H.; Rector, A.; Van Ranst, M.; Stevens, H. Rolling-circle amplification of viral DNA genomes using phi29 polymerase. *Trends Microbiol.* **2009**, *17*, 205–211. [CrossRef] [PubMed]

22. Schopf, E.; Fischer, O.N.; Chen, Y.; Tok, J.B.H. Sensitive and selective viral DNA detection assay via microbead-based rolling circle amplification. *Bioorg. Med. Chem. Lett.* **2008**, *18*, 5871–5874. [CrossRef] [PubMed]

23. Schopf, E.; Chen, Y. Attomole DNA detection assay via rolling circle amplification and single molecule detection. *Anal. Biochem.* **2010**, *397*, 115–117. [CrossRef] [PubMed]

24. Thomas, D.C.; Nardone, G.A.; Randall, S.K. Amplification of padlock probes for DNA diagnostics by cascade rolling circle amplification or the polymerase chain reaction. *Arch. Pathol. Lab. Med.* **1999**, *123*, 1170–1176. [PubMed]

25. Christian, A.T.; Pattee, M.S.; Attix, C.M.; Reed, B.E.; Sorensen, K.J.; Tucker, J.D. Detection of DNA point mutations and mRNA expression levels by rolling circle amplification in individual cells. *Proc. Natl. Acad. Sci. USA* **2001**, *98*, 14238–14243. [CrossRef] [PubMed]

26. Lagunavicius, A.; Merkiene, E.; Kiveryte, Z.; Savaneviciute, A.; Zimbaite-Ruskuliene, V.; Radzvilavicius, T.; Janulaitis, A. Novel application of Phi29 DNA polymerase: RNA detection and analysis in vitro and in situ by target RNA-primed RCA. *RNA* **2009**, *15*, 765–771. [CrossRef] [PubMed]

27. Zhou, Y.; Calciano, M.; Hamann, S.; Leamon, J.H.; Strugnell, T.; Christian, M.W.; Lizardi, P.M. In situ detection of messenger RNA using digoxigenin-labeled oligonucleotides and rolling circle amplification. *Exp. Mol. Pathol.* **2001**, *70*, 281–288. [CrossRef] [PubMed]

28. Zhao, H.; Ma, X.; Li, M.; Zhou, D.; Xiao, P.; Lu, Z. Analysis of CpG island methylation using rolling circle amplification (RCA) product microarray. *J. Biomed. Nanotechnol.* **2011**, *7*, 292–299. [CrossRef] [PubMed]

29. Qi, X.; Bakht, S.; Devos, K.M.; Gale, M.D.; Osbourn, A. L-RCA (ligation-rolling circle amplification): A general method for genotyping of single nucleotide polymorphisms (SNPs). *Nucleic Acids Res.* **2001**, *29*, e116. [CrossRef] [PubMed]

30. Pickering, J.; Bamford, A.; Godbole, V.; Briggs, J.; Scozzafava, G.; Roe, P.; Wheeler, C.; Ghouze, F.; Cuss, S. Integration of DNA ligation and rolling circle amplification for the homogeneous, end-point detection of single nucleotide polymorphisms. *Nucleic Acids Res.* **2002**, *30*, e60. [CrossRef] [PubMed]

31. Tang, Z.Y.; Cheng, Y.Q.; Du, Q.; Zhang, H.X.; Li, Z.P. Integration of rolling circle amplification and cationic conjugated polymer for the homogeneous detection of single nucleotide polymorphisms. *Chin. Sci. Bull.* **2011**, *56*, 3247–3252. [CrossRef]

32. Zhang, S.; Wu, Z.; Shen, G.; Yu, R. A label-free strategy for SNP detection with high fidelity and sensitivity based on ligation-rolling circle amplification and intercalating of methylene blue. *Biosens. Bioelectron.* **2009**, *24*, 3201–3207. [CrossRef] [PubMed]

33. Deng, K.; Li, C.; Huang, H.; Li, X. Rolling circle amplification based on signal-enhanced electrochemical DNA sensor for ultrasensitive transcription factor detection. *Sens. Actuators B Chem.* **2017**, *238*, 1302–1308. [CrossRef]

34. Meng, F.; Miao, P.; Wang, B.; Tang, Y.; Yin, J. Identification of glutathione by voltammetric analysis with rolling circle amplification. *Anal. Chim. Acta* **2016**, *943*, 58–63. [CrossRef] [PubMed]

35. Shi, H.; Mao, X.; Chen, X.; Wang, Z.; Wang, K.; Zhu, X. The analysis of proteins and small molecules based on sterically tunable nucleic acid hyperbranched rolling circle amplification. *Biosens. Bioelectron.* **2017**, *91*, 136–142. [CrossRef] [PubMed]

36. Ding, C.; Liu, H.; Wang, N.; Wang, Z. Cascade signal amplification strategy for the detection of cancer cells by rolling circle amplification and nanoparticles tagging. *Chem. Commun.* **2012**, *48*, 5019–5021. [CrossRef] [PubMed]

37. Maruyama, F.; Kenzaka, T.; Yamaguchi, N.; Tani, K.; Nasu, M. Visualization and enumeration of bacteria carrying a specific gene sequence by in situ rolling circle amplification. *Appl. Environ. Microbiol.* **2005**, *71*, 7933–7940. [CrossRef] [PubMed]

38. Ali, M.M.; Li, F.; Zhang, Z.; Zhang, K.; Kang, D.K.; Ankrum, J.A.; Chris Le, X.; Zhao, W. Rolling circle amplification: A versatile tool for chemical biology, materials science and medicine. *Chem. Soc. Rev.* **2014**, *43*, 3324–3341. [CrossRef] [PubMed]

39. Doherty, A.J.; Dafforn, T.R. Nick Recognition by DNA Ligases. *J. Mol. Biol.* **2000**, *296*, 43–56. [CrossRef] [PubMed]

40. Doherty, A.J.; Suh, S.W. Structural and mechanistic conservation in DNA ligases. *Nucleic Acids Res.* **2000**, *28*, 4051–4058. [CrossRef] [PubMed]

41. Lehman, I. DNA Iigase: Structure mechanism, function. *Science* **1974**, *186*, 790–797. [CrossRef] [PubMed]

42. Blundred, R.M.; Stewart, G.S. DNA double-strand break repair, immunodeficiency and the RIDDLE syndrome. *Expert Rev. Clin. Immunol.* **2011**, *7*, 169–185. [CrossRef] [PubMed]

43. Yu, J.-C.; Ding, S.; Chang, C.H.; Kuo, S.H.; Chan, S.T.; Hsu, G.C.; Hsu, H.M.; Hou, M.F.; Jung, L.Y.; Cheng, C.W.; et al. Genetic susceptibility to the development and progression of breast cancer associated with polymorphism of cell cycle and ubiquitin ligase genes. *Carcinogenesis* **2009**, *30*, 1562–1570. [CrossRef] [PubMed]

44. Siribal, S.; Weinfeld, M.; Karimi-Busheri, F.; Mark Glover, J.N.; Bernstein, N.K.; Aceytuno, D.; Chavalitshewinkoon-Petmitr, P. Molecular characterization of Plasmodium falciparum putative polynucleotide kinase/phosphatase. *Mol. Biochem. Parasitol.* **2011**, *180*, 1–7. [CrossRef] [PubMed]

45. Allinson, S.L. DNA end-processing enzyme polynucleotide kinase as a potential target in the treatment of cancer. *Future Oncol.* **2010**, *6*, 1031–1042. [CrossRef] [PubMed]

46. Freschauf, G.K.; Karimi-Busheri, F.; Ulaczyk-Lesanko, A.; Mereniuk, T.R.; Ahrens, A.; Koshy, J.M.; Rasouli-Nia, A.; Pasarj, P.; Holmes, C.F.B.; Rininsland, F.; et al. Identification of a small molecule inhibitor of the human DNA repair enzyme polynucleotide kinase/phosphatase. *Cancer Res.* **2009**, *69*, 7739–7746. [CrossRef] [PubMed]

47. Jiang, H.-X.; Kong, D.-M.; Shen, H.-X. Amplified detection of DNA ligase and polynucleotide kinase/phosphatase on the basis of enrichment of catalytic G-quadruplex DNAzyme by rolling circle amplification. *Biosens. Bioelectron.* **2014**, *55*, 133–138. [CrossRef] [PubMed]

48. Bodrossy, L.; Sessitsch, A. Oligonucleotide microarrays in microbial diagnostics. *Curr. Opin. Microbiol.* **2004**, *7*, 245–254. [CrossRef] [PubMed]

49. Eriksson, R.; Jobs, M.; Ekstrand, C.; Ullberg, M.; Herrmann, B.; Landegren, U.; Nilsson, M.; Blomberg, J. Multiplex and quantifiable detection of nucleic acid from pathogenic fungi using padlock probes, generic real time PCR and specific suspension array readout. *J. Microbiol. Methods* **2009**, *78*, 195–202. [CrossRef] [PubMed]

50. Atkins, S.D.; Clark, I.M. Fungal molecular diagnostics: A mini review. *J. Appl. Genet.* **2004**, *45*, 3–15. [PubMed]

51. Cho, S.-N.; Brennan, P.J. Tuberculosis: Diagnostics. *Tuberculosis* **2007**, *87*, S14–S17. [CrossRef] [PubMed]

52. López, M.M.; Bertolini, E.; Olmos, A.; Caruso, P.; Gorris, M.T.; Llop, P.; Penyalver, R.; Cambra, M. Innovative tools for detection of plant pathogenic viruses and bacteria. *Int. Microbiol.* **2003**, *6*, 233–243. [CrossRef] [PubMed]

53. Manso, J.; Mena, M.L.; Yanez-Sedeno, P.; Pingarrón, J.M. Bienzyme amperometric biosensor using gold nanoparticle-modified electrodes for the determination of inulin in foods. *Anal. Biochem.* **2008**, *375*, 345–353. [CrossRef] [PubMed]

54. Homola, J. Surface plasmon resonance sensors for detection of chemical and biological species. *Chem. Rev.* **2008**, *108*, 462–493. [CrossRef] [PubMed]

55. Cosnier, S.; Mailley, P. Recent advances in DNA sensors. *Analyst* **2008**, *133*, 984–991. [CrossRef] [PubMed]

56. Shi, D.; Huang, J.; Chuai, Z.; Chen, D.; Zhu, X.; Wang, H.; Peng, J.; Wu, H.; Huang, Q.; Fu, W. Isothermal and rapid detection of pathogenic microorganisms using a nano-rolling circle amplification-surface plasmon resonance biosensor. *Biosens. Bioelectron.* **2014**, *62*, 280–287. [CrossRef] [PubMed]

57. Daniel, D.; Lalitha, R. Tumor markers—A bird's eye view. *J. Oral Maxillofac. Surg. Med. Pathol.* **2016**, *28*, 475–480. [CrossRef]

58. De Rancher, M.-A.R.; Oudart, J.B.; Maquart, F.X.; Monboisse, J.C.; Ramont, L. Evaluation of Lumipulse® G1200 for the measurement of six tumor markers: Comparison with AIA® 2000. *Clin. Biochem.* **2016**, *49*, 1302–1306. [CrossRef] [PubMed]

59. Chung, S.; Moon, J.M.; Ban, C.; Shim, Y.B. A Simple and Fast SELEX Using an Alternating Current Potential Modulated Microfluidic Channel and an Evaluation of Sensing Ability of Aptamers. In *Meeting Abstracts*; The Electrochemical Society: Pennington, NJ, USA, 2016.

60. Mu, Q.; Annapragada, A.; Srivastava, M.; Thiviyanathan, V.; Li, X.; Gorenstein, D.; Annapragada, A.; Vigneswaran, N. Conjugate-SELEX, a novel screening method, identifies aptamers that deliver payload to the cytosol of target cells. *Cancer Res.* **2016**, *76*, 3913. [CrossRef]

61. Sanghavi, B.J.; Moore, J.A.; Chávez, J.L.; Hagen, J.A.; Kelley-Loughnane, N.; Chou, C.F.; Swami, N.S. Aptamer-functionalized nanoparticles for surface immobilization-free electrochemical detection of cortisol in a microfluidic device. *Biosens. Bioelectron.* **2016**, *78*, 244–252. [CrossRef] [PubMed]

62. Théodorou, I.; Quang, N.N.; Gombert, K.; Thézé, B.; Lelandais, B.; Ducongé, F. In Vitro and In Vivo Imaging of Fluorescent Aptamers. In *Nucleic Acid Aptamers: Selection, Characterization, and Application*; Springer: New York, NY, USA, 2016; pp. 135–150.

63. Wu, L.; Qi, P.; Fu, X.; Liu, H.; Li, J.; Wang, Q.; Fan, H. A novel electrochemical PCB77-binding DNA aptamer biosensor for selective detection of PCB77. *J. Electroanal. Chem.* **2016**, *771*, 45–49. [CrossRef]

64. Zhang, S.-B.; Zheng, L.Y.; Hu, X.; Shen, G.Y.; Liu, X.W.; Shen, G.L.; Yu, R.Q. Highly Sensitive Fluorescent Aptasensor for Thrombin Detection Based on Competition Triggered Rolling Circle Amplification. *Chin. J. Anal. Chem.* **2015**, *43*, 1688–1694. [CrossRef]

65. Kerman, K.; Ozkan, D.; Kara, P.; Meric, B.; Gooding, J.J.; Ozsoz, M. Voltammetric determination of DNA hybridization using methylene blue and self-assembled alkanethiol monolayer on gold electrodes. *Anal. Chim. Acta* **2002**, *462*, 39–47. [CrossRef]

66. Wang, Q.; Zheng, H.; Gao, X.; Lin, Z.; Chen, G. A label-free ultrasensitive electrochemical aptameric recognition system for protein assay based on hyperbranched rolling circle amplification. *Chem. Commun.* **2013**, *49*, 11418–11420. [CrossRef] [PubMed]

67. Alves-Balvedi, R.P.; Caetano, L.P.; Madurro, J.M.; Brito-Madurro, A.G. Use of 3,3′,5,5′ tetramethylbenzidine as new electrochemical indicator of DNA hybridization and its application in genossensor. *Biosens. Bioelectron.* **2016**, *85*, 226–231. [CrossRef] [PubMed]

68. Berg, H.; Horn, G.; Luthardt, U.; Ihn, W. Interaction of anthracycline antibiotics with biopolymers: Part V. Polarographic behavior and complexes with DNA. *Bioelectrochem. Bioenerget.* **1981**, *8*, 537–553. [CrossRef]

69. Zhang, Y.; Zhang, K.; Ma, H. Electrochemical DNA biosensor based on silver nanoparticles/poly (3-(3-pyridyl) acrylic acid)/carbon nanotubes modified electrode. *Anal. Biochem.* **2009**, *387*, 13–19. [CrossRef] [PubMed]

70. Lu, L.; Liu, B.; Zhao, Z.; Ma, C.; Luo, P.; Liu, C.; Xie, G. Ultrasensitive electrochemical immunosensor for HE4 based on rolling circle amplification. *Biosens. Bioelectron.* **2012**, *33*, 216–221. [CrossRef] [PubMed]

71. Yi, X.; Li, L.; Peng, Y.; Guo, L. A universal electrochemical sensing system for small biomolecules using target-mediated sticky ends-based ligation-rolling circle amplification. *Biosens. Bioelectron.* **2014**, *57*, 103–109. [CrossRef] [PubMed]

72. Latchman, D.S. Transcription factors: An overview. *Int. J. Biochem. Cell Biol.* **1997**, *29*, 1305–1312. [CrossRef]

73. Rosenbauer, F.; Tenen, D.G. Transcription factors in myeloid development: Balancing differentiation with transformation. *Nat. Rev. Immunol.* **2007**, *7*, 105–117. [CrossRef] [PubMed]

74. Engelkamp, D.; van Heyningen, V. Transcription factors in disease. *Curr. Opin. Genet. Dev.* **1996**, *6*, 334–342. [CrossRef]

75. Zhang, Y.; Ma, F.; Tang, B.; Zhang, C. Recent advances in transcription factor assays in vitro. *Chem. Commun.* **2016**, *52*, 4739–4748. [CrossRef] [PubMed]

76. Garner, M.M.; Revzin, A. A gel electrophoresis method for quantifying the binding of proteins to specific DNA regions: Application to components of the *Escherichia coli* lactose operon regulatory system. *Nucleic Acids Res.* **1981**, *9*, 3047–3060. [CrossRef] [PubMed]

77. Galas, D.J.; Schmitz, A. DNAase footprinting a simple method for the detection of protein-DNA binding specificity. *Nucleic Acids Res.* **1978**, *5*, 3157–3170. [CrossRef] [PubMed]

78. Burnette, W.N. "Western blotting": Electrophoretic transfer of proteins from sodium dodecyl sulfate-polyacrylamide gels to unmodified nitrocellulose and radiographic detection with antibody and radioiodinated protein A. *Anal. Biochem.* **1981**, *112*, 195–203. [CrossRef]

79. Li, C.; Qiu, X.; Hou, Z.; Deng, K. A dumbell probe-mediated rolling circle amplification strategy for highly sensitive transcription factor detection. *Biosens. Bioelectron.* **2015**, *64*, 505–510. [CrossRef] [PubMed]

80. Liang, Y.; Ridzon, D.; Wong, L.; Chen, C. Characterization of microRNA expression profiles in normal human tissues. *BMC Genom.* **2007**, *8*. [CrossRef] [PubMed]

81. Ambros, V. The functions of animal microRNAs. *Nature* **2004**, *431*, 350–355. [CrossRef] [PubMed]

82. Heneghan, H.M.; Miller, N.; Lowery, A.J.; Sweeney, K.J.; Newell, J.; Kerin, M.J. Circulating microRNAs as novel minimally invasive biomarkers for breast cancer. *Ann. Surg.* **2010**, *251*, 499–505. [CrossRef] [PubMed]

83. Li, C.; Feng, Y.; Coukos, G.; Zhang, L. Therapeutic microRNA strategies in human cancer. *AAPS J.* **2009**, *11*, 747–757. [CrossRef] [PubMed]

84. Zhu, W.; Qin, W.; Atasoy, U.; Sauter, E.R. Circulating microRNAs in breast cancer and healthy subjects. *BMC Res. Notes* **2009**, *2*. [CrossRef] [PubMed]

85. Stenvang, J.; Silahtaroglu, A.N.; Lindow, M.; Elmen, J.; Kauppinen, S. The utility of LNA in microRNA-based cancer diagnostics and therapeutics. In *Seminars in Cancer Biology*; Elsevier: Amsterdam, The Netherlands, 2008.

86. Cho, W.C. MicroRNAs: Potential biomarkers for cancer diagnosis, prognosis and targets for therapy. *Int. J. Biochem. Cell Biol.* **2010**, *42*, 1273–1281. [CrossRef] [PubMed]

87. Li, J.; Tan, S.; Kooger, R.; Zhang, C.; Zhang, Y. MicroRNAs as novel biological targets for detection and regulation. *Chem. Soc. Rev.* **2014**, *43*, 506–517. [CrossRef] [PubMed]

88. Volinia, S.; Calin, G.A.; Liu, C.G.; Ambs, S.; Cimmino, A.; Petrocca, F.; Visone, R.; Iorio, M.; Roldo, C.; Ferracin, M.; et al. A microRNA expression signature of human solid tumors defines cancer gene targets. *Proc. Natl. Acad. Sci. USA* **2006**, *103*, 2257–2261. [CrossRef] [PubMed]

89. Válóczi, A.; Hornyik, C.; Varga, N.; Burgyán, J.; Kauppinen, S.; Havelda, Z. Sensitive and specific detection of microRNAs by northern blot analysis using LNA-modified oligonucleotide probes. *Nucleic Acids Res.* **2004**, *32*, e175. [CrossRef] [PubMed]

90. Chen, C.; Ridzon, D.A.; Broomer, A.J.; Zhou, Z.; Lee, D.H.; Nguyen, J.T.; Barbisin, M.; Xu, N.L.; Mahuvakar, V.R.; Andersen, M.R.; et al. Real-time quantification of microRNAs by stem–loop RT–PCR. *Nucleic Acids Res.* **2005**, *33*, e179. [CrossRef] [PubMed]

91. Li, W.; Ruan, K. MicroRNA detection by microarray. *Anal. Bioanal. Chem.* **2009**, *394*, 1117–1124. [CrossRef] [PubMed]

92. Bi, S.; Li, L.; Cui, Y. Exonuclease-assisted cascaded recycling amplification for label-free detection of DNA. *Chem. Commun.* **2012**, *48*, 1018–1020. [CrossRef] [PubMed]

93. Wang, M.; Fu, Z.; Li, B.; Zhou, Y.; Yin, H.; Ai, S. One-step, ultrasensitive, and electrochemical assay of microRNAs based on T7 exonuclease assisted cyclic enzymatic amplification. *Anal. Chem.* **2014**, *86*, 5606–5610. [CrossRef] [PubMed]

94. Liu, Y.Q.; Zhang, M.; Yin, B.C.; Ye, B.C. Attomolar ultrasensitive microRNA detection by DNA-scaffolded silver-nanocluster probe based on isothermal amplification. *Anal. Chem.* **2012**, *84*, 5165–5169. [CrossRef] [PubMed]

95. Bi, S.; Cui, Y.; Dong, Y.; Zhang, N. Target-induced self-assembly of DNA nanomachine on magnetic particle for multi-amplified biosensing of nucleic acid, protein, and cancer cell. *Biosens. Bioelectron.* **2014**, *53*, 207–213. [CrossRef] [PubMed]

96. Liu, H.; Li, L.; Duan, L.; Wang, X.; Xie, Y.; Tong, L.; Wang, Q.; Tang, B. High specific and ultrasensitive isothermal detection of microRNA by padlock probe-based exponential rolling circle amplification. *Anal. Chem.* **2013**, *85*, 7941–7947. [CrossRef] [PubMed]

97. Deng, R.; Tang, L.; Tian, Q.; Wang, Y.; Lin, L.; Li, J. Toehold-initiated Rolling Circle Amplification for Visualizing Individual MicroRNAs In Situ in Single Cells. *Angew. Chem. Int. Ed.* **2014**, *53*, 2389–2393. [CrossRef] [PubMed]

98. JamesáYang, C. A T7 exonuclease-assisted cyclic enzymatic amplification method coupled with rolling circle amplification: A dual-amplification strategy for sensitive and selective microRNA detection. *Chem. Commun.* **2014**, *50*, 1576–1578.

99. Li, D.; Cheng, W.; Yan, Y.; Zhang, Y.; Yin, Y.; Ju, H.; Ding, S. A colorimetric biosensor for detection of attomolar microRNA with a functional nucleic acid-based amplification machine. *Talanta* **2016**, *146*, 470–476. [CrossRef] [PubMed]

100. Gao, X. The Progress Study of Gastric Cancer and Tumor Associated Protein. *Asian Case Rep. Oncol.* **2016**, *5*, 61–71. [CrossRef]

101. Olmsted, J. Affinity purification of antibodies from diazotized paper blots of heterogeneous protein samples. *J. Biol. Chem.* **1981**, *256*, 11955–11957. [PubMed]

102. Stavitsky, A.B.; Jarchow, C. Micromethods for the study of proteins and antibodies I. Procedure and general applications of hemagglutination and hemagglutination-inhibition reactions with tannic acid and protein-treated red blood cells. *J. Immunol.* **1954**, *72*, 360–367. [PubMed]

103. Savran, C.A.; Knudsen, S.M.; Ellington, A.D.; Manalis, S.R. Micromechanical detection of proteins using aptamer-based receptor molecules. *Anal. Chem.* **2004**, *76*, 3194–3198. [CrossRef] [PubMed]

104. Eissa, S.; Ng, A.; Siaj, M.; Zourob, M. Selection, Characterization, and Application of High Affinity Microcystin-Targeting Aptamers in a Graphene-Based Biosensing Platform. In *Meeting Abstracts*; The Electrochemical Society: Pennington, NJ, USA, 2015.

105. Chen, I.H.; Horikawa, S.; Du, S.; Liu, Y.; Wikle, H.C.; Barbaree, J.M.; Chin, B.A. Thermal Stability of Phage Peptide Probes vs. Aptamer for Salmonella Detection on Magnetoelastic Biosensors Platform. *ECS Trans.* **2016**, *75*, 165–173. [CrossRef]

106. Acharya, G.; Chang, C.L.; Doorneweerd, D.D.; Vlashi, E.; Henne, W.A.; Hartmann, L.C.; Low, P.S.; Savran, C.A. Immunomagnetic diffractometry for detection of diagnostic serum markers. *J. Am. Chem. Soc.* **2007**, *129*, 15824–15829. [CrossRef] [PubMed]

107. Lee, J.; Icoz, K.; Roberts, A.; Ellington, A.D.; Savran, C.A. Diffractometric detection of proteins using microbead-based rolling circle amplification. *Anal. Chem.* **2010**, *82*, 197–202. [CrossRef] [PubMed]

108. Noskovicova, N.; Petřek, M.; Eickelberg, O.; Heinzelmann, K. Platelet-derived growth factor signaling in the lung. From lung development and disease to clinical studies. *Am. J. Respir. Cell Mol. Biol.* **2015**, *52*, 263–284. [CrossRef] [PubMed]

109. Kuai, J.; Mosyak, L.; Brooks, J.; Cain, M.; Carven, G.J.; Ogawa, S.; Ishino, T.; Tam, M.; Lavallie, E.R.; Yang, Z.; et al. Characterization of binding mode of action of a blocking anti-platelet-derived growth factor (PDGF)-B monoclonal antibody, MOR8457, reveals conformational flexibility and avidity needed for PDGF-BB to bind PDGF receptor-β. *Biochemistry* **2015**, *54*, 1918–1929. [CrossRef] [PubMed]

110. Guo, L.; Hao, L.; Zhao, Q. An aptamer assay using rolling circle amplification coupled with thrombin catalysis for protein detection. *Anal. Bioanal. Chem.* **2016**, *408*, 4715–4722. [CrossRef] [PubMed]

111. Jiang, W.; Liu, L.; Zhang, L.; Guo, Q.; Cui, Y.; Yang, M. Sensitive immunosensing of the carcinoembryonic antigen utilizing aptamer-based in-situ formation of a redox-active heteropolyacid and rolling circle amplification. *Microchim. Acta* **2017**. [CrossRef]

112. Risch, N.; Merikangas, K. The future of genetic studies of complex human diseases. *Science* **1996**, *273*, 1516–1517. [CrossRef] [PubMed]

113. Fang, Y.; Orner, B.P. Induction of pluripotency in fibroblasts through the expression of only four nuclear proteins. *ACS Chem. Biol.* **2006**, *1*, 557–558. [CrossRef] [PubMed]

114. Zhang, J.; Chua, L.S.; Lynn, D.M. Multilayered thin films that sustain the release of functional DNA under physiological conditions. *Langmuir* **2004**, *20*, 8015–8021. [CrossRef] [PubMed]

115. Miao, W.; Bard, A.J. Electrogenerated chemiluminescence. 77. DNA hybridization detection at high amplification with [Ru(bpy)3]$^{2+}$-containing microspheres. *Anal. Chem.* **2004**, *76*, 5379–5386. [CrossRef] [PubMed]

116. Ding, C.; Wang, N.; Zhang, J.; Wang, Z. Rolling circle amplification combined with nanoparticle aggregates for highly sensitive identification of DNA and cancercells. *Biosens. Bioelectron.* **2013**, *42*, 486–491. [CrossRef] [PubMed]

117. Akbar, S.; Anwar, A.; Kanwal, Q. Electrochemical determination of folic acid: A short review. *Anal. Biochem.* **2016**, *510*, 98–105. [CrossRef] [PubMed]

118. Li, D.; Ma, Y.; Zhang, Y.; Lin, Z. Fluorescence biosensor for folate receptors in cancer cells based on terminal protection and hyperbranched rolling circle amplification. *Anal. Methods* **2016**, *8*, 6231–6235. [CrossRef]

14

A Systematic Review and Meta-Analysis of the In Vivo Haemodynamic Effects of Δ^9-Tetrahydrocannabinol

Salahaden R. Sultan [1,2], Sophie A. Millar [1] (iD), Saoirse E. O'Sullivan [1] and Timothy J. England [1,*] (iD)

1   Division of Medical Sciences & Graduate Entry Medicine, School of Medicine, University of Nottingham, Derby DE22 3DT, UK; mzxss4@nottingham.ac.uk (S.R.S.); stxsamil@nottingham.ac.uk (S.A.M.); mbzso@nottingham.ac.uk (S.E.O.)
2   Faculty of Applied Medical Sciences, King Abdulaziz University, Jeddah 21589, Saudi Arabia
*   Correspondence: timothy.england@nottingham.ac.uk

Abstract: Δ^9-Tetrahydrocannabinol (THC) has complex effects on the cardiovascular system. We aimed to systematically review studies of THC and haemodynamic alterations. PubMed, Medline, and EMBASE were searched for relevant studies. Changes in blood pressure (BP), heart rate (HR), and blood flow (BF) were analysed using the Cochrane Review Manager Software. Thirty-one studies met the eligibility criteria. Fourteen publications assessed BP (number, $n = 541$), 22 HR ($n = 567$), and 3 BF ($n = 45$). Acute THC dosing reduced BP and HR in anaesthetised animals (BP, mean difference (MD) -19.7 mmHg, $p < 0.00001$; HR, MD -53.49 bpm, $p < 0.00001$), conscious animals (BP, MD -12.3 mmHg, $p = 0.0007$; HR, MD -30.05 bpm, $p < 0.00001$), and animal models of stress or hypertension (BP, MD -61.37 mmHg, $p = 0.03$) and increased cerebral BF in murine stroke models (MD 32.35%, $p < 0.00001$). Chronic dosing increased BF in large arteries in anaesthetised animals (MD 21.95 mL/min, $p = 0.05$) and reduced BP in models of stress or hypertension (MD -22.09 mmHg, $p < 0.00001$). In humans, acute administration increased HR (MD 8.16 bpm, $p < 0.00001$). THC acts differently according to species and experimental conditions, causing bradycardia, hypotension and increased BF in animals; and causing increased HR in humans. Data is limited, and further studies assessing THC-induced haemodynamic changes in humans should be considered.

Keywords: Δ^9-Tetrahydrocannabinol; THC; cardiovascular system; blood pressure; heart rate; blood flow

1. Introduction

Δ^9-Tetrahydrocannabinol (THC) is the most abundant and widely studied phytocannabinoid, first discovered in 1964 [1]. THC is a partial agonist of both cannabinoid receptors CB_1 and CB_2 and other targets including G protein-coupled receptors GPR55 and GPR18 [2–4]. THC possesses interesting therapeutic potential as an antiemetic, appetite stimulant, and analgesic, and for the treatment of glaucoma, epilepsy, Parkinson's disease, and multiple sclerosis [5–7]. THC has been shown to be effective against refractory nausea and vomiting in cancer patients undergoing chemotherapy [8]. However, its use as a therapeutic agent is limited by its recognised psychogenic side effects including hallucinations, euphoria, dizziness, mood changes, nausea, and fatigue [8–10].

THC has numerous cardiovascular effects in animals and humans. In vitro studies have shown that THC causes endothelium-independent vasorelaxation of rabbit superior mesenteric arteries [11] and vasorelaxation of the rat mesenteric artery through sensory nerves via a CB_1 and CB_2 receptor-independent mechanism [12]. Other studies have found THC to activate a G protein-coupled receptor, inhibit calcium channels, and activate potassium channels in the rat mesenteric vasculature [13] and to cause endothelium-dependent and time-dependent vasorelaxation in the rat aorta [14,15]. In contrast, other studies have shown that THC causes vasoconstriction in guinea pig pulmonary arteries [16], rat mesenteric arteries and aorta [14,17], and rabbit ear arteries [18].

In vivo studies have reported different haemodynamic responses post-THC. An acute administration of THC caused hypotension and bradycardia in anesthetised dogs (intravenously; i.v.), conscious bats (intraperitoneal; i.p.), and humans (oral) [19–21]. In contrast, tachycardia and hypertension were reported in rats after i.p. administration of THC [22,23]. More complex effects on BP were induced by THC in anaesthetised rats [24]. The available evidence to date suggests that THC alters the haemodynamics in animals and humans, albeit with conflicting results variable with species, route of administration, and experimental conditions. Therefore, the aim this study was to systematically review and meta-analyse the in vivo literature assessing the effects of THC on the cardiovascular system in all species under different conditions.

2. Results

From the initial 2743 search results, 1935 relevant publications were identified and evaluated from three databases (Medline, EMBASE, and PubMed). Of these, 30 articles met the inclusion criteria and 1 article was added manually (Figure 1). A summary of the data extracted from the included studies is shown in Table 1.

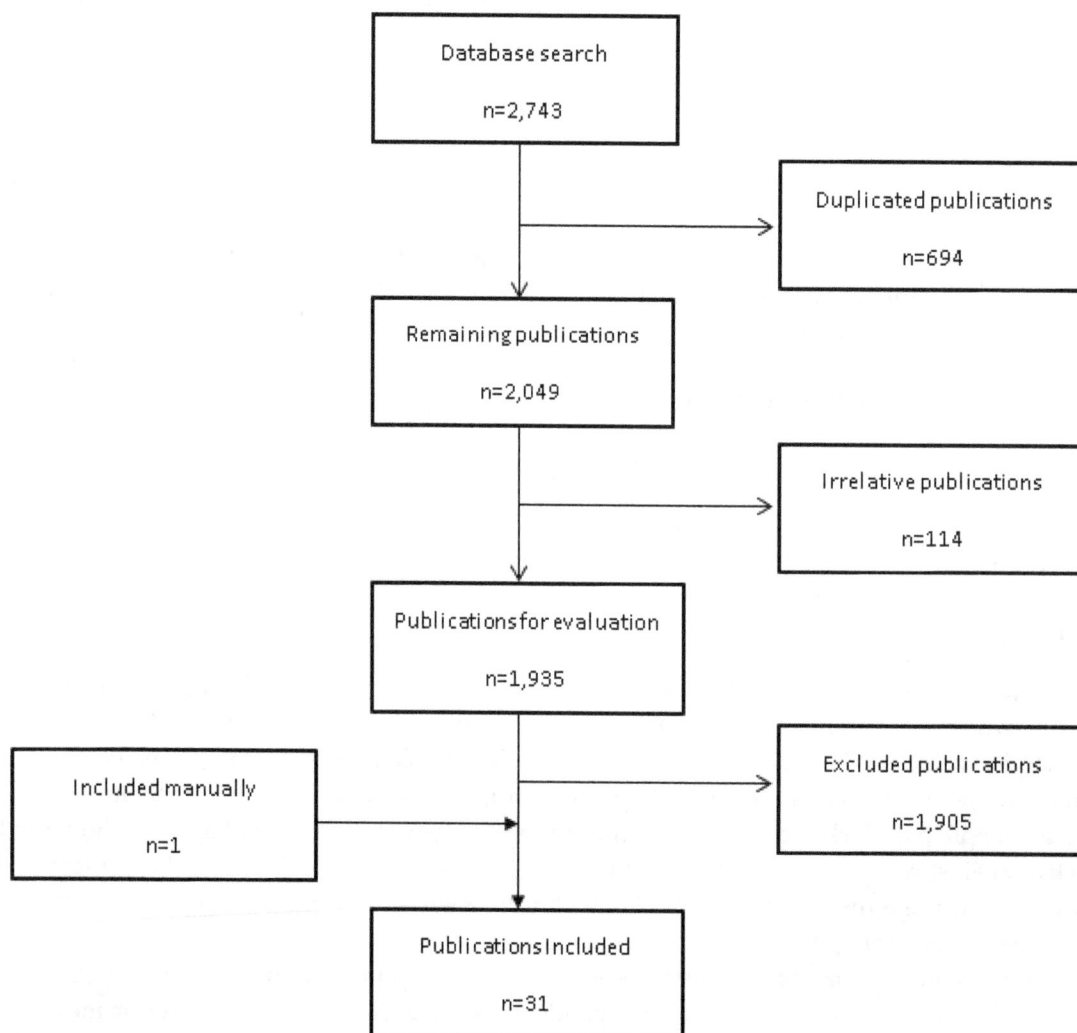

Figure 1. Flow chart for study retrieval and selection.

Table 1. Summary of the included studies divided according to the experimental conditions.

Author & Year	Study Description	Species, Model (Anaesthetic & Route)	Sample Size	THC Dose	THC Route	Time of THC Administration	Time of Haemodynamic Measurements	Basal Parameters*	Outcomes and Comments
									Anaesthetised animals
Cavero 1972 [25]	Investigate the haemodynamic effects of THC	Dogs Anaesthetised (pentobarbital, iv)	11	2.5 mg/kg	i.v.	Post-anaesthesia	Continues for 30 m post-drug	-	THC altered distribution of regional BF, and reduced HR and BP.
Cavero 1973a [26]	Investigate the haemodynamic effects of THC	Dogs Anaesthetised (pentobarbital, iv)	23	39 µg/kg–2.5 mg/kg	i.v.	Post-anaesthesia	Continues for 2 h post-drug	C: HR:169, BP:91.7; T: HR:165.7, BP:93.5	THC caused reduction in HR and BP mediated via central nervous system.
Cavero 1973b [27]	Characterise the mechanism of action of THC on HR	Dogs Anaesthetised (pentobarbital, iv)	29	39 µg/kg–5 mg/kg	i.v.	Post-anaesthesia	Continues for 140 m post-drug	-	THC induced reduction in HR through alteration of autonomic innervation to myocardium.
Cavero 1974 [19]	Investigate the effect of THC on venous return	Dogs (heart bypass) Anaesthetised (dibucaine, spinal)	8	2.5 mg/kg	i.v.	Post-anaesthesia	Pre-drug and continues for 30 m post-drug	C: HR:156, BP:85.8; T: HR:147, BP:85.	THC caused reduction in HR and BP, and reduced venous return.
Daskalopoulos 1975 [28]	Investigate the mechanism of THC on CV system	Cats Anaesthetised (urethane, iv)	40	30–300 µg/kg	i.v.	Post-anaesthesia	20 m post-drug	-	THC reduced HR and BP mediated via central nervous system.
Adams 1976 [29]	Examined the CV effects of THC	Rats Anaesthetised (urethane, ip)	72	0.1–3 mg/kg	i.v.	Post-anaesthesia	Continues for 30 min post-drug	C: HR:316.2, BP:76.2; T: HR:314.8, BP:73.5.	THC caused reduction in HR and biphasic BP response (↑ BP followed by ↓ BP), suggesting that THC depressed CV reflex functions.
Jandhyala 1976 [30]	Evaluated possible interaction with THC on HR	Dogs Anaesthetised (pentobarbital)	12	1 mg/kg	s.c.	Twice/day for 7 days Pre-anaesthesia	On the 7th day post-anaesthesia	-	Chronic THC antagonised the elevation in HR induced by the anaesthetic agent via vagal stimulation.
Jandhyala 1977 [31]	Determined chronic administration of THC on CV function	Dogs Anaesthetised (pentobarbital)	16	1 mg/kg	s.c.	Twice/day for 7 days Pre-anaesthesia	On the 7th day post-anaesthesia	-	Chronic THC had no effect on haemodynamics.
Jandhyala 1978 [32]	Investigated prolonged THC effects on CV system	Dogs Anaesthetised (pentobarbital)	16	2 mg/kg	s.c.	Single dose per day for 35 days	On the 35th day post-anaesthesia	-	Chronic THC increased BF in femoral and mesenteric arteries with no effect on HR or BP.
McConnell 1978 [33]	Examined the effects of THC on salivary flow	Cats Anaesthetised (urethane & pentobarbital, ip)	20	0.1–2 mg/kg	i.v.	Post-anaesthesia	Continues for 1 h post-drug	-	THC had no effect in stimulated salivary flow of cats. THC caused a reduction in HR and BP.

Table 1. *Cont.*

Author & Year	Study Description	Species, Model (Anaesthetic & Route)	Sample Size	THC Dose	THC Route	Time of THC Administration	Time of Haemodynamic Measurements	Basal Parameters*	Outcomes and Comments
Anaesthetised animals									
Siqueira 1979 [24]	Clarify the triple BP response post-THC	Rats Anaesthetised (urethane, ip)	50	1–10 mg/kg	i.v.	Post-anaesthesia	Continues for 70 m post-drug	-	THC induced triphasic BP response (↓ BP via vagal stimulation, then ↑ BP not dependent on sympathetic activity followed by ↓ BP due to central decrease in sympathetic tone).
Kawasaki 1980 [23]	Investigated the effect of THC on the CV system and behavior changes	Rats Anaesthetised (urethane, ip)	29	1–5 mg/kg	i.v.	Post-anaesthesia	Continues for 70 m post-drug	-	THC induced CV effects (↓ HR and ↑ BP) through vagal activity, and influence behavior changes to brain stimulation.
Schmeling 1981 [34]	Investigated the effect of THC on hypothalamus	Cats Anaesthetised (urethane, ip)	12	2 mg/kg	i.v.	Post-anaesthesia	Continues for 30 m post-drug	-	THC produced significant reductions in HR and BP and attenuated the pressor response threshold suggesting that THC reduces sympathetic activity.
Estrada 1987 [35]	Investigated the CV effects of THC	Rats Anaesthetised (pentobarbital, ip)	28	0.078–5 mg/kg	i.v.	Post-anaesthesia	3–12 min post-drug	-	THC produced adverse effects on the CV system (↓ HR and ↓ BP)
Krowicki 1999 [36]	Investigated whether CB₁ activation by THC inhibits gastric motor function	Rats Anaesthetised (ketamine and xylazine)	36	0.02–2 mg/kg	i.v.	Post-anaesthesia	Continues for 10 m post-drug	-	THC decreased gastric motor function, HR, and BP via autonomic effects mediated by CB₁.
Conscious animals									
Kaymakcalan 1974 [37]	Investigated chronic effects of THC on HR	Rats Conscious	20	10 mg/kg	s.c.	Single dose per day for 16 days	Hourly interval to 6 h on the 1st, 4th, 8th and 16th days	-	THC produced marked reduction in HR
Borgen 1974 [38]	Examined possible interaction of CBD on THC effects	Rabbits Conscious	8	3 mg/kg	i.v.	Pre-test	Pre-drug and hourly interval to 7 h post-drug	C: HR:264; T: HR:276	CBD reduced the hypothermic effect of THC and attenuated the depressant effects of THC on respiration, rectal temperature and HR
Brown 1974 [20]	Investigated CV response to THC	Rats Conscious	12	100 and 200 mg/kg	ip.	Pre-test	Pre-drug and continues for 145 m post-drug	C: HR:436, BP:101; T: HR:390, BP:114	THC induced hypothermia and reduction in HR and BP.

Table 1. *Cont.*

Author & Year	Study Description	Species, Model (Anaesthetic & Route)	Sample Size	THC Dose	THC Route	Time of THC Administration	Time of Haemodynamic Measurements	Basal Parameters *	Outcomes and Comments
Conscious animals									
Osgood 1977 [22]	Investigated THC effects on HR	Rats Conscious	18	0.5 mg/kg	i.p.	Pre-test	Continues for 30 m post-drug	-	THC had minimal effect on BP and caused an increase in HR, which may be related to central mediation release of epinephrine from adrenal gland.
Kawasaki 1980 [23]	Investigated the effects of THC on the CV system and behavior changes	Rats Conscious	21	4–8 mg/kg	i.p.	Pre-test	Continues for 2 h post-drug	-	THC induced CV effects (↓ HR and ↑ BP) through vagal activity, and influenced behavior changes to brain stimulation.
Matsuzaki 1987 [39]	Examined the effects of THC on EEG, body temperature, and HR	Monkeys Conscious	6	0.4–4 mg/kg	i.p.	Pre-test	Continues for 5 h post-drug	-	THC induced reduction in HR and hypothermia and induced responses of EGG along with behavioral depression and alertness.
Hayakawa 2007a [40]	Investigated CBD and THC effects on ischemic brain damage	Stroke Mice Conscious	17	10 mg/kg	i.p.	Pre, 3 and 4 h post-occlusion, and 1 and 2 h post-reperfusion	BP and HR: pre-reperfusion. CBF: continued 4 h post-occlusion and 1 post-reperfusion	-	Pre and post-ischemic treatment with CBD induced neuroprotection, whereas only preischemic treatment with THC induced neuroprotection. THC increased CBF with no effects on BP or HR
Hayakawa 2007b [41]	Explored the development of tolerance of THC and CBD neuroprotection	Stroke Mice Conscious	7	10 mg/kg	i.p.	Pre-occlusion and 3 h post-occlusion. Single dose per day for 14 days	During 4 h and on day 14 post-occlusion	-	Repeated treatment with CBD, but not THC, induced neuroprotection with development of tolerance. THC increased CBF on day 1 only with no effects on BP or HR.
Stress and hypertensive animal models									
Williams 1973 [42]	Studied the effects of THC on BP	Rats Stress	30	20 mg/kg	s.c.	Single dose per day for 4 days	Pre-drug, 4 h, 48 and 96 h post-drug	C: BP:128; T: BP:129	THC reduced BP
Birmingham 1973 [43]	Studies the effects of THC on BP	Rats Hypertensive	10	3 mg/kg	i.p.	Single dose per day for 7 days	Hourly to 5 h for 7 days	-	THC reduced BP
Kosersky 1978 [44]	Examined the antihypertensive effects of THC	Rats Hypertensive	12	25 mg/kg	Oral	Single dose per day for 10 days	4 h and every day for 14 days post-drug	-	THC effectively reduced BP to the same degree over the treatment period.

Table 1. *Cont.*

Author & Year	Study Description	Species, Model (Anaesthetic & Route)	Sample Size	THC Dose	THC Route	Time of THC Administration	Time of Haemodynamic Measurements	Basal Parameters*	Outcomes and Comments
					Humans				
Karniol 1973 [45]	Compared the effects of 8-THC and 9-THC	Human Healthy	21	5-20 mg	Inhale	Pre-test	Avrg. of 20 m post-drug	C: HR:82; T: HR:85	9-THC was twice as active as 8-THC in increasing HR and caused more subjective symptoms.
Karniol 1975 [46]	Examined the interaction between THC and CBN	Human Healthy	5 (M)	25 mg	Oral	Pre-test	50, 70 and 160 m post-drug	-	THC induced increase in HR and psychological effects. No change on THC effects when combined with CBN
Zimmer 1976 [47]	Examined changes of somatic parameters post-THC	Human Healthy	36	250 µg/kg	Oral	Pre-test	Pre-drug and 4 h post-drug	C: HR:87.9, BP:127.5; T: HR:89, BP:123	THC raised HR with no changes on other parameters including BP
Haney 2007 [48]	Determined the effects of naltrexone in combination with THC	Human Healthy	21 (11 M & 10 F)	2.5-10 mg	Oral	Pre-test	Continues for 6 h post-drug	-	Naltrexone enhanced intoxication effects of THC; THC increased HR
Beaumont 2009 [21]	Evaluated whether THC has inhibitory effect on transient esophageal sphincter	Human Healthy	18 (M)	10 and 20 mg	Oral	Pre-test	Continues for 4 h post-drug	C: HR:59; T: HR:59	THC inhibited the increased induced meal transient esophageal sphincter relaxation. THC increased HR and decreased BP
Klooker 2011 [49]	Assessed the effect of THC on rectal sensation	Human Healthy and IBD	10 and 12	5 and 10 mg	Oral	Pre-test	Continues for 105 m post-drug	-	THC had no effect on rectal perception to distension. THC increased HR with no effect on BP

Abbreviations: BP: blood pressure, BF: Blood flow, C: control group, CB$_1$: cannabinoid receptor 1, CBD: Cannabidiol, CBF: cerebral blood flow, CBN: cannabinol, CV: cardiovascular, D: THC treated group, F: females, G: gender, h: hour(s), HR: heart rate, , IBD: inflammatory bowel disease i.p.: intraperitoneal, i.v.: intravenous, M: males, m: minute(s), s.c.: Subcutaneous, T: treatment group, THC: Δ^9-Tetrahydrocannabinol. ↑: increased, ↓: decreased. * Basal parameters values before intervention (i.e., anaesthetic agents or THC). The units of the parameters are HR: beats/m, BP: mmHg, BF: mL/m.

2.1. Effect of THC Treatment on Haemodynamics

2.1.1. Anaesthetised Animals

Fifteen publications [19,23–36] assessed the effect of THC administration in three anaesthetised species (rats, dogs, and cats, $n = 664$). THC significantly reduced BP and HR after acute dosing (BP, MD -19.7 mmHg, 95%CI -26.16, -13.25, $p < 0.00001$; HR, MD -53.49 bpm, 95%CI -65.9, -41.07, $p < 0.00001$, Figure 2A,B). A cross-species analysis revealed that THC responses in the three species were significantly different in both BP ($p < 0.00001$) and HR ($p = 0.01$) (Figure 2A,B), and acute THC significantly reduced BP in rats and cats, but not in anesthetised dogs ($p = 0.18$, Figure 2A).

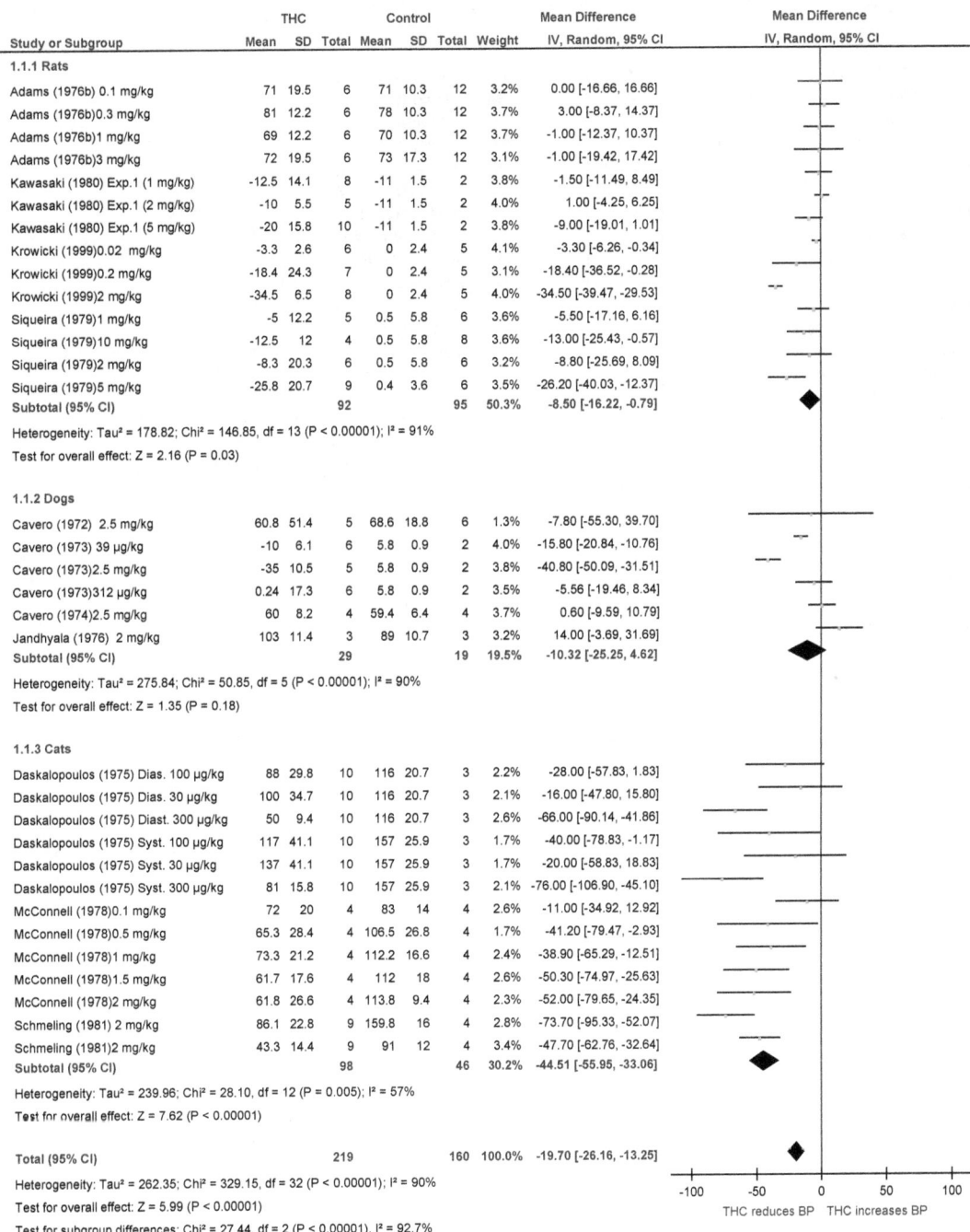

Study or Subgroup	THC Mean	SD	Total	Control Mean	SD	Total	Weight	Mean Difference IV, Random, 95% CI
1.1.1 Rats								
Adams (1976b) 0.1 mg/kg	71	19.5	6	71	10.3	12	3.2%	0.00 [-16.66, 16.66]
Adams (1976b) 0.3 mg/kg	81	12.2	6	78	10.3	12	3.7%	3.00 [-8.37, 14.37]
Adams (1976b) 1 mg/kg	69	12.2	6	70	10.3	12	3.7%	-1.00 [-12.37, 10.37]
Adams (1976b) 3 mg/kg	72	19.5	6	73	17.3	12	3.1%	-1.00 [-19.42, 17.42]
Kawasaki (1980) Exp.1 (1 mg/kg)	-12.5	14.1	8	-11	1.5	2	3.8%	-1.50 [-11.49, 8.49]
Kawasaki (1980) Exp.1 (2 mg/kg)	-10	5.5	5	-11	1.5	2	4.0%	1.00 [-4.25, 6.25]
Kawasaki (1980) Exp.1 (5 mg/kg)	-20	15.8	10	-11	1.5	2	3.8%	-9.00 [-19.01, 1.01]
Krowicki (1999) 0.02 mg/kg	-3.3	2.6	6	0	2.4	5	4.1%	-3.30 [-6.26, -0.34]
Krowicki (1999) 0.2 mg/kg	-18.4	24.3	7	0	2.4	5	3.1%	-18.40 [-36.52, -0.28]
Krowicki (1999) 2 mg/kg	-34.5	6.5	8	0	2.4	5	4.0%	-34.50 [-39.47, -29.53]
Siqueira (1979) 1 mg/kg	-5	12.2	5	0.5	5.8	6	3.6%	-5.50 [-17.16, 6.16]
Siqueira (1979) 10 mg/kg	-12.5	12	4	0.5	5.8	8	3.6%	-13.00 [-25.43, -0.57]
Siqueira (1979) 2 mg/kg	-8.3	20.3	6	0.5	5.8	6	3.2%	-8.80 [-25.69, 8.09]
Siqueira (1979) 5 mg/kg	-25.8	20.7	9	0.4	3.6	6	3.5%	-26.20 [-40.03, -12.37]
Subtotal (95% CI)			92			95	50.3%	-8.50 [-16.22, -0.79]
Heterogeneity: Tau² = 178.82; Chi² = 146.85, df = 13 (P < 0.00001); I² = 91%								
Test for overall effect: Z = 2.16 (P = 0.03)								
1.1.2 Dogs								
Cavero (1972) 2.5 mg/kg	60.8	51.4	5	68.6	18.8	6	1.3%	-7.80 [-55.30, 39.70]
Cavero (1973) 39 µg/kg	-10	6.1	6	5.8	0.9	2	4.0%	-15.80 [-20.84, -10.76]
Cavero (1973) 2.5 mg/kg	-35	10.5	6	5.8	0.9	2	3.8%	-40.80 [-50.09, -31.51]
Cavero (1973) 312 µg/kg	0.24	17.3	6	5.8	0.9	2	3.5%	-5.56 [-19.46, 8.34]
Cavero (1974) 2.5 mg/kg	60	8.2	4	59.4	6.4	4	3.7%	0.60 [-9.59, 10.79]
Jandhyala (1976) 2 mg/kg	103	11.4	3	89	10.7	3	3.2%	14.00 [-3.69, 31.69]
Subtotal (95% CI)			29			19	19.5%	-10.32 [-25.25, 4.62]
Heterogeneity: Tau² = 275.84; Chi² = 50.85, df = 5 (P < 0.00001); I² = 90%								
Test for overall effect: Z = 1.35 (P = 0.18)								
1.1.3 Cats								
Daskalopoulos (1975) Dias. 100 µg/kg	88	29.8	10	116	20.7	3	2.2%	-28.00 [-57.83, 1.83]
Daskalopoulos (1975) Dias. 30 µg/kg	100	34.7	10	116	20.7	3	2.1%	-16.00 [-47.80, 15.80]
Daskalopoulos (1975) Diast. 300 µg/kg	50	9.4	10	116	20.7	3	2.6%	-66.00 [-90.14, -41.86]
Daskalopoulos (1975) Syst. 100 µg/kg	117	41.1	10	157	25.9	3	1.7%	-40.00 [-78.83, -1.17]
Daskalopoulos (1975) Syst. 30 µg/kg	137	41.1	10	157	25.9	3	1.7%	-20.00 [-58.83, 18.83]
Daskalopoulos (1975) Syst. 300 µg/kg	81	15.8	10	157	25.9	3	2.1%	-76.00 [-106.90, -45.10]
McConnell (1978) 0.1 mg/kg	72	20	4	83	14	4	2.6%	-11.00 [-34.92, 12.92]
McConnell (1978) 0.5 mg/kg	65.3	28.4	4	106.5	26.8	4	1.7%	-41.20 [-79.47, -2.93]
McConnell (1978) 1 mg/kg	73.3	21.2	4	112.2	16.6	4	2.4%	-38.90 [-65.29, -12.51]
McConnell (1978) 1.5 mg/kg	61.7	17.6	4	112	18	4	2.6%	-50.30 [-74.97, -25.63]
McConnell (1978) 2 mg/kg	61.8	26.6	4	113.8	9.4	4	2.3%	-52.00 [-79.65, -24.35]
Schmeling (1981) 2 mg/kg	86.1	22.8	9	159.8	16	4	2.8%	-73.70 [-95.33, -52.07]
Schmeling (1981) 2 mg/kg	43.3	14.4	9	91	12	4	3.4%	-47.70 [-62.76, -32.64]
Subtotal (95% CI)			98			46	30.2%	-44.51 [-55.95, -33.06]
Heterogeneity: Tau² = 239.96; Chi² = 28.10, df = 12 (P = 0.005); I² = 57%								
Test for overall effect: Z = 7.62 (P < 0.00001)								
Total (95% CI)			219			160	100.0%	-19.70 [-26.16, -13.25]
Heterogeneity: Tau² = 262.35; Chi² = 329.15, df = 32 (P < 0.00001); I² = 90%								
Test for overall effect: Z = 5.99 (P < 0.00001)								
Test for subgroup differences: Chi² = 27.44, df = 2 (P < 0.00001), I² = 92.7%								

Mean Difference IV, Random, 95% CI
-100 -50 0 50 100
THC reduces BP   THC increases BP

(A)

Figure 2. *Cont.*

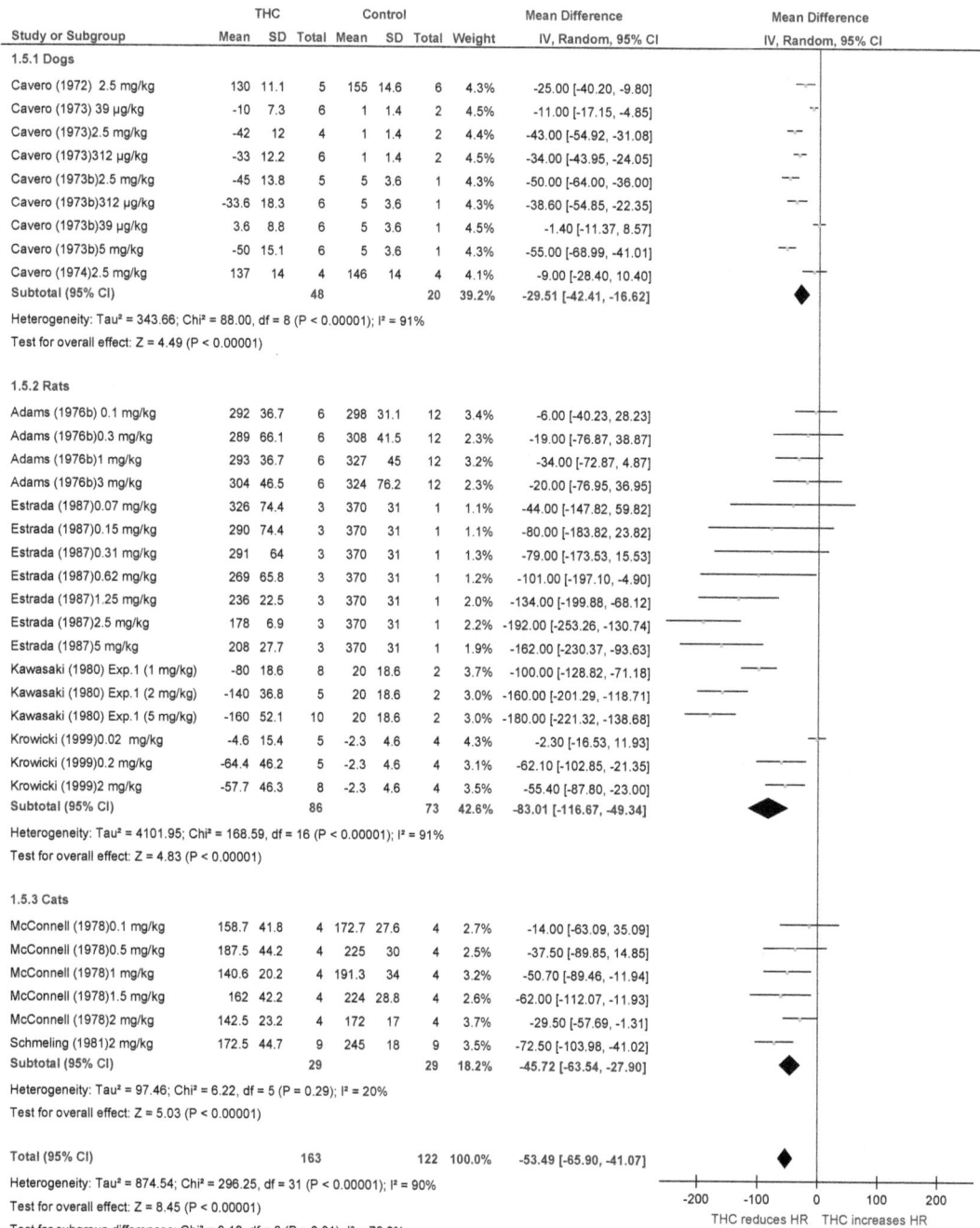

Study or Subgroup	THC Mean	SD	Total	Control Mean	SD	Total	Weight	Mean Difference IV, Random, 95% CI
1.5.1 Dogs								
Cavero (1972) 2.5 mg/kg	130	11.1	5	155	14.6	6	4.3%	-25.00 [-40.20, -9.80]
Cavero (1973) 39 µg/kg	-10	7.3	6	1	1.4	2	4.5%	-11.00 [-17.15, -4.85]
Cavero (1973)2.5 mg/kg	-42	12	4	1	1.4	2	4.4%	-43.00 [-54.92, -31.08]
Cavero (1973)312 µg/kg	-33	12.2	6	1	1.4	2	4.5%	-34.00 [-43.95, -24.05]
Cavero (1973b)2.5 mg/kg	-45	13.8	5	5	3.6	1	4.3%	-50.00 [-64.00, -36.00]
Cavero (1973b)312 µg/kg	-33.6	18.3	6	5	3.6	1	4.3%	-38.60 [-54.85, -22.35]
Cavero (1973b)39 µg/kg	3.6	8.8	6	5	3.6	1	4.5%	-1.40 [-11.37, 8.57]
Cavero (1973b)5 mg/kg	-50	15.1	6	5	3.6	1	4.3%	-55.00 [-68.99, -41.01]
Cavero (1974)2.5 mg/kg	137	14	4	146	14	4	4.1%	-9.00 [-28.40, 10.40]
Subtotal (95% CI)			48			20	39.2%	-29.51 [-42.41, -16.62]
Heterogeneity: Tau² = 343.66; Chi² = 88.00, df = 8 (P < 0.00001); I² = 91%								
Test for overall effect: Z = 4.49 (P < 0.00001)								
1.5.2 Rats								
Adams (1976b) 0.1 mg/kg	292	36.7	6	298	31.1	12	3.4%	-6.00 [-40.23, 28.23]
Adams (1976b)0.3 mg/kg	289	66.1	6	308	41.5	12	2.3%	-19.00 [-76.87, 38.87]
Adams (1976b)1 mg/kg	293	36.7	6	327	45	12	3.2%	-34.00 [-72.87, 4.87]
Adams (1976b)3 mg/kg	304	46.5	6	324	76.2	12	2.3%	-20.00 [-76.95, 36.95]
Estrada (1987)0.07 mg/kg	326	74.4	3	370	31	1	1.1%	-44.00 [-147.82, 59.82]
Estrada (1987)0.15 mg/kg	290	74.4	3	370	31	1	1.1%	-80.00 [-183.82, 23.82]
Estrada (1987)0.31 mg/kg	291	64	3	370	31	1	1.3%	-79.00 [-173.53, 15.53]
Estrada (1987)0.62 mg/kg	269	65.8	3	370	31	1	1.2%	-101.00 [-197.10, -4.90]
Estrada (1987)1.25 mg/kg	236	22.5	3	370	31	1	2.0%	-134.00 [-199.88, -68.12]
Estrada (1987)2.5 mg/kg	178	6.9	3	370	31	1	2.2%	-192.00 [-253.26, -130.74]
Estrada (1987)5 mg/kg	208	27.7	3	370	31	1	1.9%	-162.00 [-230.37, -93.63]
Kawasaki (1980) Exp.1 (1 mg/kg)	-80	18.6	8	20	18.6	2	3.7%	-100.00 [-128.82, -71.18]
Kawasaki (1980) Exp.1 (2 mg/kg)	-140	36.8	5	20	18.6	2	3.0%	-160.00 [-201.29, -118.71]
Kawasaki (1980) Exp.1 (5 mg/kg)	-160	52.1	10	20	18.6	2	3.0%	-180.00 [-221.32, -138.68]
Krowicki (1999)0.02 mg/kg	-4.6	15.4	5	-2.3	4.6	4	4.3%	-2.30 [-16.53, 11.93]
Krowicki (1999)0.2 mg/kg	-64.4	46.2	5	-2.3	4.6	4	3.1%	-62.10 [-102.85, -21.35]
Krowicki (1999)2 mg/kg	-57.7	46.3	8	-2.3	4.6	4	3.5%	-55.40 [-87.80, -23.00]
Subtotal (95% CI)			86			73	42.6%	-83.01 [-116.67, -49.34]
Heterogeneity: Tau² = 4101.95; Chi² = 168.59, df = 16 (P < 0.00001); I² = 91%								
Test for overall effect: Z = 4.83 (P < 0.00001)								
1.5.3 Cats								
McConnell (1978)0.1 mg/kg	158.7	41.8	4	172.7	27.6	4	2.7%	-14.00 [-63.09, 35.09]
McConnell (1978)0.5 mg/kg	187.5	44.2	4	225	30	4	2.5%	-37.50 [-89.85, 14.85]
McConnell (1978)1 mg/kg	140.6	20.2	4	191.3	34	4	3.2%	-50.70 [-89.46, -11.94]
McConnell (1978)1.5 mg/kg	162	42.2	4	224	28.8	4	2.6%	-62.00 [-112.07, -11.93]
McConnell (1978)2 mg/kg	142.5	23.2	4	172	17	4	3.7%	-29.50 [-57.69, -1.31]
Schmeling (1981)2 mg/kg	172.5	44.7	9	245	18	9	3.5%	-72.50 [-103.98, -41.02]
Subtotal (95% CI)			29			29	18.2%	-45.72 [-63.54, -27.90]
Heterogeneity: Tau² = 97.46; Chi² = 6.22, df = 5 (P = 0.29); I² = 20%								
Test for overall effect: Z = 5.03 (P < 0.00001)								
Total (95% CI)			163			122	100.0%	-53.49 [-65.90, -41.07]
Heterogeneity: Tau² = 874.54; Chi² = 296.25, df = 31 (P < 0.00001); I² = 90%								
Test for overall effect: Z = 8.45 (P < 0.00001)								
Test for subgroup differences: Chi² = 9.18, df = 2 (P = 0.01), I² = 78.2%								

Mean Difference IV, Random, 95% CI
-200 -100 0 100 200
THC reduces HR   THC increases HR

(B)

Figure 2. Changes in (**A**) BP and (**B**) HR induced by acute THC dosing in anaesthetised animals.

Chronic THC administration (7–35 days) tended to increase mesenteric, femoral, and renal BF ($p = 0.05$, Figure 3C) with no significant effect on HR or BP. Heterogeneity was statistically significant for BP and HR measurements after acute THC dosing ($p < 0.00001$; $I^2 = 90\%$) and for BP after chronic THC dosing (BP, $p = 0.03$, $I^2 = 72\%$).

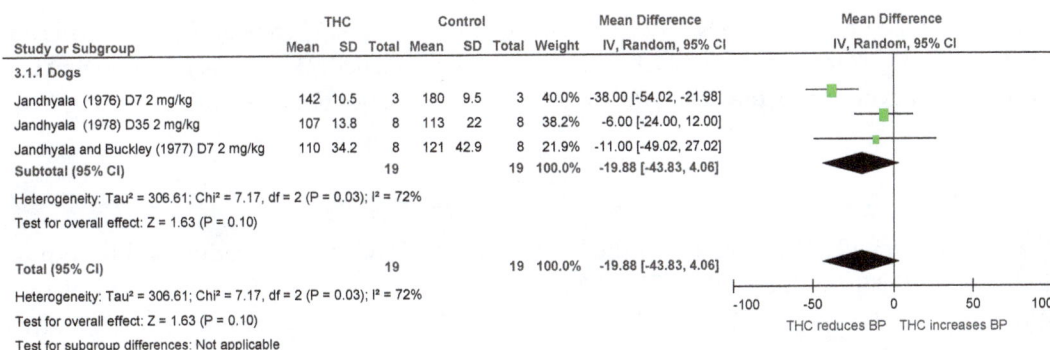

(A)

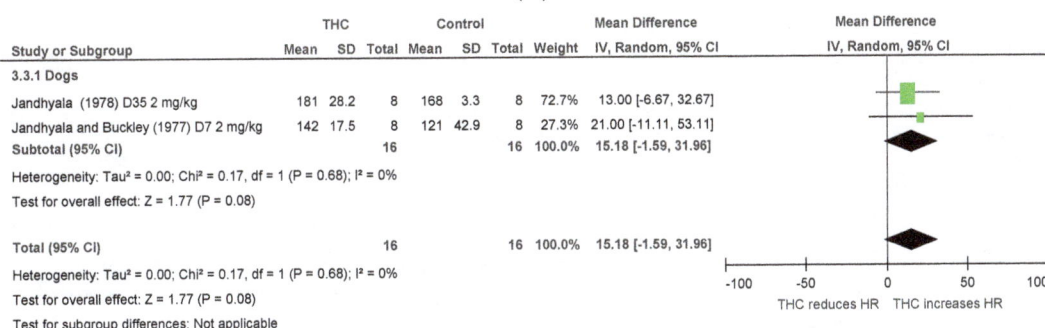

(B)

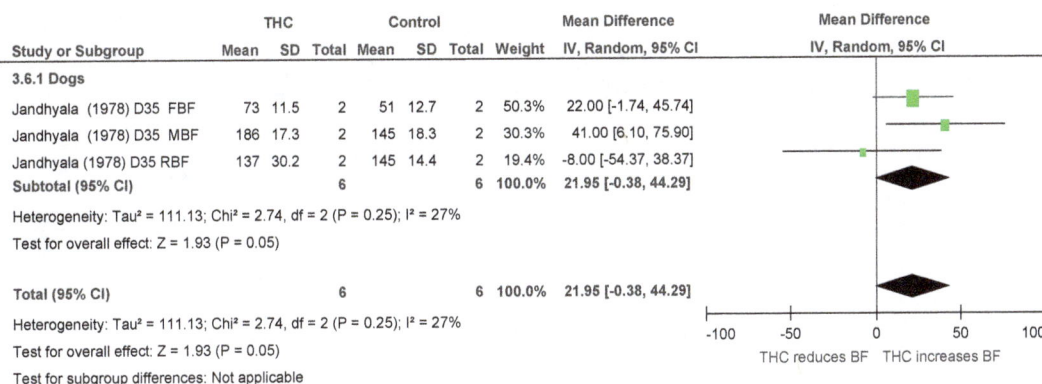

(C)

Figure 3. Changes in (**A**) blood pressure, (**B**) heart rate, and (**C**) blood flow (BF) induced by chronic THC dosing in anaesthetised animals.

2.1.2. Conscious Animals

Eight publications [20,22,23,37–41] assessed the effect of THC administration in five conscious species, including rats, bats, mice, rabbits, and monkeys ($n = 170$). THC significantly reduced BP and HR after acute dosing (BP, MD -12.3 mmHg, 95%CI -19.42, -5.18, $p = 0.0007$; HR, MD -30.05 bpm, 95%CI -38.47, -21.64, $p < 0.00001$, Figure 4A,B), and significantly increased CBF in murine models of stroke (BF, MD 32.35%, 95%CI 23.81, 40.88, $p < 0.00001$, Figure 4C). A cross-species analysis revealed that acute THC did not affect BP in bats ($p = 0.36$) and rats ($p = 0.11$) (Figure 4B). Heterogeneity was statistically significant for BP and HR measurements after acute THC dosing (BP, $p < 0.00001$, $I^2 = 83\%$; HR, $p < 0.00001$, $I^2 = 87\%$), but not in BF ($p = 0.5$, $I^2 = 0\%$).

2.1.3. Conscious Animal Models of Stress or Hypertension

Two publications [43,44] assessed the effect of THC administration on BP in hypertensive rats ($n = 22$), and one [42] in a rat model of stress ($n = 30$). Acute and chronic (4–10 days) THC dosing significantly reduced BP (acute THC, MD −61.37 mmHg, 95% CI −117.56, −5.17, $p = 0.03$, Figure 5A; chronic THC, MD −22.09 mmHg, 95% CI −30.61, −13.58, $p < 0.00001$, Figure 5B). Heterogeneity was statistically significant after acute dosing ($p < 0.00001$, $I^2 = 99\%$), but not after chronic dosing ($p = 0.69$, $I^2 = 0\%$).

2.1.4. Human Studies

Six publications [21,45–49] assessed the acute effect of THC administration on HR in humans ($n = 150$), no studies examined BP or BF. THC significantly increased HR after acute dosing (HR, MD 8.16 bpm, 95% CI 4.99, 11.33, $p < 0.00001$, Figure 6). Heterogeneity was statistically significant ($p < 0.00001$; $I^2 = 76\%$).

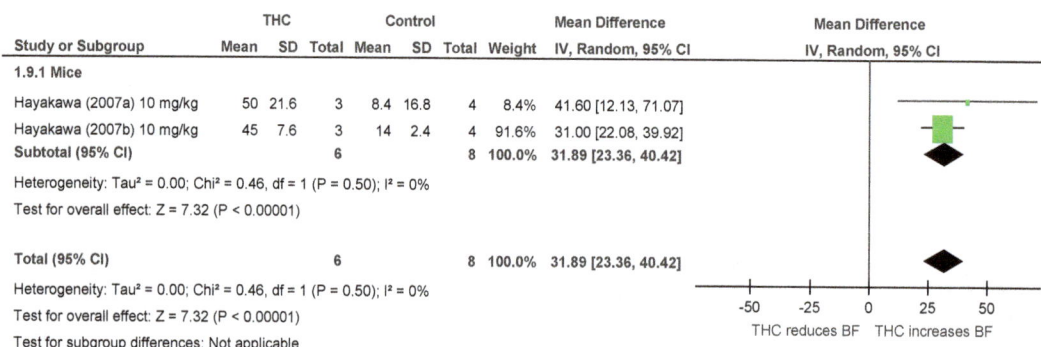

(A)

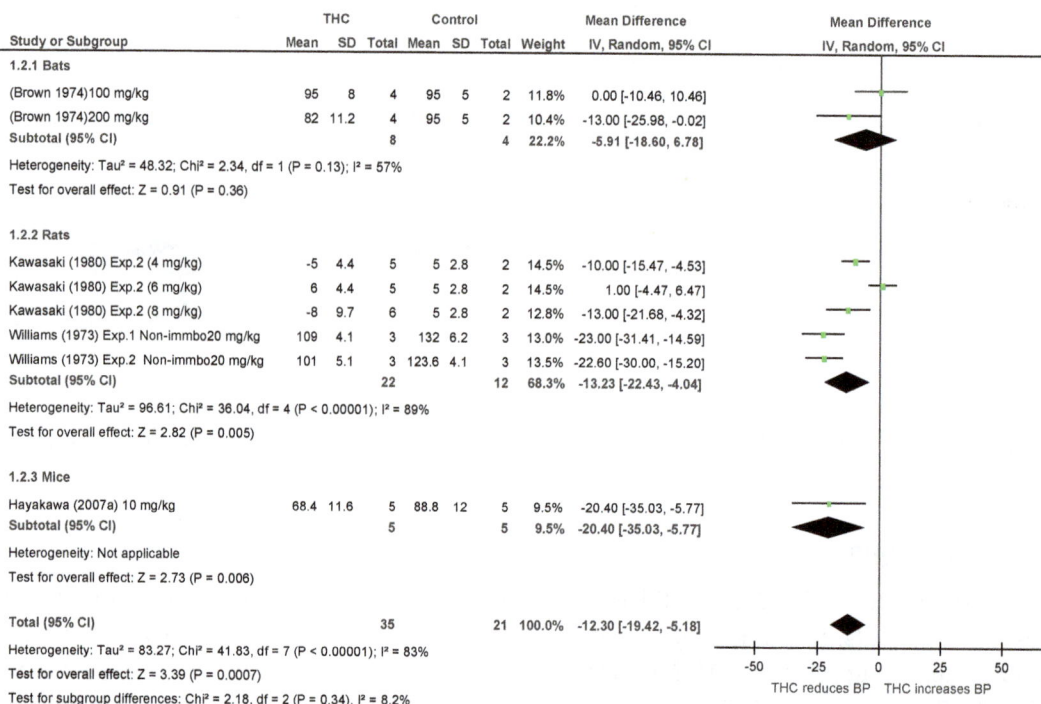

(B)

Figure 4. *Cont.*

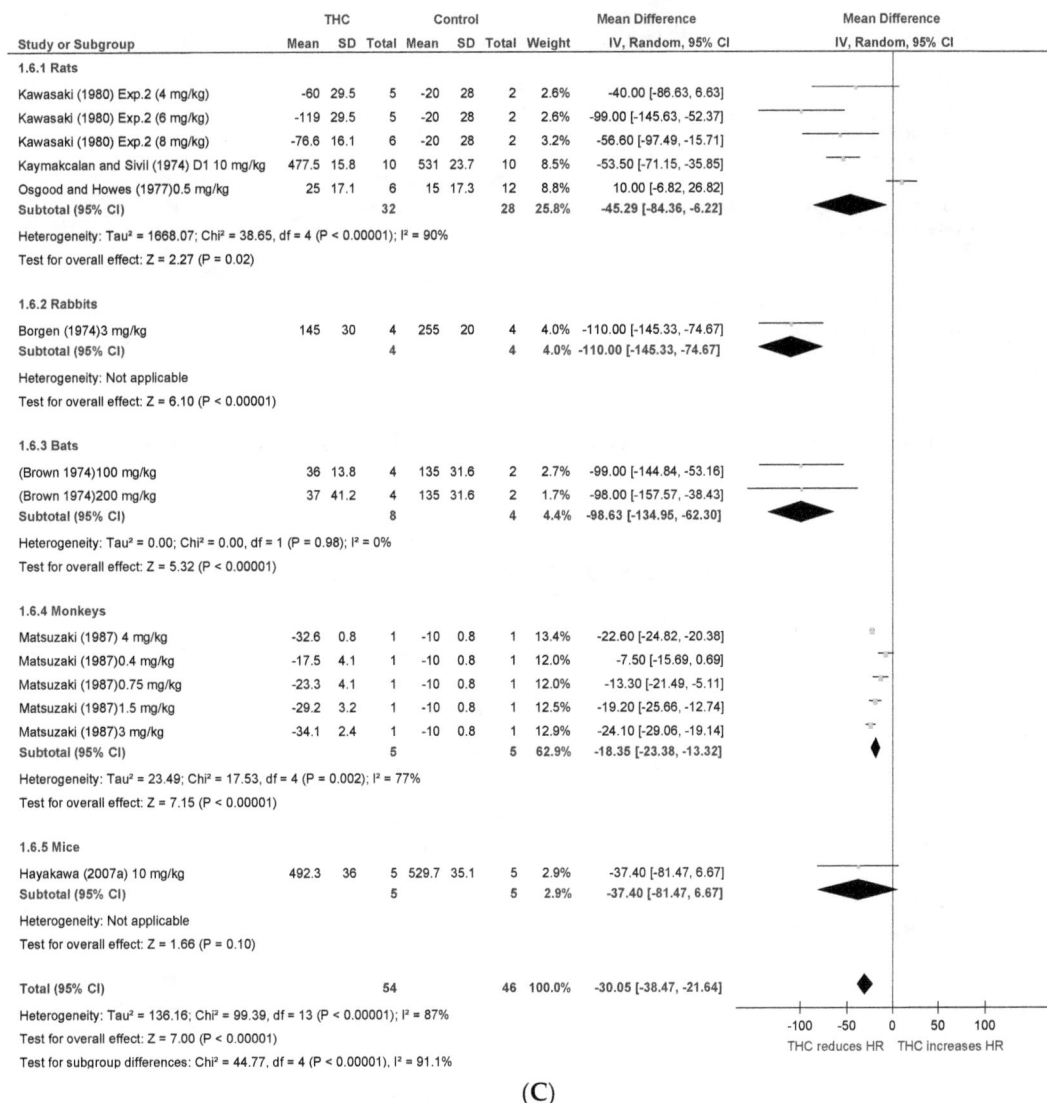

(C)

Figure 4. Changes in (**A**) BP, (**B**) HR, and (**C**) blood flow induced by acute THC dosing in conscious animals.

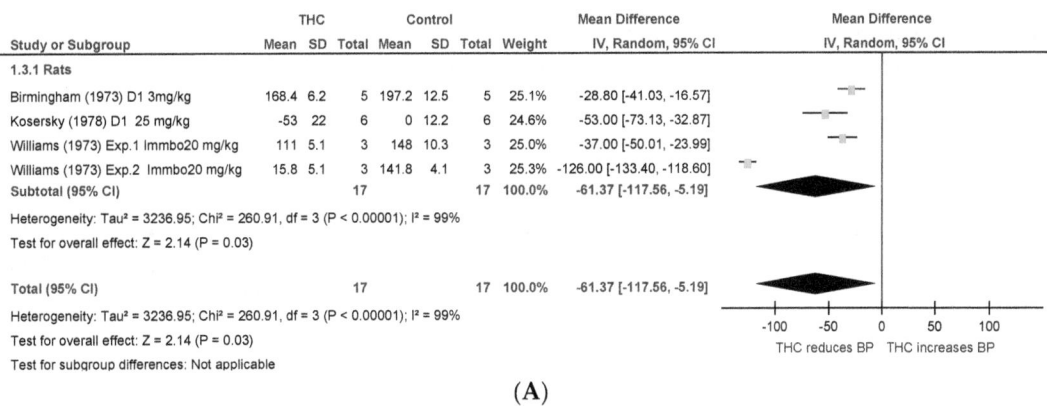

(A)

Figure 5. *Cont.*

Study or Subgroup	THC Mean	SD	Total	Control Mean	SD	Total	Weight	Mean Difference IV, Random, 95% CI
3.4.1 Rats								
Birmingham (1973) D7 3mg/kg	164.2	9.3	5	184.2	15.6	5	28.6%	-20.00 [-35.92, -4.08]
Kosersky (1978) D10 25 mg/kg	-32	17.1	6	-1	12.2	6	25.7%	-31.00 [-47.81, -14.19]
Williams (1973) Exp.1 D4 Immbo20 mg/kg	130	8.3	3	148	10.3	3	32.3%	-18.00 [-32.97, -3.03]
Williams (1973) Exp.2 D4 Immbo20 mg/kg	133	13.5	3	152.4	15.5	3	13.4%	-19.40 [-42.66, 3.86]
Subtotal (95% CI)			17			17	100.0%	-22.09 [-30.61, -13.58]
Heterogeneity: Tau² = 0.00; Chi² = 1.48, df = 3 (P = 0.69); I² = 0%								
Test for overall effect: Z = 5.09 (P < 0.00001)								
Total (95% CI)			17			17	100.0%	-22.09 [-30.61, -13.58]
Heterogeneity: Tau² = 0.00; Chi² = 1.48, df = 3 (P = 0.69); I² = 0%								
Test for overall effect: Z = 5.09 (P < 0.00001)								
Test for subgroup differences: Not applicable								

(B)

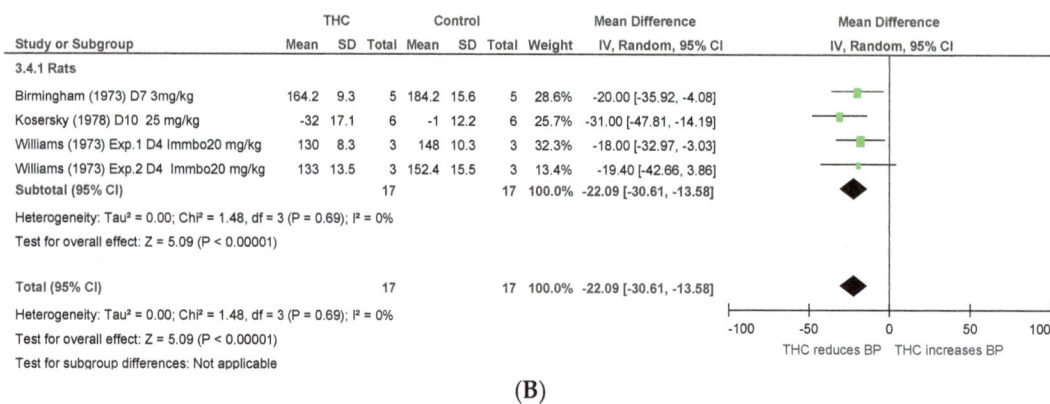

Figure 5. Changes in BP induced by (**A**) acute and (**B**) chronic THC dosing in animal models of stress or hypertension.

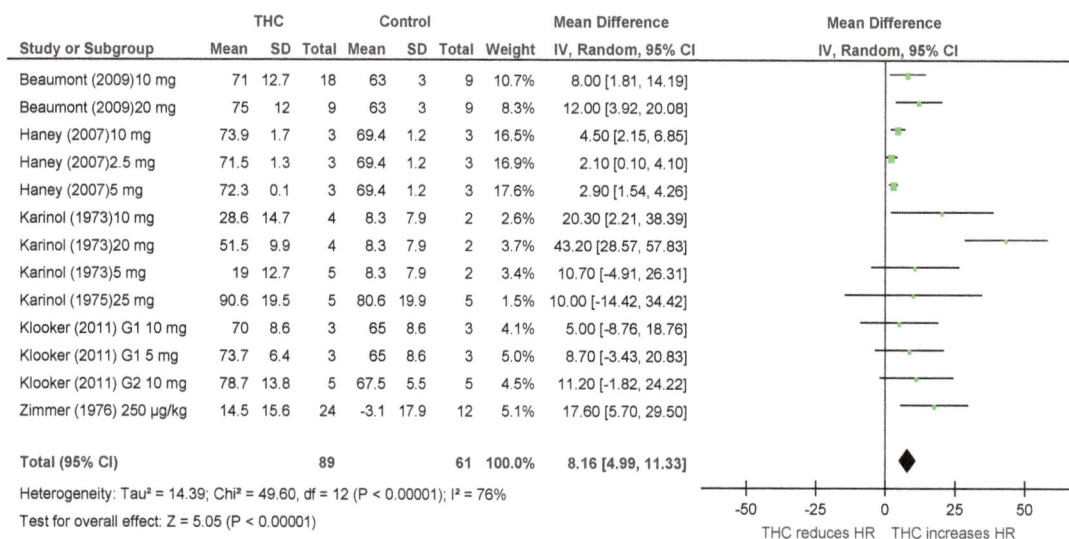

Study or Subgroup	THC Mean	SD	Total	Control Mean	SD	Total	Weight	Mean Difference IV, Random, 95% CI
Beaumont (2009)10 mg	71	12.7	18	63	3	9	10.7%	8.00 [1.81, 14.19]
Beaumont (2009)20 mg	75	12	9	63	3	9	8.3%	12.00 [3.92, 20.08]
Haney (2007)10 mg	73.9	1.7	3	69.4	1.2	3	16.5%	4.50 [2.15, 6.85]
Haney (2007)2.5 mg	71.5	1.3	3	69.4	1.2	3	16.9%	2.10 [0.10, 4.10]
Haney (2007)5 mg	72.3	0.1	3	69.4	1.2	3	17.6%	2.90 [1.54, 4.26]
Karinol (1973)10 mg	28.6	14.7	4	8.3	7.9	2	2.6%	20.30 [2.21, 38.39]
Karinol (1973)20 mg	51.5	9.9	4	8.3	7.9	2	3.7%	43.20 [28.57, 57.83]
Karinol (1973)5 mg	19	12.7	5	8.3	7.9	2	3.4%	10.70 [-4.91, 26.31]
Karinol (1975)25 mg	90.6	19.5	5	80.6	19.9	5	1.5%	10.00 [-14.42, 34.42]
Klooker (2011) G1 10 mg	70	8.6	3	65	8.6	3	4.1%	5.00 [-8.76, 18.76]
Klooker (2011) G1 5 mg	73.7	6.4	3	65	8.6	3	5.0%	8.70 [-3.43, 20.83]
Klooker (2011) G2 10 mg	78.7	13.8	5	67.5	5.5	5	4.5%	11.20 [-1.82, 24.22]
Zimmer (1976) 250 µg/kg	14.5	15.6	24	-3.1	17.9	12	5.1%	17.60 [5.70, 29.50]
Total (95% CI)			89			61	100.0%	8.16 [4.99, 11.33]
Heterogeneity: Tau² = 14.39; Chi² = 49.60, df = 12 (P < 0.00001); I² = 76%								
Test for overall effect: Z = 5.05 (P < 0.00001)								

Figure 6. Changes in HR induced by acute THC dosing in humans.

2.2. Dose–Response to THC

Doses ranging from 0.0003 to 770 mg were used in different species. The animal analyses showed a trend in the reduction of BP with higher THC doses ($p = 0.07$), with no change in HR. In humans, THC caused dose-dependent tachycardia ($p = 0.01$) (Figure 7).

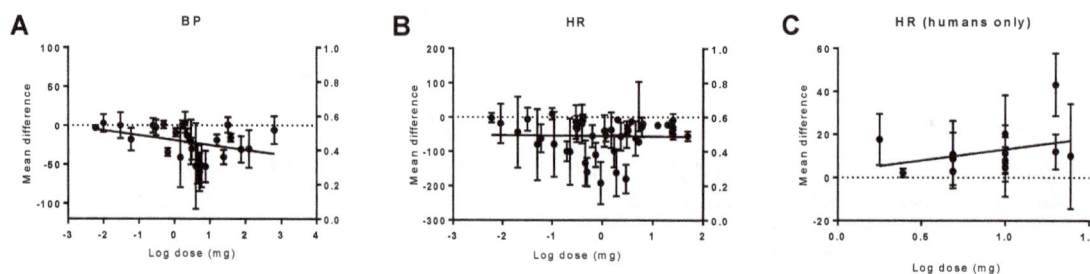

Figure 7. The effect of different THC doses on haemodynamic responses in vivo. The mean difference (MD) in animals' blood pressure (BP, (**A**)), animals' heart rate (HR, (**B**)), or heart rate (in humans only) ($p = 0.01$) (HR, (**C**)) is plotted against the log dose (mg) for each study. Error bars represent 95% confidence intervals (CI). Near-significant and significant dose-dependent effects on the blood pressure in animals ($p = 0.07$) and on the HR in humans ($p = 0.01$).

2.3. Quality

Among the 31 included publications, 6 publications used randomisation in their design and reported blinding assessment of outcome and measurements. Twenty publications assessed more than one outcome, 19 conducted dose–response relationships, 26 assessed a time window for intervention, 11 measured outcomes >24 h post-drug, and no publications provided incomplete data. There was no significant relationship between the quality score and any outcome (Spearman's rho coefficient of BP 0.22, $p = 0.09$; HR 0.27, $p = 0.07$ and BF 0.58, $p = 0.3$).

2.4. Publication Bias

Egger's test showed that bias was present in all studies except in studies in anaesthetised animals, conscious animals ($p = 0.001$), animal models of stress or hypertension (C) ($p = 0.001$), and humans (D) ($p < 0.0001$) (Appendix A, Figure A1).

3. Discussion

The aim of this study was to determine the effect of THC on haemodynamics in vivo in animals and cannabis-naïve humans. Our analysis has shown that an acute dosing of THC reduced BP and HR, and increased BF in animals of different models. Chronic dosing of THC tended to increase BF in anaesthetised animals and reduced BP in animal models of stress or hypertension. The data concerning the effects of THC in humans was limited to HR only, revealing a dose-dependent increase, suggesting further work is required to determine the full haemodynamic effects of acute and chronic THC administration in humans, especially given the different effects of THC on HR observed across species.

Our meta-analysis showed that acute THC dosing in anaesthetised animals reduced BP and HR, while a subgroup analysis revealed that there was no effect on BP or HR of anaesthetised dogs. However, Cavero et al. (1972, 1973, 1974) reported that intravenous administration of THC induced hypotension and bradycardia in dogs anaesthetised with pentobarbital caused by a reduction in the cardiac output and venous return mediated by the autonomic system [19,25–27]. Similarly, Schmeling reported that the reduction in sympathetic activity induced by THC in cats may cause hypotension and bradycardia [34]. It is suggested that the vagus nerve and the sympathetic outflow play a role in these effects induced by THC [36] and can be inhibited by the administration of a CB_1 antagonist [50]. The administration of THC for seven days subcutaneously reduced the increase in HR induced by pentobarbital anaesthetic agent in dogs, suggesting that THC antagonises the pentobarbital effect on the parasympathetic system (inhibiting the vagal tone) [30]. In rats anesthetised with pentobarbital, hypotension was reported after the administration of THC [35]; on the contrary, hypertension was reported in rats anesthetised with urethane post-THC [36], suggesting that THC may act differently with different anaesthetic agents. These studies suggest that the effects of THC in anaesthetised animals (hypotension and bradycardia) are induced through a central mechanism via the activation of CB_1 receptors.

In conscious animals under normal conditions, THC caused a variety of effects: hypotension was observed in bats, an effect which may be related to a change in venous activity [20], whereas another study in rats reported that THC induced tachycardia and hypertension, which are centrally mediated by increasing the level of adrenaline in the circulation [22]. However, studies in rat models of stress and hypertension, showed that THC lowered BP effectively [42–44]. The mechanism of the antihypertensive effect of THC in these models still needs to be studied.

Our meta-analysis in cannabis-naïve humans highlighted the limited number of studies investigating the effect of THC in humans (6 publications, $n = 123$ participants) with insufficient data to meta-analyse BP or regional BF. Studies in cannabis-naïve volunteers showed that the administration of THC orally or by inhalation caused tachycardia [46–49,51]. Tachycardia is also reported in humans after smoking cannabis [52–54] which may indicate that tachycardia induced post-cannabis smoking is caused by THC. The increase in HR caused by THC can be inhibited by CB_1 antagonism [55], suggesting that CB_1 activation may play a role in the haemodynamic effect of THC in humans. A greater number of studies investigating the haemodynamic effect of THC and its mechanisms under normal and pathological conditions in humans are required.

Several studies have reported that phytocannabinoids such as cannabidiol (CBD) may alter the effect of THC. For example, Borgen and Davis suggested that CBD may act as a potential antagonist of the THC effect on HR in rabbits and rats [38] and protects against some of the negative effects of THC in humans with potentially opposite effects on regional brain functions [56,57]. The combination of CBD and THC such as in Sativex®, a licenced agent for the symptomatic treatment of spasticity in multiple sclerosis, has shown that CBD inhibits the tachycardia effect induced by THC in humans [58].

Dose–response analyses showed a relationship between THC dose and effect size on BP, but not HR, in different animal models, and on human HR. Dose-dependent effects on BP were also observed post-THC in anaesthetized rats [24,36], cats [28], and dogs [26]. A dose of 100 and 200 mg caused a dose-dependent reduction on the BP of conscious bats, but not on HR [20]. HR dose-dependent reduction was reported in anaesthetized dogs [26,27] and conscious monkeys [39]. In human studies, doses between 2.5 and 25 mg were used. A dose-dependent increase in HR was observed in humans after oral THC administration of 5, 10, and 20 mg [21,49]. Over-intoxication has been reported after 20 mg of oral administration of THC in 5 of 21 healthy volunteers [48].

There are a number of limitations to consider in this analysis. First, the principal intention of 10 of the included studies was not to assess the cardiovascular effects of THC administration; therefore, the data extracted through secondary haemodynamic outcomes in this meta-analysis is for hypothesis-generating purposes. Second, the results should be interpreted with caution because of the heterogeneity between studies in terms of THC dose, time, and route of administration; the responses to THC will clearly be dependent upon peak plasma concentration, which are not easily comparable across studies. Indeed, a significant statistical heterogeneity was observed in the majority of the meta-analyses. Third, only 6 out of 31 articles used randomisation and described a masked assessment of outcomes, factors that can influence the reported outcomes. However, we found no significant correlation between study quality and effect size in this review.

In conclusion, this study has summarised the in vivo cardiovascular effects of THC administration. Our analysis demonstrates that THC acts differently according to species, causing tachycardia in humans, and bradycardia, hypotension, and an increase in regional BF in animals under different conditions. THC may be a potential future treatment for cardiovascular disorders, though its use as a single agent will be limited by CB_1 mediated psychogenic side effects, events that could be counterbalanced with other agents such as CBD. Data from human studies using THC alone is limited to heart rate only, thereby further good quality, randomised, blinded studies investigating the haemodynamic effects of THC in humans should be considered.

4. Materials and Methods

4.1. Search Strategy

All studies investigating the haemodynamic effects of THC (including BP, HR, and BF) were searched for (until April 2017) in Medline, EMBASE, and PubMed. Search keywords included: Δ^9-Tetrahydrocannabinol, Tetrahydrocannabinol, THC, Dronabinol, Marinol, Nabilone, Namisol, cardiovascular, blood pressure, systolic, diastolic, hypertension, hypotension, heart rate, tachycardia, bradycardia, blood flow, haemodynamic, vasodilation, vasorelaxation, and vasoconstriction. References from the included studies were also hand-searched.

Prespecified inclusion and exclusion criteria were used to prevent bias; the studies had to be in vivo, assess haemodynamics (BP, HR or BF), be original articles, be controlled studies, and use cannabis-naïve participants. Therefore, the exclusion criteria were: *in vitro* studies, mixtures of Δ^9-THC with other cannabis extracts, studies investigating the interaction of THC with other drugs or cannabinoids, studies not assessing haemodynamics (BP, HR, or BF), review articles, editorials, and uncontrolled studies.

4.2. Data Acquisition

Data on BP (mmHg), HR (beats per minute, bpm), and BF (% change from baseline or mL/min) were extracted from the included papers, and the changes in haemodynamics 2 h post-drug after acute THC dosing were used for the analyses. This time point was selected as the peak plasma time is between 30 min and 4 h after oral administration and it was the most common time point when haemodynamics were measured throughout the articles. If there were no measurements taken at this time point (2 h post-drug), the closest time point to 2 h was used for the analyses. In chronic studies, the measurements taken at the end of the studies were used for the analyses. If the exact number of animals used in each drug group was not available, the lowest number of animals within the range given was used for the experimental group (THC), and the highest number was used for the control group. If a crossover design was used in a study, the total number of humans was distributed equally to the two groups. Articles were excluded if data were not available. Grab application (version 1.5) was used to extract values from the figures given in published articles if no values were stated within the text. If the published articles used multiple groups (e.g., to assess dose-dependent effects) with one control group, then the number of humans or animals per control group was divided into the number of comparison groups. For the dose–response analysis, the total dose of the drug administrated up to the time when the haemodynamics was measured was used.

4.3. Quality

Eight-point criteria derived from Stroke Therapy Academic Industry Recommendations (STAIR) [59–61] and the Cochrane collaborations tool [62] were used to identify the risk of bias. Each of the following criteria was equal to 1 point: randomisation, blinding of outcome assessment, blinding of personnel and participant, assessment of more than one outcome, dose–response relationship, therapeutic time window, assessment of outcome >24 h, and incomplete outcome data.

4.4. Data Analysis

The studies were divided into acute and chronic groups. The data from human and animal studies were analysed separately. The animals were divided into two groups, anaesthetised and conscious, as the autonomic nervous system may respond differently in the two conditions [63], then grouped before the analysis in normal and abnormal (i.e., models of stress or hypertension) models and then subgrouped by species (mice, rats, dogs, etc.). For the THC dose–response analysis, the data were grouped according to the endpoint (BP, HR, or BF), and then subgrouped according to the dose. The data from each group were analysed as forest plots using the Cochrane Review Manager software (Version 5.3. Copenhagen: The Nordic Cochrane Centre, The Cochrane Collaboration, 2014), and as funnel plots using Stata (StataCorp. 2009. Stata Statistical Software: Release 11. College Station, TX, USA). Funnel plot asymmetry (publication bias) was assessed by Egger's test [64]. Stata was also used for meta-regression that described the relationship between THC dose and effect size. PRISM 7 (GraphPad, Software, La Jolla, CA, USA) was used to produce the figures of dose–response. Since heterogeneity was expected between the study protocols (different species, models, dose, and time) random-effect models were used. The results of continuous data are expressed as mean difference (MD) with 95% confidence intervals (CIs). The studies were weighted by sample size, and statistical significance was set at $p <0.05$.

Author Contributions: T.J.E. and S.E.O. conceived and designed the experiments; S.R.S. and S.A.M. collected and analyzed the data; all authors wrote and revised the manuscript.

Conflicts of Interest: The authors declare no conflict of interest.

Appendix A

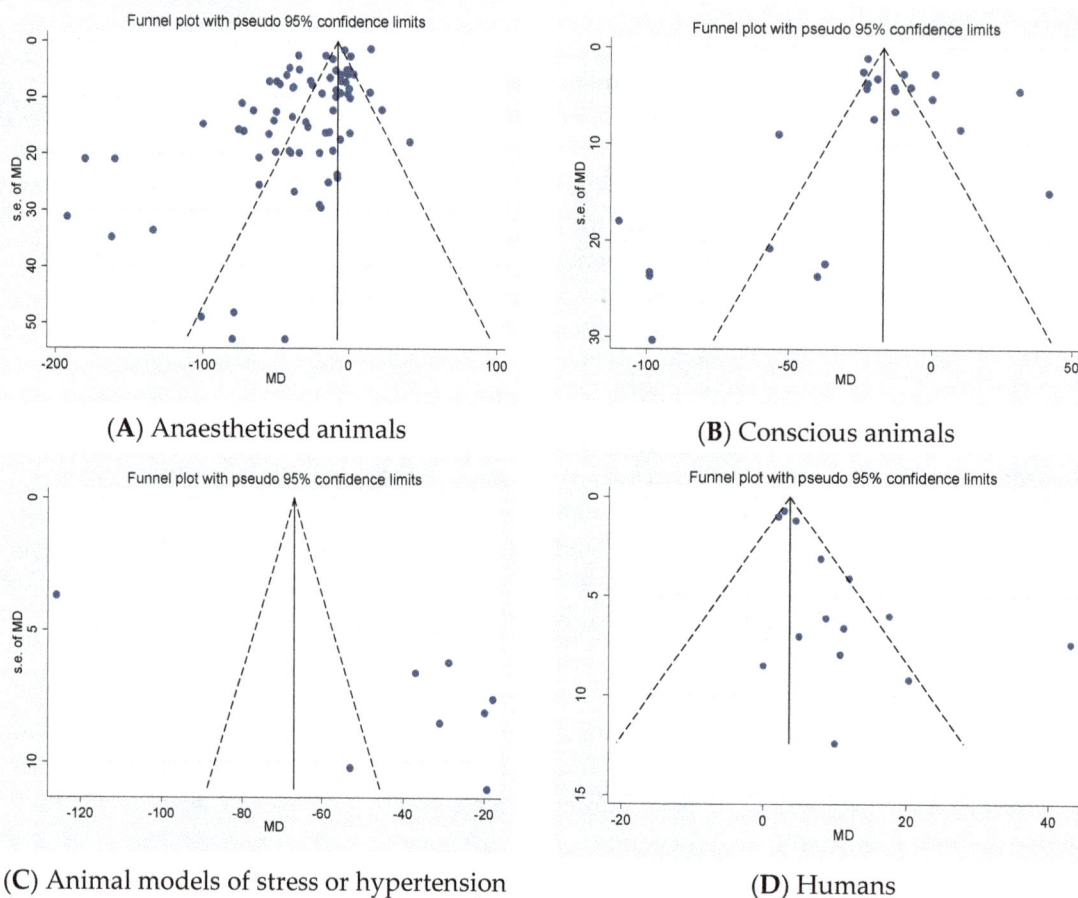

(**A**) Anaesthetised animals

(**B**) Conscious animals

(**C**) Animal models of stress or hypertension

(**D**) Humans

Figure A1. Funnel plots for each outcome evaluating the publication bias. The standard error (SE) of the mean difference (MD) in haemodynamics (MD, *y* axis) for each study is plotted against its effect size (*horizontal* axis). There was significant bias in conscious animals (**B**) ($p = 0.001$), animal models of stress or hypertension (**C**) ($p = 0.001$), and humans (**D**) ($p < 0.0001$). No significant bias in anaesthetised animals (**A**).

References

1. Gaoni, Y.; Mechoulam, R. Isolation, Structure, and Partial Synthesis of an Active Constituent of Hashish. *J. Am. Chem. Soc.* **1964**, *86*, 1646–1647. [CrossRef]
2. Pertwee, R.G. Pharmacological actions of cannabinoids. *Handb. Exp. Pharmacol.* **2005**, *20*, 1–51.
3. Ryberg, E.; Larsson, N.; Sjögren, S.; Hjorth, S.; Hermansson, N.O.; Leonova, J.; Elebring, T.; Nilsson, K.; Drmota, T.; Greasley, P.J. The orphan receptor GPR55 is a novel cannabinoid receptor. *Br. J. Pharmacol.* **2007**, *152*, 1092–1101. [CrossRef] [PubMed]
4. McHugh, D.; Page, J.; Dunn, E.; Bradshaw, H.B. Delta(9)-Tetrahydrocannabinol and N-arachidonyl glycine are full agonists at GPR18 receptors and induce migration in human endometrial HEC-1B cells. *Br. J. Pharmacol.* **2012**, *165*, 2414–2424. [CrossRef] [PubMed]
5. Ben Amar, M. Cannabinoids in medicine: A review of their therapeutic potential. *J. Ethnopharmacol.* **2006**, *105*, 1–25. [CrossRef] [PubMed]
6. Lastres-Becker, I.; Molina-Holgado, F.; Ramos, J.A.; Mechoulam, R.; Fernandez-Ruiz, J. Cannabinoids provide neuroprotection against 6-hydroxydopamine toxicity in vivo and in vitro: Relevance to Parkinson's disease. *Neurobiol. Dis.* **2005**, *19*, 96–107. [CrossRef] [PubMed]

7.   Buccellato, E.; Carretta, D.; Utan, A.; Cavina, C.; Speroni, E.; Grassi, G.; Candeletti, S.; Romualdi, P. Acute and chronic cannabinoid extracts administration affects motor function in a CREAE model of multiple sclerosis. *J Ethnopharmacol.* **2011**, *133*, 1033–1038. [CrossRef] [PubMed]

8.   Whiting, P.F.; Wolff, R.F.; Deshpande, S.; Di Nisio, M.; Duffy, S.; Hernandez, A.V.; Keurentjes, J.C.; Lang, S.; Misso, K.; Ryder, S.; et al. Cannabinoids for Medical Use: A Systematic Review and Meta-analysis. *JAMA* **2015**, *313*, 2456–2473. [CrossRef] [PubMed]

9.   Todaro, B. Cannabinoids in the treatment of chemotherapy-induced nausea and vomiting. *J. Natl. Compr. Cancer Netw.* **2012**, *10*, 487–492. [CrossRef]

10. Abrams, D.I.; Guzman, M. Cannabis in cancer care. *Clin. Pharmacol. Ther.* **2015**, *97*, 575–586. [CrossRef] [PubMed]

11. Fleming, I.; Schermer, B.; Popp, R.; Busse, R. Inhibition of the production of endothelium-derived hyperpolarizing factor by cannabinoid receptor agonists. *Br. J. Pharmacol.* **1999**, *126*, 949–960. [CrossRef] [PubMed]

12. Zygmunt, P.M.; Andersson, D.A.; Högestätt, E.D. Δ^9Tetrahydrocannabinol and Cannabinol Activate Capsaicin-Sensitive Sensory Nerves via a CB1 and CB2 Cannabinoid Receptor-Independent Mechanism. *J. Neurosci.* **2002**, *22*, 4720–4727. [PubMed]

13. O'Sullivan, S.E.; Kendall, D.A.; Randall, M.D. The effects of $\Delta(9)$-tetrahydrocannabinol in rat mesenteric vasculature, and its interactions with the endocannabinoid anandamide. *Br. J. Pharmacol.* **2005**, *145*, 514–526. [CrossRef] [PubMed]

14. O'Sullivan, S.E.; Kendall, D.A.; Randall, M.D. Vascular effects of delta 9-tetrahydrocannabinol (THC), anandamide and N-arachidonoyldopamine (NADA) in the rat isolated aorta. *Eur. J. Pharmacol* **2005**, *507*, 211–221. [CrossRef] [PubMed]

15. O'Sullivan, S.E.; Tarling, E.J.; Bennett, A.J.; Kendall, D.A.; Randall, M.D. Novel time-dependent vascular actions of Delta9-tetrahydrocannabinol mediated by peroxisome proliferator-activated receptor gamma. *Biochem. Biophys. Res. Commun.* **2005**, *337*, 824–831. [CrossRef] [PubMed]

16. Kaymakcalan, S.; Turker, R.K. The evidence of the release of prostaglandin-like material from rabbit kidney and guinea-pig lung by (minus)-trans-delta9-tetrahydrocannabinol. *J. Pharm. Pharmacol.* **1975**, *27*, 564–568. [CrossRef] [PubMed]

17. Duncan, M.; Kendall, D.A.; Ralevic, V. Characterization of cannabinoid modulation of sensory neurotransmission in the rat isolated mesenteric arterial bed. *J. Pharmacol. Exp. Ther.* **2004**, *311*, 411–419. [CrossRef] [PubMed]

18. Barbosa, P.P.; Lapa, A.J.; Lima-Landman, M.T.; Valle, J.R. Vasoconstriction induced by delta 9-tetrahydrocannabinol on the perfused rabbit ear artery. *Arch. Int. Pharmacodyn. Ther.* **1981**, *252*, 253–261. [PubMed]

19. Cavero, I.; Lokhandwala, M.F.; Buckley, J.P.; Jandhyala, B.S. The effect of $(-)$-Δ^9-trans-tetrahydrocannabinol on myocardial contractility and venous return in anesthetized dogs. *Eur. J. Pharmacol.* **1974**, *29*, 74–82. [CrossRef]

20. Brown, D.J.; Miller, F.N.; Longnecker, D.E.; Greenwald, E.K.; Harris, P.D.; Forney, R.B. The influence of delta 9-tetrahydrocannabinol on cardiovascular and subcutaneous microcirculatory systems in the bat. *J. Pharmacol. Exp. Ther.* **1974**, *188*, 624–629. [PubMed]

21. Beaumont, H.; Jensen, J.; Carlsson, A.; Ruth, M.; Lehmann, A.; Boeckxstaens, G. Effect of delta9-tetrahydrocannabinol, a cannabinoid receptor agonist, on the triggering of transient lower oesophageal sphincter relaxations in dogs and humans. *Br. J. Pharmacol.* **2009**, *156*, 153–162. [CrossRef] [PubMed]

22. Osgood, P.F.; Howes, J.F. Δ^9-tetrahydrocannabinol and dimethylheptylpyran induced tachycardia in the conscious rat. *Life Sci.* **1977**, *21*, 1329–1335. [CrossRef]

23. Kawasaki, H.; Watanabe, S.; Oishi, R.; Ueki, S. Effects of delta-9-tetrahydrocannabinol on the cardiovascular system, and pressor and behavioral responses to brain stimulation in rats. *Jpn. J. Pharmacol.* **1980**, *30*, 493–502. [CrossRef] [PubMed]

24. Siqueira, S.W.; Lapa, A.J.; Ribeiro do Valle, J. The triple effect induced by delta 9-tetrahydrocannabinol on the rat blood pressure. *Eur. J. Pharmacol.* **1979**, *58*, 351–357. [CrossRef]

25. Cavero, I.; Ertel, R.; Buckley, J.P.; Jandhyala, B.S. Effects of $(-)$-Δ^9-trans-tetrahydrocannabinol on regional blood flow in anesthetized dogs. *Eur. J. Pharmacol.* **1972**, *20*, 373–376. [CrossRef]

26. Cavero, I.; Buckley, J.P.; Jandhyala, B.S. Hemodynamic and myocardial effects of (−)-Δ9-trans-tetrahydrocannabinol in anesthetized dogs. *Eur. J. Pharmacol.* **1973**, *24*, 243–251. [CrossRef]

27. Cavero, I.; Solomon, T.; Buckley, J.P.; Jandhyala, B.S. Studies on the bradycardia induced by (−)-delta9-trans-tetrahydrocannabinol in anesthetized dogs. *Eur. J. Pharmacol.* **1973**, *22*, 263–269. [CrossRef]

28. Daskalopoulos, N.; Schmitt, H.; Laubie, M. Action of delta 9 tetrahydrocannabinol on the central cardiovascular regulation: Mechanism and localization. *Lencephale* **1975**, *1*, 121–132.

29. Adams, M.D.; Earnhardt, J.T.; Dewey, W.L.; Harris, L.S. Vasoconstrictor actions of delta8- and delta9-tetrahydrocannabinol in the rat. *J. Pharmacol. Exp. Ther.* **1976**, *196*, 649–656. [PubMed]

30. Jandhyala, B.S.; Malloy, K.P.; Buckley, J.P. Effects of chronic administration of delta9-tetrahydrocannabinol on the heart rate of mongrel dogs. *Res. Commun. Chem. Pathol. Pharmacol.* **1976**, *14*, 201–204. [PubMed]

31. Jandhyala, B.S.; Buckley, J.P. Autonomic and cardiovascular effects of chronic delta9-tetrahydrocannabinol administration in mongrel dogs. *Res. Commun. Chem. Pathol. Pharmacol.* **1977**, *16*, 593–607. [PubMed]

32. Jandhyala, B.S. Effects of prolonged administration of delta 9-tetrahydrocannabinol on the autonomic and cardiovascular function and regional hemodynamics in mongrel dogs. *Res. Commun. Chem. Pathol. Pharmacol.* **1978**, *20*, 489–508. [PubMed]

33. McConnell, W.R.; Dewey, W.L.; Harris, L.S.; Borzelleca, J.F. A study of the effect of delta 9-tetrahydrocannabinol (delta 9-THC) on mammalian salivary flow. *J. Pharmacol. Exp. Ther.* **1978**, *206*, 567–573. [PubMed]

34. Schmeling, W.T.; Hosko, M.J.; Hardman, H.F. Potentials evoked in the intermediolateral column by hypothalamic stimulation—Suppression by Δ9-tetrahydrocannabinol. *Life Sci.* **1981**, *29*, 673–680. [CrossRef]

35. Estrada, U.; Brase, D.A.; Martin, B.R.; Dewey, W.L. Cardiovascular effects of delta 9- and delta 9(11)-tetrahydrocannabinol and their interaction with epinephrine. *Life Sci.* **1987**, *41*, 79–87. [CrossRef]

36. Krowicki, Z.K.; Moerschbaecher, J.M.; Winsauer, P.J.; Digavalli, S.V.; Hornby, P.J. Delta9-tetrahydrocannabinol inhibits gastric motility in the rat through cannabinoid CB1 receptors. *Eur. J. Pharmacol.* **1999**, *371*, 187–196. [CrossRef]

37. Kaymakcalan, S.; Sivil, S. Lack of tolerance to the bradycardic effect of delta 9-trans-tetrahydrocannabinol in rats. *Pharmacology* **1974**, *12*, 290–295. [PubMed]

38. Borgen, L.A.; Davis, W.M. Cannabidiol interaction with delta9-tetrahydrocannabinol. *Res. Commun. Chem. Pathol. Pharmacol.* **1974**, *7*, 663–670. [PubMed]

39. Matsuzaki, M.; Casella, G.A.; Ratner, M. delta 9-Tetrahydrocannabinol: EEG changes, bradycardia and hypothermia in the rhesus monkey. *Brain Res. Bull.* **1987**, *19*, 223–229. [CrossRef]

40. Hayakawa, K.; Mishima, K.; Nozako, M.; Hazekawa, M.; Irie, K.; Fujioka, M.; Orito, K.; Abe, K.; Hasebe, N.; Egashira, N.; et al. Delayed treatment with cannabidiol has a cerebroprotective action via a cannabinoid receptor-independent myeloperoxidase-inhibiting mechanism. *J. Neurochem.* **2007**, *102*, 1488–1496. [CrossRef] [PubMed]

41. Hayakawa, K.; Mishima, K.; Nozako, M.; Ogata, A.; Hazekawa, M.; Liu, A.X.; Fujioka, M.; Abe, K.; Hasebe, N.; Egashira, N.; et al. Repeated treatment with cannabidiol but not Delta9-tetrahydrocannabinol has a neuroprotective effect without the development of tolerance. *Neuropharmacology* **2007**, *52*, 1079–1087. [CrossRef] [PubMed]

42. Williams, R.B.; Ng, L.K.Y.; Lamprecht, F.; Roth, K.; Kopin, I.J. Δ9-Tetrahydrocannabinol: A hypotensive effect in rats. *Psychopharmacologia* **1973**, *28*, 269–274. [CrossRef] [PubMed]

43. Birmingham, M.K. Reduction by 9-tetrahydrocannabinol in the blood pressure of hypertensive rats bearing regenerated adrenal glands. *Br. J. Pharmacol.* **1973**, *48*, 169–171. [CrossRef] [PubMed]

44. Kosersky, D.S. Antihypertensive effects of delta9-tetrahydrocannabinol. *Arch. Int. Pharmacodyn. Ther.* **1978**, *233*, 76–81. [PubMed]

45. Karniol, I.G.; Carlini, E.A. Comparative Studies in Man and in Laboratory Animals on Δ^8-and Δ^9-trans-Tetrahydrocannabinol. *Pharmacology* **1973**, *9*, 115–126. [CrossRef] [PubMed]

46. Karniol, I.G.; Shirakawa, I.; Takahashi, R.N.; Knobel, E.; Musty, R.E. Effects of delta9-tetrahydrocannabinol and cannabinol in man. *Pharmacology* **1975**, *13*, 502–512. [CrossRef] [PubMed]

47. Zimmer, B.D.; Bickel, P.; Dittrich, A. Changes of simple somatic parameters by delta-9-trans-tetrahydrocannabinol (delta-9-THC) in a double-blind-study. Short communication. *Arzneimittelforschung* **1976**, *26*, 1614–1616. [PubMed]

48. Haney, M. Opioid antagonism of cannabinoid effects: Differences between marijuana smokers and nonmarijuana smokers. *Neuropsychopharmacology* **2007**, *32*, 1391–1403. [CrossRef] [PubMed]

49. Klooker, T.K.; Leliefeld, K.E.; Van Den Wijngaard, R.M.; Boeckxstaens, G.E. The cannabinoid receptor agonist delta-9-tetrahydrocannabinol does not affect visceral sensitivity to rectal distension in healthy volunteers and IBS patients. *Neurogastroenterol. Motil.* **2011**, *23*, 30–35. [CrossRef] [PubMed]

50. Lake, K.D.; Compton, D.R.; Varga, K.; Martin, B.R.; Kunos, G. Cannabinoid-induced hypotension and bradycardia in rats mediated by CB1-like cannabinoid receptors. *J. Pharmacol. Exp. Ther.* **1997**, *281*, 1030–1037. [PubMed]

51. Strougo, A.; Zuurman, L.; Roy, C.; Pinquier, J.L.; van Gerven, J.M.; Cohen, A.F.; Schoemaker, R.C. Modelling of the concentration—Effect relationship of THC on central nervous system parameters and heart rate—Insight into its mechanisms of action and a tool for clinical research and development of cannabinoids. *J. Psychopharmacol.* **2008**, *22*, 717–726. [CrossRef] [PubMed]

52. Schwope, D.M.; Bosker, W.M.; Ramaekers, J.G.; Gorelick, D.A.; Huestis, M.A. Psychomotor performance, subjective and physiological effects and whole blood Delta(9)-tetrahydrocannabinol concentrations in heavy, chronic cannabis smokers following acute smoked cannabis. *J. Anal. Toxicol.* **2012**, *36*, 405–412. [CrossRef] [PubMed]

53. Mathew, R.J.; Wilson, W.H.; Humphreys, D.; Lowe, J.V.; Wiethe, K.E. Middle cerebral artery velocity during upright posture after marijuana smoking. *Acta Psychiatr. Scand.* **1992**, *86*, 173–178. [CrossRef] [PubMed]

54. Mathew, R.J.; Wilson, W.H.; Humphreys, D.F.; Lowe, J.V.; Wiethe, K.E. Changes in middle cerebral artery velocity after marijuana. *Biol. Psychiatry* **1992**, *32*, 164–169. [CrossRef]

55. Klumpers, L.E.; Roy, C.; Ferron, G.; Turpault, S.; Poitiers, F.; Pinquier, J.L.; van Hasselt, J.G.; Zuurman, L.; Erwich, F.A.; van Gerven, J.M. Surinabant, a selective cannabinoid receptor type 1 antagonist, inhibits Delta9-tetrahydrocannabinol-induced central nervous system and heart rate effects in humans. *Br. J. Clin. Pharmacol.* **2013**, *76*, 65–77. [CrossRef] [PubMed]

56. Bhattacharyya, S.; Morrison, P.D.; Fusar-Poli, P.; Martin-Santos, R.; Borgwardt, S.; Winton-Brown, T.; Nosarti, C.; CM, O.C.; Seal, M.; Allen, P.; et al. Opposite effects of delta-9-tetrahydrocannabinol and cannabidiol on human brain function and psychopathology. *Neuropsychopharmacology* **2010**, *35*, 764–774. [CrossRef] [PubMed]

57. Niesink, R.J.; van Laar, M.W. Does Cannabidiol Protect Against Adverse Psychological Effects of THC? *Front. Psychiatry* **2013**, *4*, 130. [CrossRef] [PubMed]

58. Karniol, I.G.; Shirakawa, I.; Kasinski, N.; Pfeferman, A.; Carlini, E.A. Cannabidiol interferes with the effects of delta 9-tetrahydrocannabinol in man. *Eur. J. Pharmacol.* **1974**, *28*, 172–177. [CrossRef]

59. Stroke Therapy Academic Industry Roundtable. Recommendations for standards regarding preclinical neuroprotective and restorative drug development. *Stroke* **1999**, *30*, 2752–2758.

60. England, T.J.; Hind, W.H.; Rasid, N.A.; O'Sullivan, S.E. Cannabinoids in experimental stroke: A systematic review and meta-analysis. *J. Cereb. Blood Flow Metab.* **2015**, *35*, 348–358. [CrossRef] [PubMed]

61. Sultan, S.R.; Millar, S.A.; England, T.J.; O'Sullivan, S.E. A Systematic Review and Meta-Analysis of the Haemodynamic Effects of Cannabidiol. *Front. Pharmacol.* **2017**, *8*, 81. [CrossRef] [PubMed]

62. Higgins, J.P.; Altman, D.G.; Gotzsche, P.C.; Juni, P.; Moher, D.; Oxman, A.D.; Savovic, J.; Schulz, K.F.; Weeks, L.; Sterne, J.A.; et al. The Cochrane Collaboration's tool for assessing risk of bias in randomised trials. *BMJ* **2011**, *343*, 889–893. [CrossRef] [PubMed]

63. Neukirchen, M.; Kienbaum, P. Sympathetic nervous system: Evaluation and importance for clinical general anesthesia. *Anesthesiology* **2008**, *109*, 1113–1131. [CrossRef] [PubMed]

64. Egger, M.; Davey Smith, G.; Schneider, M.; Minder, C. Bias in meta-analysis detected by a simple, graphical test. *BMJ* **1997**, *315*, 629–634. [CrossRef] [PubMed]

15

Endocannabinoids in Body Weight Control

Henrike Horn †, Beatrice Böhme †, Laura Dietrich and Marco Koch *

Institute of Anatomy, Medical Faculty, University of Leipzig, 04103 Leipzig, Germany;
Henrike.Horn@medizin.uni-leipzig.de (H.H.); Beatrice.Schuetzelt@medizin.uni-leipzig.de (B.B.);
lauri.dietrich@yahoo.de (L.D.)
* Correspondence: marco.koch@medizin.uni-leipzig.de
† These authors contributed equally.

Abstract: Maintenance of body weight is fundamental to maintain one's health and to promote longevity. Nevertheless, it appears that the global obesity epidemic is still constantly increasing. Endocannabinoids (eCBs) are lipid messengers that are involved in overall body weight control by interfering with manifold central and peripheral regulatory circuits that orchestrate energy homeostasis. Initially, blocking of eCB signaling by first generation cannabinoid type 1 receptor (CB1) inverse agonists such as rimonabant revealed body weight-reducing effects in laboratory animals and men. Unfortunately, rimonabant also induced severe psychiatric side effects. At this point, it became clear that future cannabinoid research has to decipher more precisely the underlying central and peripheral mechanisms behind eCB-driven control of feeding behavior and whole body energy metabolism. Here, we will summarize the most recent advances in understanding how central eCBs interfere with circuits in the brain that control food intake and energy expenditure. Next, we will focus on how peripheral eCBs affect food digestion, nutrient transformation and energy expenditure by interfering with signaling cascades in the gastrointestinal tract, liver, pancreas, fat depots and endocrine glands. To finally outline the safe future potential of cannabinoids as medicines, our overall goal is to address the molecular, cellular and pharmacological logic behind central and peripheral eCB-mediated body weight control, and to figure out how these precise mechanistic insights are currently transferred into the development of next generation cannabinoid medicines displaying clearly improved safety profiles, such as significantly reduced side effects.

Keywords: body weight; obesity; anorexia; cancer cachexia; endocannabinoids; cannabinoid type 1 receptor; CB1; allosteric CB1 ligands

1. Introduction

It has evolved in human and most other species that the body weight remains relatively constant for most of the lifetime. In other words, an individual able to balance the body weight long-term was successful and survived, most likely because body weight stability would ultimately have guaranteed a sustained energy supply [1]. Even before becoming adults, species-specific interrelations exist between body weight gain and longitudinal growth during pre-and postnatal development [2]. Thus, when occurring in physiological ranges, body weight development and maintenance are fundamental to maintain health and to promote longevity, while underweight, overweight, and specifically obesity in childhood, adolescence and adulthood are associated with adverse health consequences throughout the life course [3].

At first glance, the present body weight calculation of an individual mostly reflects the latest intake, storage and expenditure of energy. Indeed, the control of energy metabolism strongly accounts for the individual's body weight [4]. In this, various regulatory circuits in the central nervous system (CNS) and the periphery orchestrate the maintenance of energy homeostasis. First of all, energy intake in terms of food ingestion is supervised in the CNS. Here, environmental and metabolic information is received, integrated and finally transformed into generation of physiological behaviors such as food foraging and energy expenditure in order to provide the energy required for differentiation, growth, regeneration and maintenance of all cells, tissues and organs of the body [5].

1.1. Overeating and Obesity—What Is the Evolutionary Benefit of Fat Storage?

Assuming that the presence of sufficient food represented a selective pressure in evolution, one beneficial adaptation apparently was the opportunity to long-term store excess of energy in the body's fat depots [6]. Accordingly, so-called "pro-feeding" regulatory circuitries, in which energy consumption dominates energy expenditure, evolved as an indispensable prerequisite allowing for the storage of energy [7]. Besides food scarcity, also other selective pressures would have been accounted for these beneficial adaptations. These include the avoidance of predators and that the immune system was able to use the internal energy resources to overcome debilitating diseases such as infections [8]. However, since food is sufficiently available in today's world, the aforementioned pro-feeding behavioral outcome in which overeating is favored over fasting, in combination with continuous reduction in physical activity, has led to a global obesity epidemic within the last century [9]. Since obesity is a major risk factor for severe secondary diseases such as type 2 diabetes, cardiovascular and neurological diseases and certain kinds of cancer, basic research and clinical studies are dedicating a lot of efforts in order to develop weight loss strategies and obesity therapeutics.

1.2. The Endocannabinoid System—A Reliable Partner in Body Weight Control?

One important prerequisite to develop therapeutic interventions such as anti-obesity drugs is the discovery and better understanding of the cellular and molecular elements of the pro-feeding circuitries in our body. Interestingly, one class of endogenous signaling molecules, the so-called endocannabinoids (eCBs), was identified as a highly conserved group of molecules that significantly contributes to metabolic control. Compared to the millennia-old use of cannabis, which is one of the oldest crops cultivated by humankind, the understanding of the basic mechanisms underlying eCB action is a very recent achievement. First uses of hemp for its fibers and as a food source in China can be traced back as far as 6000 years, a first documentation of using cannabis as a medical remedy putatively dates back more than 4000 years [10]. Recreational and medical cannabis use throughout history can be found in many cultures and all over the world [11,12]. However, starting only slightly more than 50 years ago, with the isolation and structural elucidation of cannabidiol [13] and tetrahydrocannabinol (THC) [14,15], the cannabinoid signaling system causing the well-known and medically appreciated effects of Cannabis sativa was revealed piecemeal by the scientific community [16]. After decades of pioneering the uncovering of the cannabinoid system, Mechoulam stated that "[C]annabinoids represent a medicinal treasure trove which waits to be discovered." [17]. In this article we will review the involvement of the endocannabinoid system (ECS) in body weight control both centrally and peripherally, arguing that cannabinoids and congeners represent compounds and targets of promising potential for the treatment of eating disorders and metabolic disturbances.

1.3. Biochemistry of the Endocannabinoid System—An Outline

Evidence that cannabinoids act through a receptor in the brain was found in the late eighties of the last century [18]. The two cannabinoid type 1 (CB1) and 2 (CB2) receptors are G protein-coupled receptors (GPCRs) expressed in virtually all tissues of the body. While CB1 is more abundant in the CNS, CB2 is the predominant cannabinoid receptor in the periphery, especially in cells of the immune system [19,20]. Four years after the discovery of the receptors, the first endogenous ligand for cannabinoid receptors, N-arachidonoylethanolamine (anandamide, AEA), was identified [21] and later supplemented by 2-arachidonylglycerol (2-AG) [22], marking the breakthrough that initiated a whole new field of research investigating the ECS [23].

Many endogenous and synthetic compounds that are part of or interfere with the ECS have been identified and developed (reviewed in [16,24,25]), offering insights into the mechanisms of eCB signaling as well as bearing potential for future treatments. Even though more eCBs have been found, AEA and 2-AG remain the best-characterized representatives. Synthesis, signaling and degradation of these two compounds are visualized in Figure 1.

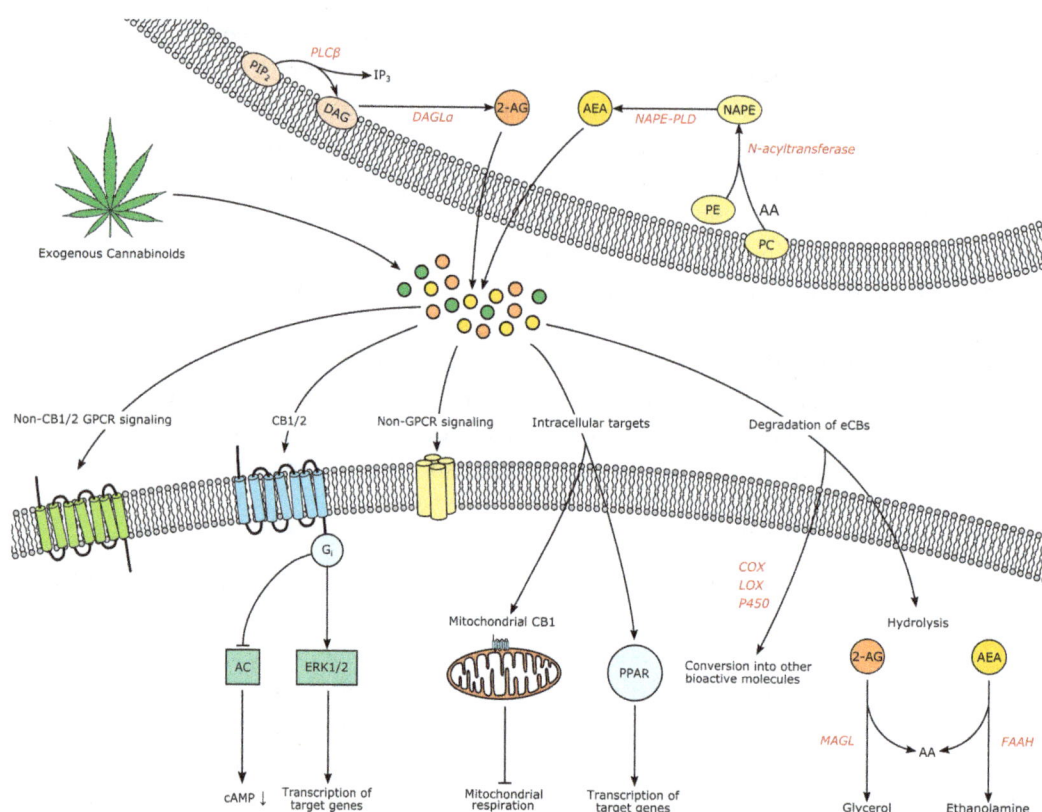

Figure 1. The endocannabinoids (eCBs) AEA and 2-AG are produced on demand from lipid precursors and released to the extracellular space. Endogenous and exogenous cannabinoids act through the same signaling systems: Binding to Gi-coupled receptors CB1 or CB2 modulates intracellular cascades and leads for example to the inhibition of adenylyl cyclase (AC) or the regulation of transcription through extracellular signal-regulated kinases (ERKs). Alternative receptors are non-CB1/2 GPCRs, non-GPCRs like TRPV1 and, intracellularly, mitochondrial CB1 (mtCB1) and peroxisome proliferator-activated receptors (PPARs). Signaling is terminated through hydrolysis, but eCBs might also serve as substrates for cyclooxygenases (COXs), lipoxygenases (LOXs) or cytochromes P450 (P450), yielding additional bioactive compounds. Note that all illustrated processes do not have to take place in distinct cells as autocrine eCB signaling has been shown as well. Abbreviations: PIP2 phosphatidylinositol 4,5-bisphosphate, IP3 inositol-1,4,5-trisphosphat, DAG Diacylglycerol, PLC phospholipase C, DAGL diacylglycerol lipase, 2-AG 2-arachidonylglycerol, PC phosphatidylcholine, PE phosphatidylethanolamine, AA arachidonic acid, NAPE N-arachidonoyl phosphatidylethanolamine, NAPE-PLD NAPE-specific phospholipase D, MAGL monoacylglycerol lipase, FAAH fatty acid amide hydrolase.

Both lipophilic molecules are synthesized from membrane phospholipids on demand upon intracellular Ca^{2+}-elevation, following concomitant activation of receptors [26,27]. The precursor of AEA is N-arachidonoyl phosphatidylethanolamine (NAPE), formed by the transfer of arachidonic acid from phosphaditylcholine to phosphatidylethanolamine by an enzyme yet to be characterized, followed by formation of AEA by NAPE-specific phospholipase D (NAPE-PLD) [25]. However, additional alternative pathways have been suggested [28]. AEA and 2-AG do not seem to be complementary: decreased brain levels of AEA after global NAPE-PLD-knockout did not increase 2-AG in the CNS, except for the brainstem [29]. Leishman et al. demonstrated that knockout of NAPE-PLD causes extensive lipidome changes beyond N-acetylethanolamines, for example the elevation of prostaglandins, providing strong evidence for the underappreciated complexity of the ECS and its relationship to other lipid messenger systems [29].

For the synthesis of 2-AG, phoshpholipase C β catalyzes the hydrolysis of phosphatidylinositol 4,5-bisphosphate to diacylglycerol, which serves as the substrate for diacylglycerol lipases (DAGL) α and β [25]. Signaling of AEA is terminated through uptake and intracellular degradation by fatty acid amide hydrolase (FAAH), while 2-AG is degraded by monoacylglycerol lipase (MAGL) [25]. Compared to classical neurotransmitters and -modulators, eCB transport mechanisms are less well understood. The existence of eCB transporters controlling release and uptake is under debate [30–33]. Due to their hydrophobic nature, eCBs are dependent on binding proteins in aqueous environments, such as albumin [34]. However, how eCBs travel into, through and out of the extracellular space remains enigmatic. As all processes influencing the temporospatial characteristics of eCB signaling constitute potential drug targets, research elucidating these processes is imperatively needed.

In the classical view, activation of CB1 and CB2 leads to G_i-mediated inhibition of adenylyl cyclase and a subsequent closure of calcium and opening of potassium channels, underlying the proposed retrograde mode of eCB signaling in the CNS: activated postsynaptic neurons release eCBs, which lower presynaptic intracellular Ca^{2+} and therefore decrease the probability of transmitter release. Depending on the nature of the presynaptic cell, this process is known as 'depolarization-induced suppression of excitation' (DSE) or 'inhibition' (DSI) [35]. However, more signaling pathways have been discovered, for example activation of the mitogen-activated protein kinase (MAPK) cascades that control cell proliferation, differentiation and death [36]. The eCB signaling has the potential to alter transcription through the MAPK pathway synergistically with other neuropeptides [37]. Also, the universal coupling to G_i did not remain unchallenged [36,38], non-retrograde pathways have been identified, such as autocrine inhibition [39], and non-CB1/2 signaling has been discovered, for example through the cation channel transient receptor potential vanilloid 1 (TRPV1), through peroxisome proliferator-activated receptors (PPAR) and potentially through additional GPCRs like GPR55 [40]. Interestingly, CB1 is also located in mitochondria of neural cells (termed "mtCB1"), and the activation of mtCB1 decreases mitochondrial activity and respiration and therefore affects neuronal activity [41]. Additionally, it is now clear that glia is also involved in CNS eCB signaling [42]. Both microglia and astrocytes are expressing receptors and enzymes involved in eCB signaling [43–45], further shaping the activity of brain circuits through eCBs [46]. Yet, despite the complexity of the ECS and the myriad of unanswered questions, anatomical and functional studies lead to an extensive insight into eCB involvement in physiology and pathology [47]. Prompted by the traditional knowledge that the consumption of THC usually increases appetite even in sated states, it was found that one of the pivotal roles of eCBs is in the control of appetite, feeding and subsequently body weight [48]. In the following sections, we will elucidate the eCB-driven neuromodulation of the underlying brain circuits.

2. Endocannabinoids in Central Control of Body Weight

Eating can be seen as the orchestrated output of the nervous system after integrating humoral and neuronal signals balancing energy needs against energy reserves, processing sensory cues, as well as the motivational and emotional state of an individual—constantly weighing in feeding against other survival needs. The classical view distinguishes homeostatic (sustenance-driven) and hedonic (reward-driven) feeding. Simply put, homeostatic feeding will halt once the organism is replete with energy and nutrients, while hedonic feeding might continue. However, all feeding behavior of higher organisms is influenced by brain regions that process reward, centers that integrate aversion versus preference and circuits that make predictions about the future need and availability of food while constantly evaluating hormonal and neuronal feedback from the periphery. Both "hedonic" and "homeostatic" circuitries are intricately interwoven as evidence accumulates that brain regions that have been classically viewed as predominantly involved in homeostatic feeding are influenced by higher corticolimbic and "hedonic" areas of the brain and vice versa [49,50].

In an "obesigenic" environment of easy accessibility and high nutritional density of food, preponderance of the hedonic aspects of feeding without restriction may lead to overeating and obesity [51,52]. To our knowledge, there are no accounts for an obesity epidemic in wildlife, while for humans (as well as for their domestic animals)—in many regions of the world—efforts to obtain calorie-dense, rewarding food are reduced to a minimum and competition for food is virtually absent, and thus, the hard-wired, pro-feeding circuits seemingly promote obesity. One of the important actuators in these circuits and bearers of hope as therapeutic targets are eCBs.

The eCB involvement in body weight control is already shaped early in life: interestingly, in several mammalian species' milks, including human, 2-AG, the endogenous FAAH-inhibitor oleamide and other eCB-like compounds were found [53]. Furthermore, CB1 seems to be involved in suckling, as blocking CB1 using rimonabant within the first postnatal hours and days of mouse pups prevents milk intake [54]—an effect which is also seen in CB1-knockout (CB1$^{-/-}$) mice on the first postnatal day. However, CB1$^{-/-}$ mice start suckling eventually on postnatal day two or three, suggesting a compensatory mechanism [55]. When mouse pups were orally administered AEA during the nursing period, they exhibited higher body weight, increased fat amount, insulin resistance and higher levels of CB1 expression in adipose tissue in adult life [56,57] as well as altered CB1 signaling in the hypothalamus [58]. However, in this case—as in many studies—central and peripheral effects cannot be clearly distinguished: Is altered hypothalamic eCB signaling the cause or the result of the observed metabolic effects? Infant THC exposure through breastfeeding has been associated with sedation and impaired motor development [59], altered metabolic states have not been described, but it is uncertain whether these effects were considered.

The crucial role of eCBs in the control of body weight has been further demonstrated in global CB1$^{-/-}$ mice, where caloric intake and body weight are significantly lower than in control mice [60] and global CB1$^{-/-}$ mice are resistant to diet-induced obesity (DIO) under a high fat diet (HFD) [61]. On the other hand, globally CB1-deficient mice show significantly reduced life span without any apparent pathology and the cause has not been elucidated [62]. In view of the market withdrawal of Rimonabant as an anti-obesity drug, better knowledge of eCB actions throughout the body are required, especially a separation between central and peripheral effects and a distinction between cause and consequence. Thus, many efforts are still being undertaken to probe eCB signaling in more confined brain regions and organs—in order to understand the underlying mechanisms and provide safe and efficient drug therapies.

2.1. Feeling Hungry or Sated: Peripheral Signals and the Hypothalamus

Behaviors associated with feeding often begin with one central feeling that has the power to override all other undertakings of an organism: hunger, an unpleasant feeling of energy need or, complementary, "appetite", the desire to eat. Initiated by humoral signals such as ghrelin, hypoglycemia and a decline in leptin, activities of neural ensembles throughout the brain prepare the body for one of the most fundamental behavioral patterns: seek food, acquire food, ingest food and digest food. Additionally, numerous autonomous and unconscious processes take place that adjust the body for a state of nutritional deficiency—reduced energy expenditure on the one hand, motivational and sensory focusing towards food intake in anticipation of the rewarding experience on the other hand.

2.2. The Hypothalamus Is a Gate for Feeding Behavior

The hypothalamus is considered a center of prime importance in the integration and control of bodily functions essential for survival such as circadian rhythm, body temperature, plasmaosmolarity, as well as feeding. Since a profuse regulation of hypothalamic activity by eCBs has been shown [9,63], we want to put a special emphasis on this circuitry. In order to exert their integrative role in feeding control, hypothalamic neurons show ample expression of receptors for hormones and nutrients and are extensively connected to other brain regions involved in feeding.

Hypothalamic neurons occupy a domain especially suitable for sensing blood-borne signals: due to the close proximity to the median eminence (ME), a highly vascularized circumventricular organ lacking the blood-brain barrier (BBB), neurons in this region have direct access to the bloodstream. Anatomically and functionally, one can distinguish more than ten nuclei within the hypothalamus, zoned into an anterior (or "preoptic"), medial (or "tuberal") and posterior hypothalamus—due to the scope of this review, we will focus on the areas involved in feeding, which are mainly located in the tuberal zone—for a thorough primer on the hypothalamus, see [64]. Basically, a local ECS relevant for body weight control is present in numerous of these specific hypothalamic nuclei. Autonomous, hypothalamic and reward-related feeding areas show a complex pattern of interconnectivity, which remains to be fully disentangled. Some important feeding-related connections discussed here are visualized in Figure 2. For example, the arcuate nucleus (ARC) sends output to other hypothalamic feeding centers: Ventro—and dorsomedial hypothalamus (VMH, DMH), paraventricular nucleus (PVN) and lateral hypothalamus (LH). At the same time, all aforementioned nuclei receive input from the nucleus of the solitary tract (NTS) as well as from the parabrachial nucleus (PBN). Conversely, LH, PBN and NTS are sending output to nucleus accumbens (NAcc) and limbic areas for processes involving reward and motivation, as well as to motor and autonomic areas, for example to the dorsal nucleus of the vagus nerve (DVN). Furthermore, ARC and PVH also send long-range connections to PBN and autonomic motor centers [64].

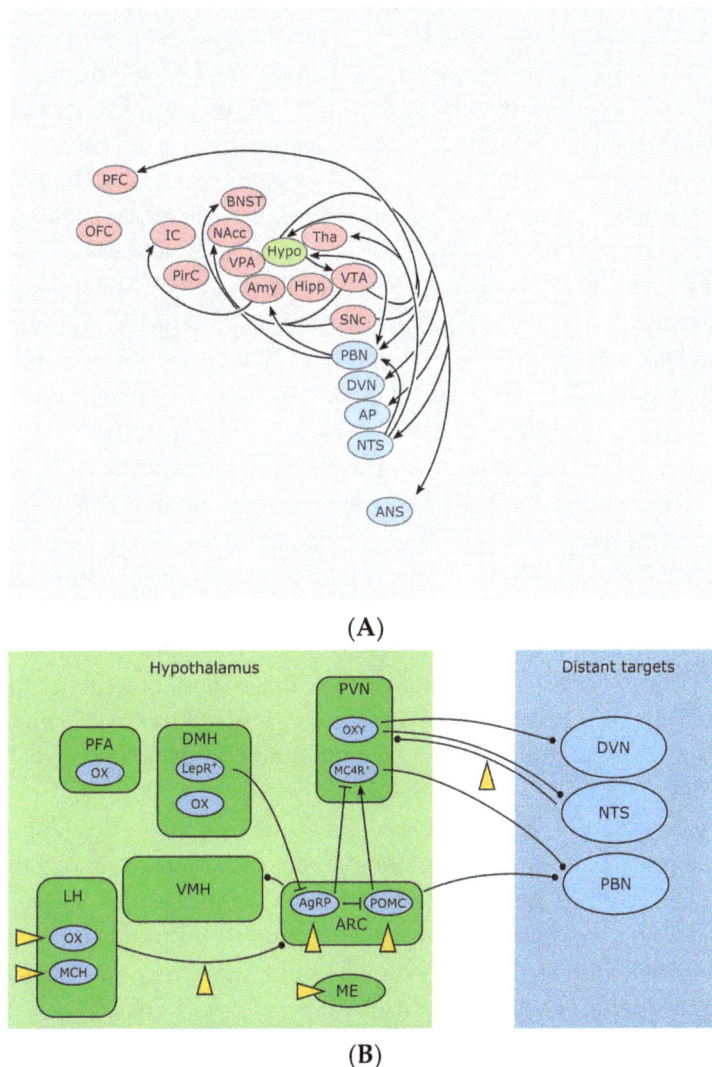

(A)

(B)

Figure 2. (A) Brain regions where the ECS influences different aspects of feeding.

Blue: autonomous "hotspots" that convey sensory and visceral information from the periphery to the CNS and vice versa. Green: the hypothalamus is of pivotal significance for the integration of humoral and neuronal signals that evaluate the calorie supply of the whole body. Red: areas especially important for motivation, decision-making, emotion and reward—influencing complex behaviors such as foraging and the choice of food. Abbreviations: PFC prefrontal cortex, OFC orbitofrontal cortex, IC insular cortex, PirC piriform cortex, BNST bed nucleus of the stria terminalis, NAcc nucleus accumbens, VPA ventral pallidum, Amy amygdala, Hypo hypothalamus, Tha thalamus, Hipp hippocampus, VTA ventrotegmental area, SNc substantia nigra, pars compacta, PBN parabrachial nucleus, DVN dorsal nucleus of the vagus nerve, AP area postrema, NTS Nucleus of the solitary tract, ANS autonomic nervous system. (**B**) Pathways and cell types of hypothalamic circuits and their distant connections with the autonomous system. endocannabinoid system (ECS) targets marked by yellow arrowheads. Abbreviations: PFA perifornical area, LH lateral hypothalamus, DMH dorsomedial hypothalamus, VMH ventromedial hypothalamus, PVN paraventricular nucleus, ARC arcuate nucleus, ME median eminence, OX orexin, MCH melanin-concentrating hormone, LEPR leptin receptor, OXY oxytocin, MCR4 melanocortin type 4 receptor, DVN dorsal nucleus of the vagus nerve, NTS nucleus of the solitary tract, PBN parabrachial nucleus.

Located in close proximity to the third ventricle, the ARC contains two reciprocally active neuron populations: ventromedially located Agouti-related peptide (AgRP)/neuropeptide Y (NPY) and dorsolaterally located proopiomelanocortin (POMC) neurons, whose activity codes for hunger and satiety, respectively [65]. ARC neurons assess the caloric need of the body through humoral as well as neuronal signals. Ghrelin activates AgRP/NPY neurons and induces feeding [66]. Leptin depolarizes POMC neurons in the ARC while hyperpolarizing AgRP/NPY neurons [67]. Following fasting, AgRP/NPY neurons are active. During refeeding, a dorsolateral shift of the neuronal activity from AgRP into POMC neurons can be observed, indicating a decrease in hunger and an increase in satiety [65]. POMC and AgRP/NPY neurons innervate the same "satiety" target neurons in the PVN. These neurons express melanocortin receptor 4 (MC4R), a GPCR activated by α-melanocyte stimulating hormone, which is released by POMC neurons, while AgRP is an inverse agonist on these receptors. Additionally, AgRP/NPY neurons inhibit PVN neurons through release of GABA and NPY. The aforementioned MC4R target neurons project to PBN and, when activated, induce satiety behaviors [68]. However, the activity of ARC neurons can be disrupted by cannabinoids and induce a feeding response in a state of satiety with concomitant paradox activity of POMC neurons [48]. Furthermore, presynaptic terminals on AgRP/NPY-neurons (but not the postsynaptic cells themselves) show CB1-expression, suggesting a retrograde control of AgRP activity through eCBs [69].

Besides ARC AgRP/NPY and POMC neurons, other neuronal populations residing in the ARC are involved in feeding control, like dopaminergic neurons [70] as well as orexigenic somatostatin (SST) neurons [71]. As more than 50 transcriptionally different cell types in the ARC-ME complex alone have been identified [71], an even greater complexity of this region, potentially the hypothalamus in general, remains to be unraveled. Moreover, evidence accumulates that ARC cells serve roles beyond feeding, for instance the control of bone mass [72] or immunomodulation through T-cell activation [73] by AgRP/NPY neurons.

Animals with lesioned PVN show increased food intake and obesity [74]. The PVN contains oxytocin-producing neurons that connect to autonomic centers, which eventually send visceroefferents through the vagus nerve [75]. It has been found that oxytocin, besides its well-known functions in bonding, birth and sexuality, shapes vagal parasympathetic output, leading to a decreased food intake [76,77]. Oleoylethanolamide (OEA), a non-CB1 lipid messenger with structural similarities to AEA [78] exerted anorexigenic effects through activation of noradrenergic projections from NTS to PVN and increases oxytocin levels in PVN and supraoptic nucleus [79,80] offering a new pathway connecting the ECS with neuropeptides involved in food intake.

Integrating peripheral and central signals and information about the environment, the LH orchestrates a broad variety of homeostatic and behavioral functions, such as sleep, stress and anxiety, but also feeding and reward [81]. Cells in the LH are heterogeneous and often classified by the expression of neuropeptides. Prominent representatives are orexin/hypocretin neurons (OX) and melanin-concentrating hormone (MCH) neurons. MCH is increased during fasting [82] and overexpression of MCH leads to hyperphagia and obesity while MCH-knockout causes hypophagia and decreases body weight [83]. Orexin A and B (OX-A, OX-B) were named after their initially observed feeding-stimulating effect [84], and are solely produced in the hypothalamic LH, perifornical area (PFA) and DMH [85]. It was later found that OXs also play an important role in sleep/wakefulness [86] as patients suffering from narcolepsy lack OX expression. Cannabinoids influence the activity of LH neurons in a disparate manner: CB1 activation activates MCH neurons but inhibits OX neurons [87]. Key to this discrepancy might be the organization of the synaptic input to these cells. The innervation of OX neurons depends on the metabolic state of the animal: in lean mice, excitatory input outnumbers inhibitory synapses and the excitatory overbalance even increases after overnight fasting [88]. Expanding on this finding, a study by Cristino et al. [89,90] found that OX neurons in leptin-deficient ob/ob and DIO mice receive predominantly inhibitory input, originating from ARC AgRP/NPY neurons. The driver of this remodeling seems to be impaired leptin signaling in the ARC. At the same time, ob/ob mice show a relative overexpression of DAGLα, leading to higher levels of eCBs and a decrease in inhibitory inputs through DSI. Together with a subsequent study [91], the following mechanism was proposed: OX neurons in wildtype animals use eCB signaling as a negative feedback to dampen excitation. In ob/ob mice however, pathological wiring and enhanced eCB signaling leads to a preferential disinhibition and the relative predominance of excitatory inputs causes a positive feedback that could potentially drive eating behavior despite elevated leptin levels. No similar synaptic rearrangements were seen in MCH neurons [92]. However, in another study, MCH neurons of the LH were also shown to downregulate their inhibitory input through retrograde eCB signaling [93], while leptin—through inhibition of voltage-gated calcium channels—lowers eCB production and subsequently inhibits DSI [93]. This interaction between elevated leptin and eCB signaling could ultimately decrease food intake. Furthermore, CBs also influence the activity in LH target regions. OX-expressing neurons, among other functions, are involved in reward and motivation, as they are active during cues for rewards such as food or drugs and project to reward centers [94]. OX receptors OX1R and OX2R can be found in many brain regions, among them are prefrontal cortex (PFC), ventral tegmental area (VTA), thalamus, hypothalamus, BNST and brainstem [95]. Delivery of OX-A to the hindbrain increases meal size and frequency, potentially through blockade of amylin, a satiety-inducing pancreatic peptide, in the NTS and/or area postrema [96]. A surprising interaction between eCBs and OXs within the hypothalamus has been found by Morello et al. [37]: POMC neurons in the ARC express both CB1 and OX1R and they receive synaptic input by OX neurons of the LH. In obese mice, OX-A signaling was elevated, while POMC and α-melanocyte stimulating hormone transcripts were downregulated in POMC neurons mediated through STAT3. Interestingly, this effect required both OX-A and CB1 signaling, suggesting a potential multi-target pharmacological approach in treating obesity.

Further evidence for the synergism between OXs and eCBs has been found in projections from LH to VTA, a pathway that might be relevant for the reward-related aspects of food as well: during stress, OX-A release in VTA leads to a 2-AG/CB1-mediated dis-inhibition and subsequently to a reinstatement of cocaine-place-preference in previously extinguished mice [97]. These two examples emphasize the need for studies of feeding regulation that address interactions between neuropeptides and other neuromodulatory systems.

2.3. Peripheral Signals Extensively Influence CNS Circuits

In what follows, we will outline the central effects of feeding-related humoral signals. For the discussion of their peripheral actions, the reader is referred to the Section 3. One of the humoral factors evoking hunger is ghrelin, a peptide hormone that is released both in the gastrointestinal tract (mainly in the stomach) and the brain, for example in the hypothalamus [98]. When administered peripherally or centrally, ghrelin stimulates feeding in animals fed ad libitum, but does not further increase acute food intake in fasted or calorie-restricted animals [99]. Midbrain transection abolishes the orexigenic effect of peripherally administered ghrelin [66]. AgRP/NPY neurons are depolarized by the application of ghrelin, both indirectly due to changes in the presynaptic input and directly due to activation of currents in the cell itself [100]. Surprisingly, in CB1$^{-/-}$ mice, ghrelin does not increase feeding [101]. Furthermore, ghrelin application increases eCB levels in the PVN in wild-type, but not in CB1-knockout animals, and this increase can be turned off by CB1-blockade [101]. In addition to the hypothalamus, ghrelin acts through the activation of feeding circuits in the amygdala and the NTS, as well as through the activation of motivation- and reward-related areas such as the dopaminergic projections from VTA to the NAcc [102].

Leptin is a hormone mainly produced in the adipose tissue conveying the status of the energy reserves, acting on medium timescales (hours)—for example, leptin levels remain unchanged within the first 30 min of refeeding after a long fasting and reach control levels after 6 h [65]. While leptin deficiency strongly induces feeding and a decrease in energy expenditure [68], metabolic disorders such as obesity go along with elevated leptin levels but altered responses to leptin, often termed "leptin resistance" [103]. Extra-hypothalamic leptin effects have been found for example in the thalamus during postnatal development [104], in the VTA, where leptin decreases basal and feeding-evoked dopamine, which in turn decreases food intake [105], and in the NTS, where leptin increases pSTAT3 levels without effects on body weight and food intake [106]. It was recently shown that triglycerides cross the BBB and counteract the anorexigenic effects of leptin. Remarkably, leptin uptake in several brain regions was increased upon administration of triglycerides while at the same time leptin- and insulin resistance were observed [107]. The first observation of interactions between leptin and eCBs was made by Di Marzo et al.: Leptin-deficient ob/ob and leptin receptor-defective db/db mice show elevated hypothalamic eCB levels. Administration of leptin to ob/ob mice normalized eCB-levels [108]. When administering the CB1 inverse agonist AM251 and leptin together intraperitoneally (i.p.), food intake and body weight were reduced in rats and this effect was dependent on serotonin signaling. Interestingly, the doses used were subanorectic for each compound individually, showing a synergism between leptin and eCB signaling [109]. Additionally, leptin resistance in DIO mice could be reversed by administration of the peripheral CB1 antagonist JD5037, which surprisingly also decreased hypothalamic AEA levels and hence attenuated central CB signaling, too [110].

Cholecystokinin (CCK) is released by the duodenum during digestion of food. In addition to its effects on the gastrointestinal system, CCK may bind to vagal CCK receptors or CCK receptors 1 and 2 in the brain [111] and induce behaviors associated with satiety. Peripheral injection of CCK is associated with sated behaviors such as halted food intake, less exploration and general inactivity [112]. Following midbrain transections, the behavioral effect of peripherally administered CCK was diminished, as the autonomic neurons in the NTS were disconnected from forebrain structures such as thalamus and hypothalamus, showing that the effects of CCK are not limited to intestinal organs, nor purely autonomic [113]. CCK-expressing neurons in the NTS, as well as another dopamine β-hydroxylase-expressing population, innervate calcitonin gene-related protein expressing PBN neurons. Activation of this pathway leads to decreased food intake and body weight [114]. The CCK and eCB system have been shown to be jointly involved in learning [115] and in circuits involved in anxiety and pain [116]. A feeding-related synaptic connection depending on humoral, neuronal and eCB signaling has been studied by Khlaifia et al.: long term synaptic depression (LTD) between visceroafferent fibers and neurons of the NTS is affected by the feeding state of an animal. Following fasting, elevated ghrelin levels impair eCB-mediated LTD, which can be restored by the elevation of CCK. This mechanism can be thought of as an integrator between visceroafferents and blood-borne signals: the humoral satiety signal CCK attenuates neuronal transmission while the "hunger hormone" ghrelin leads to a more reliable conveyance of afferent signals [117]. Both humoral and neuronal pathways are linked by eCBs, underlining their importance as local modulators, especially in feeding circuits.

Neurons of the ARC and ME express insulin receptors, predominantly axonally located [118]. Insulin decreases NPY expression [119] and hyperpolarizes an insulin receptor expressing subset of POMC neurons [120], contradicting the assumption that—due to the observed anorexigenic effects of intracerebroventricularly (i.c.v.) administered insulin [119]—POMC neurons should be stimulated by insulin [121]. Most interactions between insulin and eCB signaling have been described in the periphery—see Section 3.

Glucagon-like peptide (GLP-1) is secreted postprandially in the gut and was later discovered to be also produced in a subset of neurons of the NTS, innervating hypothalamus (specifically ARC, DMH and PVN), thalamus and cortex [122]. GLP-1 receptors were also found in the BNST, central amygdala and dorsal lateral septum [123]. The identified sites of GLP-1 receptors support the putative role of GLP-1 in decreasing homeostatic and hedonic feeding [124] that have been observed behaviorally [125,126]. OEA and 2-oleoylglycerol have been shown to increase the potency of GLP-1 signaling by binding to GLP-1 directly, suggesting a potential fine-tuning mechanism for this pathway [127]. However, more research investigating the crosstalk between GLP-1 and eCBs and its functional implications, especially in vivo, has to be conducted.

Other than the outlined hormonal signaling systems, several brain regions are also capable of nutrient sensing. For some compounds, the diffusion is facilitated in areas lacking tight junctions of the BBB, for example in the ME as well as in the area postrema.

Fatty acid sensing takes place throughout the brain, is involved in many processes and interwoven with other signaling systems, especially with the ECS [128]. Dietary polyunsaturated fatty acids (PUFA) have been shown to be of importance for processes such as neuroprotection, synaptogenesis and synaptic plasticity [129]. The underlying mechanisms are on the one hand the fact that PUFAs constitute essential components of cell membranes, on the other hand because PUFAs bind to receptors such as GPCR40 and PPAR [129]. Interestingly, a close relationship between PUFA and eCB signaling has been shown. For example, a lifetime dietary deficiency of n-3 PUFAs abrogates CB1-dependent LTD in PFC and NAcc with effects on emotions, namely promotion of anxiety and depression-like behavior in rodents [130].

Protein availability is constantly monitored in the CNS through amino acid sensing. Amino acids cross the BBB through carrier proteins [131]. A substantial body of evidence supports a suggested pathway through which—during a state of deficiency—amino acid sensing neurons in the anterior piriform cortex lead to foraging for a diet that provides essential amino acids required for survival [132]. Furthermore, the i.c.v. application of leucine leads to hypophagic responses mediated by amino acid-sensing centers in the brainstem and hypothalamus [133].

Finally, glucose levels are probably the nutrient signals with the highest priority as severe hypoglycemia is a potentially life-threatening condition. Therefore, neural circuits have emerged that constantly monitor glucose levels and—in case of hypoglycemia—activate the counter-regulatory response through the sympathetic nervous system and increase the likelihood of feeding [134]. Pivotal glucose sensing centers reside in the hypothalamus and brainstem and neuronal glucose sensing has also been found in the peripheral nervous system, for example in the ganglion inferius of the vagus nerve, where almost half of the afferent neurons are either excited or inhibited by glucose [135]. Hypothalamic neurons that sense glucose are POMC and AgRP/NPY neurons of the ARC as well as MCH and OX neurons of the LH [136]. Impairment in glucose sensing mechanisms in POMC neurons, which can be caused by obesity, has been shown to be detrimental for overall regulation of blood glucose levels [137]. Also, glucose sensing is dependent on the metabolic state of the animal [138] and leptin increases glucose sensitivity [139]. Furthermore, glial cells have been shown to be involved in hypothalamic glucose sensing as well: astrocytes sense glucose levels and show altered phenotypes in response to hyperglycemia [140,141] as well as altered glucose uptake following leptin treatment [142]. Interestingly, leptin signaling and glucose sensitivity in astrocytes are linked by the ECS: ablating

CB1 in astrocytes interferes with their leptin sensitivity and alters glycogen storage [143]. Moreover, tanycytes are responsive to glucose too [144], their involvement in glucose sensing has been reviewed in [145].

2.4. "Wanting" Food: Motivation, Food Seeking and Decision-Making

Food, especially when rich in nutrients and calories, is a primary source of reward [146]—imaginably, as highly nutritious food is usually harder to obtain (e.g., collecting low-calorie plants versus hunting energy-dense game), a rewarding feeling is linked to its consumption and a strong drive to seek for and consume such food served as an evolutionary advantage, especially in respect of human brain development [147]. Reinforcing feelings are already triggered during presentation and anticipation of food intake, which are in combination with food seeking behavior often referred to as the "wanting" aspect of feeding. The "liking" component of feeding relates to the hedonic feelings of pleasure during food consumption [52,148]—often nonspecifically termed "palatability" [149]—and during food digestion. In 1996, Berridge suggested that "liking" and "wanting" are implemented by separable neural circuits and not necessarily conscious [148]. Ultimately, both liking and wanting interact to some extent and are further shaped and by learning processes as most food preferences are acquired and changed throughout life—to an extent that even innately aversive stimuli like bitterness can be overcome due to the link between their consumption and positive feelings, as in coffee, tea and beer [52].

Dopaminergic neurons of the VTA and substantia nigra, pars compacta projecting to a wide array of brain regions are—among other processes—involved in motivation and the incentive value of items and therefore part of the "wanting" system. Interactions between the ECS and dopaminergic circuits are extensive and have been reviewed in [150,151]. I.c.v. injection of ghrelin increases locomotor activity and dopamine release in the VTA, indicating an increased motivation for food seeking. These ghrelin effects can be significantly reduced by i.p. application of the CB1 inverse agonist Rimonabant, while food intake is unchanged [102]. Conversely, leptin decreases dopamine release in the VTA and reduces food intake [105]. Dopaminergic neurons themselves do not express CB1. However, CB1 is present in their GABAergic input terminals which control dopamine release [152]. Accordingly, VTA neurons showed an increased firing rate in response to exposure to synthetic CB1 agonist HU210 in the majority of cells [153].

The NAcc, part of the ventral striatum, is a key recipient of dopaminergic projections from the VTA, also receiving glutamatergic input from PFC, basolateral amygdala (BLA), hippocampus and thalamus [154]. One could think of the NAcc as a system that puts the "wanting" into action in order to achieve "liking" as it integrates diverse inputs and elicits goal-directed behavior [155]. The role of the ECS in the motivational aspects of feeding are beginning to be understood [52] and evidence exists for ECS involvement in many motivation-related areas. For example, fasting induces a strong increase in 2-AG and AEA in the forebrain components of the limbic system [156], indicating eCB modulation of the motivation to acquire food during hunger. Also, experience shapes the activity and organization of the NAcc, partially mediated by eCBs. Low-frequency stimulation of excitatory medial PFC afferents can induce CB1-dependent presynaptic LTD [157], suggesting the possibility that the ECS alters feeding behavior through motivational circuits.

Certainly, our behavior and choices are not exclusively driven by the "wanting" system, as immediate rewards always have to be weighed up against long-term goals of an individual [158]. In order to make choices that are beneficial for the survival of an organism, estimating the value of an item, such as food, is necessary for anticipating the outcome of a certain decision [159]. The orbitofrontal cortex has been suggested to encode specific information about an item and from that, infer anticipated outcomes of a choice, and is therefore, together with the adjacent PFC, involved in decision-making [160,161]. The orbitofrontal cortex encodes both information about the value of an object and value-independent, identity-specific information [159,161]. Identity-unspecific value information however seems to be represented by neurons in the ventromedial PFC in humans. Taken together, parallel circuits are involved in predicting the outcome of a decision [159]. However, in many cases, a decision cannot be easily made, for example when the number of factors to be taken into account exceeds our capacities or when there is a lack of past experience allowing for the estimation of the value of an item. At these times, "wanting" and "liking" may—often subconsciously—help guide our behavior [158]. The underlying behavioral pattern for many eating disorders such as anorexia nervosa or DIO are persistent maladaptive food choices [162]. In a rat model of binge-eating behavior, where female rats had a temporally limited access to HFD in addition to their normal diet, CB1 levels in the PFC were found to decrease in the binge-eating group [163]. Another study showed a slight decrease in PFC AEA levels in mice on HFD compared to standard diet (SD) [61]. Taken together, the ECS in the PFC seems to be downregulated under HFD. When blocking CB1 with low doses of orally administered Rimonabant in rats, food intake was preferentially suppressed for sweet food, while intake of normal chow remained unchanged [164].

The consumption of cannabis sativa has an orexigenic effect on humans, anecdotally especially for highly palatable food. In a study where subjects underwent memory testing, the intake of marshmallows increased significantly after smoking a marihuana cigarette [165]. In addition to this orexigenic effect, THC has been reported to be anorexigenic as well. Oral administration of low doses of THC increased acute food intake in rats, which was compensated by lower food intake afterwards [166], while higher i.p. doses decreased feeding [167]. This is in line with the observation that the feeding response to cannabinoids is "biphasic", where low doses of THC and AEA have an orexigenic and high doses have an anorexigenic effect [168–171]. The biphasic feeding response was also seen in sated animals and blocking CB1 with Rimonabant abolished it [171]. Noteworthy, high doses of THC not only decreased feeding but also water intake [169] and an alternative to the explanation that high levels of cannabinoids lead to a feeling of satiety is, that the preponderance of psychotropic and locomotor effects prevents animals from food and water intake (for further discussion, see Section 4. One may speculate whether the increased food intake reflects stronger "wanting" or "liking". However, evidence exists on THC-increased palatability through the activation of dopamine signaling in the NAcc [172], and by sharpening olfactory sensation [173].

2.5. The "Liking" Phase of Feeding: Food Consumption

The perception of taste is essential for the assessment of edibility of food, for the evaluation of its nutritional values as well as—ultimately—the development of food preferences through rewarding experiences and associations [174,175]. Sensory information from taste receptors (see also Section 3) is conveyed to the NTS by the hypoglossal, facial and vagus nerve. From the NTS, taste information in humans is transferred to the PBN of the reticular formation, which is involved in processes such as thermoregulation, arousal and taste and connects to other brain regions related to feeding and reward, such as hypothalamus, thalamus, amygdala and cortex [176]. The infusion of 2-AG to the PBN increases food intake preferably for sweet and fatty food but not for standard chow [177], whereas activation of μ-opioid receptors (MORs)—which show a similar distribution pattern—increased the intake of chow. Furthermore, blocking MOR did not interfere with eCB actions. Therefore, eCBs in PBN seem to constitute a selective reinforcement signal for palatable food [177]. During refeeding following a long fast, there is a significant increase in PBN activity even during the consumption of a standard chow diet [65]. From the gustatory PBN, taste information is conveyed to the NAcc, potentially linking reward to afferent taste information by increasing dopamine levels [178]. Evidence is accumulating that opioid and cannabinoid system are interacting [179]. In addition to dopaminergic control, stimulation of MOR of the NAcc increases the task-dependent consumption of palatable food, which may be caused by enhanced salience of a reward but also due to increased food seeking behavior. Caref et al. found that, when blocking MOR in the NAcc, a decreased cued approach of fatty food is only observed in sated, but not in food-restricted animals, emphasizing the state-dependency of MOR-expressing NAcc neurons promoting food seeking behavior [180]. The NAcc has been shown to express only low levels of CB1 [181] as the major population of cells, medium spiny neurons, which transfer NAcc output to other brain regions, are CB1-negative. Fast-spiking interneurons however, which provide strong inhibitory input to medium spiny neurons, express CB1 in about 40% of the cells. These CB1-expressing fast-spiking interneurons have been shown to become more excitable during cocaine withdrawal [182]. Some eating disorders seemingly share similarities with addictions, such as cravings and over-consumption of food despite knowledge about its negative effects [51]. The NAcc is involved both in reward during addiction as well as food intake. However, whether "food addiction" is a fitting term or whether overeating and binge eating are "just" physiological behaviors taken to an extreme, is debatable [183].

Parts of the "liking" aspects of food intake are processed in cortical areas, like gustatory cortices and insular cortex (IC). The secondary gustatory cortex in primates including humans is located in the orbitofrontal cortex and it connects the primary sensations of smell, taste and texture to reward values [184]. The IC receives visceral inputs through the thalamus as well as through other nuclei in midbrain and hindbrain [184]. In mice, the insular cortex, but not the adjacent somatosensory cortex, is necessary for responding to visual cues that predict food [185]. Livneh et al. found pathways that connect AgRP/NPY neurons to IC through the thalamus and BLA [185]. In the same study, Ca^{2+} imaging insular cortex neurons in wake mice revealed a broad activation pattern during visual cue and food consumption, that did not show any spatial organization. While sated mice did not consume food during presentation of the visual stimulus, chemogenetic activation of hypothalamic AgRP/NPY neurons restored the licking response, potentially mimicking a state of hunger. In the suggested pathway, AgRP/NPY neurons disinhibit BLA neurons through the paraventricular thalamus. BLA sends axon collaterals to IC, putatively providing information about the value of a cued reward [185] and this input might be enhanced during hunger. Support for involvement of the ECS in cortical sensory processing stems from studies in humans suffering from anorexia and bulimia nervosa, where an increased CB1 density in insular cortex and inferior temporal and frontal lobe was found, pointing at a potentially impaired processing of interoceptive, gustatory and reward-related behavior [186].

2.6. Digestion of Food: Induction of a Feeling of Satiety

The feeling of "satiety" can stem from different underlying causes—on the one hand from energy replenishment, for example mediated by normalized glucose levels following hypoglycemia, as well as from reaching capacity limits of the digestive tract. While the former could be described as a positive feeling of "replete" as opposed to the latter unpleasant feeling of "stuffed", we will refer to both processes as "sated".

The pivotal centers for the control of meal size and meal termination—potential readouts for satiety—lie in the brainstem, controlled by humoral and neuronal afferents from the periphery. In addition to the aforementioned taste pathways relevant during ingestion, visceral afferents from internal organs during digestion are transmitted through the vagus nerve to neurons in the NTS as well as the area postrema via glutamatergic synapses [187]. Located in the medulla oblongata, the NTS connects to forebrain regions as well as to the area postrema, which is a brain region involved in vomiting (see next section), and to the nucleus ambiguus and the dorsal nucleus of the vagal nerve [113]—which influence intestinal motility. Vagal afferents include information from intestinal stretch receptors and gut peptides such as ghrelin [66], glucagon like-peptide 1 (GLP-1), peptide YY and cholecystokinin (CCK), which bind to receptors expressed at intestinal terminals of the vagus nerve [188]; see also Section 3. A deafferentation of the vagus nerve in rats leads to increased meal sizes, which are compensated by lower meal frequency and result in a normal body weight. Furthermore, a nutrient preload of the stomach suppresses feeding just as well as in controls with intact vagal afferents. Taken together, vagal afferents are not solely necessary for the induction of satiety nor maintenance of body weight [189].

Brain regions other than hindbrain have been proposed to be involved in satiety-related signaling. In addition to its well-known functions in memory the hippocampus has been shown to be involved in the processing of signals of satiety and regulating appetite [61,190] and hippocampal changes in the ECS related to feeding have been observed: in mice on a HFD, levels of AEA and 2-AG (as well its synthesizing enzyme DAGLα) are significantly increased in hippocampus compared to SD, accompanied by a slight increase in CB1 levels in the stratum radiatum of CA1 and CA3 [61]. Hence, HFD enhances eCB signaling in the hippocampus [61]. Moreover, the observed molecular changes have a functional outcome: upon activation of a cell, DSI was stronger in HFD mice when compared to mice fed normal food [61].

2.7. In Case the Food Cannot Be Digested: Nausea and Vomiting

Nausea and subsequently vomiting are autonomous processes intended to prevent the ingestion or digestion of potentially harmful substances. These feelings can be elicited both peripherally by the GI tract or centrally, in the area postrema [191], triggered by the dorsal vagus complex. Nausea, the uncomfortable feeling that precedes vomiting, as well as vomiting are common side effects of medication and often accompany pathologies [192]. Especially in cancer, these side effects of chemotherapeutics can aggravate tumor-associated weight loss severely and hence are important symptoms to treat. Cannabis sativa has been known for its antiemetic properties for a long time [193]. However, careful examination of the underlying processes is essential, as chronic cannabis consumption lead to frequent vomiting for reasons yet unknown [194]. ECS influences on nausea and vomiting have been reviewed in [191], potential therapeutic interventions will be discussed below.

2.8. Expanding the Neurocentric View: Glia in Feeding Control

In addition to a neurocentric view on feeding circuits, glial cells recently drew increasing interest as they have been shown to participate in feeding control. Astrocytes, the most abundant type of glia in the CNS, show versatile phenotypes across brain regions and a tendency to adapt to anatomical and physiological properties of their surrounding neurons [195–197]. Due to astrocyte ability to shape synaptic transmission and neuronal activity [47,198–200] by forming close interactions with synapses (termed "tripartite synapse" [201]) and through the release of "gliotransmitters" [202,203], one can imagine that astrocytes are involved in feeding control.

Yang et al. reported that astrocytes are capable of reducing food intake through the increase in extracellular adenosine, whose A_{2A} receptor has been shown to form heteromers with CB1 [92,204]. Astrocytic adenosine release in the hypothalamus inhibits the activity of AgRP/NPY neurons of the ARC both basally as well as following ghrelin stimulation [205]. On top of this, astrocytes have been shown to be critically involved in glucose-mediated effects in the hypothalamus. The cell-specific knockout of their insulin receptors impairs glucose uptake to the CNS and leads to altered metabolism and behavior in response to glucose elevation [206,207]. The fact that hypothalamic astrocytes are important elements in hypothalamic feeding circuitry is further supported by the findings that, during postnatal development, astrocytes proliferate in response to leptin [208] and the knockout of astrocytic leptin receptor blunts leptin-induced feeding suppression and induces hyperphagia [209,210]. Providing a cellular basis for astrocyte involvement in eCB signaling, Navarrete et al. showed that astrocytes express CB1 and respond to eCBs released by neighboring pyramidal cells [43]. Another study found that astrocytic eCB sensitivity can mediate heterosynaptic long-term-potentiation (LTP) through the release of gliotransmitters, suggesting a glia-dependent pathway by which eCB signaling can affect synapses located remotely from the eCB release site [46].

Tanycytes are a specialized type of radial glia surrounding the third ventricle, making contact with both the portal capillaries and the cerebrospinal fluid. Generally, tanycytes express a broad variety of receptors for neuropeptides important for the hypothalamic feeding circuitry and distinct types of tanycytes can be distinguished—for a review on tanycytes, see [211]. Tanycytes have for example been shown to be involved in glucosensing [144,145], amino acid sensing [212] and leptin sensing [213]—in the latter study, tanycytes were shown to exert abnormal functions in leptin transport in ob/ob and DIO mice, emphasizing their critical role in a circuit that was mainly studied with a neurocentric view so far. Tanycytes show polar DAGLα-immunostaining [214], ordering investigation of tanycyte-produced eCBs and their effects on the nearby feeding circuitry [215].

Microglia are the resident macrophages in CNS parenchyma. As HFD causes an inflammatory response in the brain [216], a proliferation of microglia can be observed [217]. Blocking this microglial proliferation ameliorates HFD-induced pathologies such as adiposity and leptin resistance [217]. Moreover, microglial activation has been shown to modify neuronal activity in feeding circuits: inflammatory activation of ARC microglia changes synaptic input to and altered activity of POMC neurons, leading to a sickness behavior in mice [218]. Similarly to eCB-mediated immunomodulation in the periphery, microglia phenotypes can be altered by eCB activation as well [45], suggesting an additional pathway through which the eCB imbalance in hypothalamic feeding circuits alters neuronal activity. Buckley et al. revealed through CB2-knockout studies that the immunomodulatory effects in peripheral tissues are mediated by CB2 [219], but found that binding of a synthetic agonist was unaffected in the brain, supporting the prevalent role of CB1 in the CNS. However, it was later shown that microglia, as the principal immune cells of the CNS, do express CB2 [220,221] with functional implications both in health [222,223] and disease [224]. However, microglial expression of CB2, which is upregulated during microglial activation [225], remains difficult to visualize and quantify as basal expressions seem low and detection methods are unreliable [226]. Noteworthy, CB2 signaling was not only shown to exert an anti-inflammatory role, it also affected cognitive processes such as contextual fear memory, shown in a study by Li and Kim [223]. For further discussion of the immunomodulatory effects of eCBs see section 'The emerging role of the hepatic and pancreatic ECS in metabolic disorders'.

The evidence for glial involvement in homeostatic and feeding circuits as well as in eCB signaling, it becomes clear that research investigating the eCB involvement in body weight control should span all cell types as they potentially provide the "missing link" for the multitude of unexplained eCB effects.

2.9. Back from the Brain to the Periphery: Neuronal Output Influencing Metabolism

In the previous section, we reviewed how signals from the periphery influence the CNS and how this information is integrated and processed in a variety of circuits. As mentioned earlier, global $CB1^{-/-}$ mice do not develop an obese phenotype when fed a HFD [61]. Interestingly, following CB1-knockout specifically in GABAergic neurons, body weight on SD is equal to control mice, but on HFD, visceral fat and body weight over time are lower. As the calorie intake is equal to control animals, these GABAergic cells may be involved in a circuit that regulates energy expenditure rather than food intake [61]. Similarly, in a study by Quarta et al., the anorexic and weight decreasing effects of rimonabant were ablated in mice with a CB1-knockout directed to glutamatergic, calmodulin-dependent protein kinase-expressing cells [227]. It was shown that these mice exhibit an overactivity of the sympathetic nervous system and increased thermogenesis, mediated by a pathway from forebrain to NTS and from there to the periphery, leading to an improved metabolic profile. In what follows, we want to examine the evidence for peripheral effects of eCB signaling and the consequences for body weight control.

3. Endocannabinoids in Peripheral Body Weight Control

3.1. Peripheral eCB Signaling in Metabolic Health and Disease

From a plethora of investigations on metabolism and body weight control, it emerged that the ECS is not only a partaker in the aforementioned brain circuitries but also represents an elementary factor in numerous peripheral organs in control of energy metabolism and consequentially in the regulation of body weight. In this chapter, we will focus on the indispensable role of the ECS for the regulation of food digestion, nutrient transformation and energy expenditure due to the interactions between eCBs and signaling cascades in the gastrointestinal (GI) tract, liver, pancreas, fat depots and endocrine glands.

Basically, all compounds of the ECS described before are also present in the body's periphery. Both CB1 and CB2 show strong expression in peripheral tissues. For example, CB1 is robustly detectable in liver hepatocytes, adipocytes of white fat depots, as well as in different cell types of the GI tract, pancreas and skeletal muscles. In contrast, CB2 is predominantly expressed in immune and blood cells, where eCBs mediate immunomodulatory actions. Besides the well-established contribution of the ECS in regulation of energy metabolism in the body's periphery under physiological conditions, the overall involvement of eCBs in modulation of inflammatory events [228,229] also accounts for pathophysiological processes in metabolic diseases, such DIO or type 2 diabetes [230]. The first evidence that eCBs are important for body weight regulation via peripheral CB1 activation came from a study by Cota et al. in 2003 [231]. The lean phenotype of $CB1^{-/-}$ mice under normal chow feeding and the resistance against DIO, accompanied by maintenance of insulin sensitivity after high fat feeding, suggested that eCB signaling in DIO not only leads to hypothalamic alterations, but also to peripheral impairments in the liver, pancreas and adipocyte tissue [231]. In connection to these findings, induction of lipogenesis in adipocytes by peripheral CB1 activation was described [231] and hepatic CB1 was shown to be responsible for development of diet-induced steatosis, dyslipidemia, insulin- and leptin resistance [232–234]. In this regard, it was found that the main degrading enzymes for eCBs such as AEA and 2-AG show very high expression levels in the adipose tissue and the liver [235,236]. Moreover, the levels of eCBs in these peripheral organs depend on the nutrition state. For example, induction of DIO alters the activity of the enzymes for the synthesis and degradation of AEA and 2-AG [23,230,237–240].

These observations were accompanied by several studies in mice and rats showing that chronic treatment with rimonabant reduces body weight, independent of central regulation of food intake [241–244]. Moreover, detrimental parameters in the course of DIO, such as increased levels of blood glucose and triglycerols, as well as hyperinsulinemia and -leptinemia were reversed after treatment with CB1 inverse agonists [23,233]. Due to these findings, one major approach in obesity research is to focus on selective peripheral inverse agonists and neutral antagonists to treat obesity, in order to avoid central psychotropic side effects. This aspect will be outlined in the final chapter of this review. An overview of the peripheral effects of the ECS in DIO is shown in Figure 3.

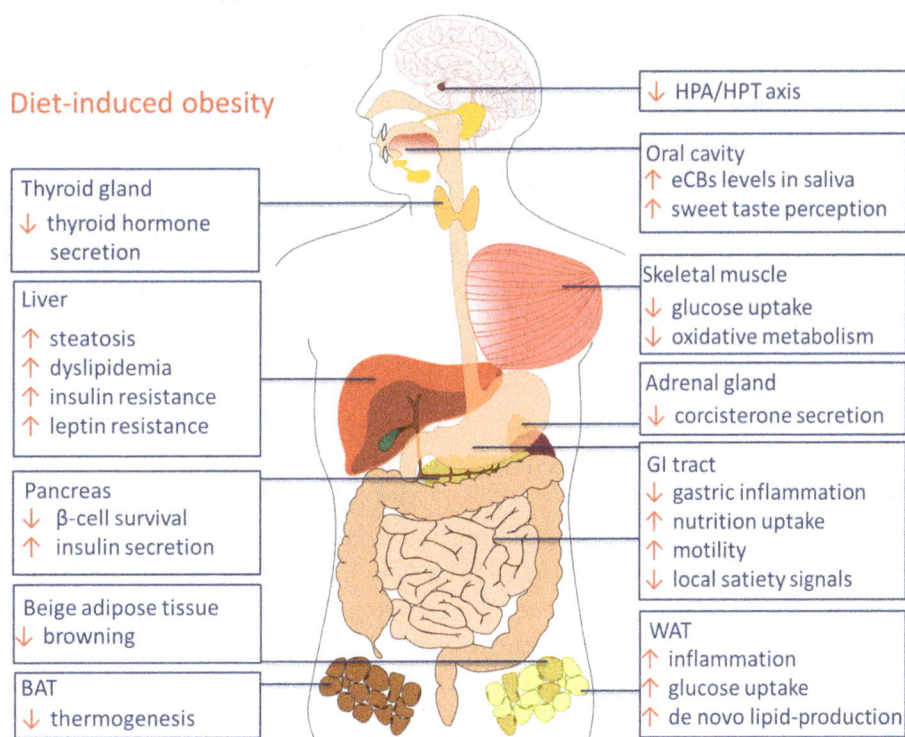

Figure 3. Peripheral effects of the ECS in diet-induced obesity. Abbreviations: BAT brown adipose tissue, HPA hypothalamic pituitary adrenal axis, HPT hypothalamic pituitary thyroid axis, GI gastrointestinal, WAT white adipose tissue.

In the upcoming sections, we will follow cannabinoid effects throughout the sequence of food intake and digestion, starting at the very first stage in the mouth, where the eCBs affect taste sensation [245–248] and influence secretion of saliva by modulation of the vegetative innervation of the salivary glands [249]. We will then follow the way of the ingested nutrients through the GI tract, and describe the role of the eCBs in the communication between the GI tract, liver, pancreas, skeletal muscles, fat depots and the brain. Finally, we will also address the role of the ECS in the neuroendocrine axes between hypothalamus, pituitary, adrenal and thyroid glands.

3.2. The ECS in The Oral Cavity: Taste Sensation and Saliva Production

Increased levels of eCBs were observed in the saliva of obese, insulin resistant individuals during fasting compared to fasting normal weight individuals [249]. Therefore, salivary eCBs might serve as biomarkers for obesity. Another group confirmed these findings and found that besides the increased levels of eCBs in the saliva of obese subjects, also the levels of uric acid and C-reactive protein were upregulated [250].

The content and composition of dietary fat plays a crucial role for the perception of taste. Fat as a primary taste quality is detected by several receptors in the oral cavity. An innate attraction to fat-rich nutrition might be due to the oro-sensory detection of dietary lipids leading to dopamine outflow in the ventral striatum. In this region of the midbrain, sensory stimuli are processed and "wanting" and "liking" (see Section 2) lead to a stimulation of increased intake of fat [251].

Experimentally, rodents showed a strong preference for diets rich in fat and containing linoleic acid. This preference is lost in knockout-mice lacking the CD36 fat receptor, which is expressed for example in taste buds [246,247]. Binding of a long-chain fatty acid at the CD36-receptor causes a signaling cascade that induces the release of neuromediators and gastrointestinal hormones [252]. The sensory information is conveyed to the NTS via the gustatory nerves and transmitted through a reflex loop via the vagus nerve to the peripheral axis where an early secretion of digestive enzymes and hormones [253,254] takes places in order to prepare the body for incoming lipids. Another study showed that the free acid component of dietary fat advanced the accumulation of eCBs in the proximal small intestine. Oleic acid and linoleic acid are the respective components of the diet, which triggered this effect [251]. The authors suggested that the fat-sensing effect mediated by CD36 and lingual lipase activity are involved in the initiation of eCB signaling in the jejunum, but this interaction must be investigated in more detail in further studies [251].

"The fatter the food, the more palatable" holds true for humans as well, and therefore, dietary fat influences our eating habits. Therefore, it is not surprising that in the "western diet" the percentage of linoleic acid raised from 1% to 8% of total energy intake in the last century, strongly contributing to the raise in obesity due to ingestion of energy dense foods [255]. Most strikingly, the content of our diet, especially the percentage of fat, and the kind of fat can influence the levels of eCBs in brain, small intestine and liver [256].

Sweet taste perception is also influenced by eCBs [245,257]. The study of Yoshida et al. showed a significantly increased activity of the chorda tympani, which innervates the anterior tongue, triggered by sweet compounds after i.p. injection of 2-AG and AEA [245]. This effect was observed 10–30 min after injection in wild type mice and was diminished to control levels 60–120 min after injection. Moreover, this effect was absent in CB1$^{-/-}$ mice [245]. This increase was only observed in response to sweet compounds, as 2-AG showed no effect on the nerve response to the other tastes qualities salty, bitter, sour or umami [245]. Moreover, many single nucleotide polymorphisms (SNPs) exist at the gene locus of the sweet receptor, leading to a high variability and consequently influence taste perception and personal food preference [174,258].

However, the perception of sweet taste is more complex due to the fact that there are many factors involved in this sensation, because paracrine and endocrine hormones influence the sensibility of the taste receptor and consequently modify the palatability of food and eating behavior. The different players in this modulation process are leptin, CCK, NPY, oxytocin, insulin, ghrelin and galanin [259]. Yoshida et al. suggest an interaction between leptin and the ECS in regard to sweet taste sensitivity, which may influence eating behavior and energy homeostasis via central and peripheral mechanisms [174,248,260]. In leptin receptor-defective (*db/db*) mice, the nerve response to sweet sensation is decreased when blocking CB1 [248]. To sum up, the ECS is of significant relevance in the oral cavity by modulation of taste sensation of sugar and fat. Finally, saliva production itself is influenced by the ECS [261,262].

3.3. The ECS in the GI Tract

All key players of the ECS are present in the stomach and intestine, allowing for the local de-novo synthesis of AEA, 2-AG and OEA. These eCBs operate in an auto-, para- and endocrine fashion. When activated by eCBs, CB1 in the GI tract induces GI motility, reduces the secretion of acid and fluid and accelerates mesenteric vasodilation [263]. Furthermore, the activated ECS mediates a reducing effect on gastric damage and intestinal inflammation [264,265]. These essential anti-inflammatory aspects of the ECS optimize the uptake of the nutrients in the GI tract. Besides CB1 and CB2, other eCB receptors exist in the GI tract, namely TRPV1 [266], the PPAR class [267], as well as GPR119 [268] and GPR55 [269]. For example, OEA, an eCB-like compound generated on demand from enterocytes, is an agonist at PPARα [270], TRPV1 channels [271] and the orphan GPCRs GPR55 and GPR119 [272], but not to CB1 and CB2 [273]. The production of OEA is induced by food intake [274] and repressed by food deprivation [275]. OEA mediates satiety by PPARα activation [276], decreases food intake and consecutively body weight gain [277]. PPARα is a nuclear receptor influencing various aspects of lipid metabolism [270]. Fu et al. suggest that satiety, induced by PPARα activation, is mediated by the reduction of nitric oxide (NO) through transcriptional downregulation of the intestinal nitric oxide synthase [270,278]. OEA also triggers the release of the anorexigenic hormone GLP-1 by binding to GPR119 of enteroendocrine L-cells [279,280].

The stomach and small intestine send humoral signals to the brain to control of energy balance, and different studies suggest that the ECS is involved in these pathways [281]. In this, the peripheral ECS in the GI tract strongly affects the secretion of classical humoral factors like ghrelin, CCK and GLP-1 [282]. The central dopamine deficiency caused by a HFD is probably linked by intestinal OEA levels [283]. Supplementation of OEA under HFD leads to restoration of dopamine levels accompanied by the intake of less palatable food with reduced fat content [283], illustrating the potential of gut-derived eCB to affect central reward circuit systems.

Conversely, the type of food which we consume, can, for its constitution of different components, influence the ECS. The study of Monteleone et al. demonstrated an increase of the 2-AG and ghrelin plasma levels of healthy volunteers when they are allowed to consume their favorite food which was mostly high in fat and sugar [284]. In experiments with rodents that had access to a diet rich in fat and sucrose, both features of the "Western diet", heightened levels of AEA and 2-AG in plasma and additionally in the jejunum were observed, accompanied with a greater portion intake and weight gain [285]. Additionally, our high-fat western diet has a high ratio of n-6/n-3 PUFAs, today the ratio is 20:1 or even higher in comparison to evolution in which the ratio was 1:1 [255]. It is thus assumed that this drastic increase goes along with the development of obesity. The ratio of n-6/n-3 PUFAs has an impact on the AEA [286,287] and 2-AG levels [288]. In an interventional study by Berge et al., obese men were supplemented with krill powder, which contains the n-3 PUFAs docosahexaenoic and eicosapentaenoic acids. This supplementation resulted in a decrease of AEA and triglyceride levels in plasma and to a reduction of ectopic fat accumulation [286]. Accordingly, animal studies showed that a diet rich in n-6 PUFA and poor in n-3 PUFA increases brain levels of AEA [287] and of 2-AG [288]. Similarly to other phospholipid-derived compounds [289,290], the underlying mechanism might be an altered availability of substrates for eCB synthesizing enzymes.

Another route through which the ECS interacts in the regulation of food intake are vagal afferents, which link the GI tract to the medulla and brainstem nuclei related to satiety to supervise the process of food digestion. After food intake, the duodenum secretes CCK, which then binds to CCK receptors located at afferent terminals of the vagus nerve [108]. The incoming signal is then transferred to the hypothalamus to reduce food intake. It was shown that upon CB1 activation, the release of CCK in the duodenum is inhibited, presumably involving enteroendocrine L-cells expressing gene transcripts for CB1 [291].

Besides these effects, eCBs also seem to interact with intestinal microbiota. The first indication that there exists a communication between the ECS and the gut microbiota was reported in 2007 [292]. The presence of the bacterial strain *Lactobacillus acidophilus* induces the expression of cannabinoid receptors and MOR in intestinal cells lowering abdominal pain in rats. Also, THC consumption affects the gut microbiome [293]—for further discussion, see the Section 4 of this review.

Together, all these findings represent an effect of diet on the ECS in the intestinal tract suggesting an association between western-style diet and the involvement of eCB signaling in hyperphagia [251,294].

3.4. Liver

Under physiological conditions, the hepatic ECS is assumed to be idle. If it reaches a pathophysiological state, as in the course of DIO, the ECS will be activated [23]. Such a pathophysiological state is for example hepatic steatosis, induced by HFD or excessive alcohol consumption. Hepatic steatosis is linked to an upregulation of liver CB1, triggered by retinoic acid, which is produced by hepatic stellate cells [295]. When activated CB1 was chronically blocked with an inverse agonist like rimonabant, the process of steatosis could be reversed [233,296].

$CB1^{-/-}$ mice show a resistance to the development DIO and to the development of the accompanying hepatic steatosis. HFD induces lipogenesis in the hepatocytes [232]. Activation of hepatic CB1 increases lipogenesis and concomitantly inhibits fatty acid oxidation, the catabolic process of lipid metabolism [233,234]. The ECS-promoted accumulation of fat in the liver depends on ATP. There is a negative correlation between the ATP content of the liver and the insulin resistance of hepatocytes and CB1 in the liver serves as an important modulator of hepatic energy status [295]. Another study showed a decreased FAAH activity in hepatic steatosis, presumably causing a rise in eCBs, especially in AEA. Monounsaturated fatty acids, which are produced by the enzyme stearoyl CoA desaturase-1, lead to a depression of FAAH activity. Stearoyl CoA desaturase-1 is an enzyme in the liver whose expression is induced upon HFD [297]. Other enzymes and proteins involved in fatty acid synthesis and consecutively the development of hepatic steatosis are upregulated by eCB-driven activation of hepatic CB1: sterol regulatory element binding transcription factor 1, fatty acid synthase and acetyl coenzyme-A carboxylase-1 [232].

A physiological key feature of the liver is the production of bile acids, which are required for absorption of ingested fats. It was shown that hepatic CB1 contributes to alcohol-induced shifts in the expression of bile acid metabolizing enzymes, involving ER-bound transcription factor Crebh (cAMP-responsive element binding protein, hepatocyte specific) as downstream CB1 effector [298]. Interestingly, the activity of NAPE-PLD, one of the key enzymes involved in biosynthesis of *N*-acetylethanolamines such as AEA, OEA and PEA, is controlled by bile acids [299,300]. Here, the binding of bile acids enhances dimer assembly of NAPE-PLD, which is required for catalytic activity. Since the various products of NAPE-PLD carry different effects on feeding and energy metabolism, for example, AEA can be orexigenic, while OEA serves as an important satiety signal, it would be interesting to see whether there exists a physiological interrelation between the ECS and bile acid composition and under which circumstances this putative interaction accounts for body weight control in healthy normal weight and obese people.

3.5. Pancreas

The pancreas secretes digestive enzymes into the duodenum. In cultured lobules and acini of guinea pig and rat pancreas, both CB1 and CB2 involvement in exocrine secretion was observed [301]. In an experimental model of acute pancreatitis, it was shown that CB2 signaling led to reduction in inflammation via MAPK signaling, finally affecting cytokine release [302]. Thus, it would be interesting to test for the functional contribution of the ECS in the exocrine part of the pancreas under normal and HFD.

Compared to the exocrine pancreas, the ECS is well known for its contribution to blood glucose control, mostly by direct interference with endocrine cell types of the pancreatic Langerhans islets [230,303]. Different studies revealed an impact of ECS on the control of β-cell function [304,305]. However, differing opinions still exist regarding which cell type in the Langerhans islets expresses which type of cannabinoid receptor. While there are studies showing that CB1 mRNA and protein are expressed in α-cells and CB2 is expressed in both α- and β-cells [239,306,307], most studies agree on the presence of eCBs and expression of CB1 in β-cells and an increase of insulin release leading to activated CB1 receptors [239,308,309].

Pancreatic β-cells influence themselves via an autocrine anti-apoptotic feedback loop: insulin binds to the insulin receptor and positively regulates the survival of β-cells. Kim et al. performed in vitro studies demonstrating that the phosphorylation of the pro-apoptotic protein B-cell lymphoma 2 (Bcl-2)-antagonist of cell death is reduced, leading to the inhibition of the insulin receptor kinase activity. The hypothesized underlying mechanism is the formation of a heteromeric complex between CB1 and the insulin receptor [310]. Also, TRPV1 was found in both α- and β-cells of mouse pancreatic islets. It was supposed that this receptor is involved in the development of the pancreas as its genetic knockout or pharmacological blockade results in an increased ratio of β- to α-cells, which finally causes an increased islet size [311].

3.6. The Emerging Role of the Hepatic and Pancreatic ECS in Metabolic Disorders

Obesity-associated inflammation in liver, pancreas and white adipose tissue (WAT), accompanied by insulin resistance and hepatic steatosis, was potentiated by pharmacological CB2 receptor activation and diminished in globally CB2-deficient mice. This suggests a selective CB2 antagonism in DIO as a potential pharmacological strategy to exert metabolic benefits [228]. However, and in contrast to that, numerous data also point toward a beneficial role of CB2 activation in metabolic control in lean as well as in obese and diabetic rodent models [230]. For instance, it was demonstrated that CB2 activation improved glucose tolerance in lean rats, supporting that CB2 is relevant for physiological control of glucose metabolism [312]. In the same study, both CB1 and CB2 were observed in rat pancreatic β- and non-β-cells, illustrating putative interactions between CB1 and CB2 in glucose homeostasis [312]. While CB1 activation contributes to body weight gain and onset of metabolic syndrome, CB2 signaling is thought to mediate contrariwise beneficial effects, aiming at anti-inflammation and reversal of metabolic syndrome [313]. Indeed, CB2 was described to increase protective effects in a model of diabetic nephropathy [229]. Altogether, once the mechanisms underlying the inflammation in metabolic organs are understood, the impaired fat metabolism in the adipose tissue could be overcome by the development of pharmaceuticals, which can treat the inflammation and repress it to a baseline level.

3.7. Skeletal Muscle

Following digestion and uptake, nutrients are utilized by muscle cells, which, as an important metabolic entity, make use of eCB signaling [314–319]. Activation of the ECS decreases insulin-stimulated glucose uptake and oxidative metabolism in human skeletal muscle [314,315]. The decrease in oxidative metabolism is caused by inhibition of substrate oxidation and inhibition of mitochondrial biogenesis, similarly to results obtained in liver and adipose tissue [320]. The negative correlation between the activated ECS and insulin is triggered by an impact of CB1 on the PI 3-kinase/PKB and on the Raf-MEK1/2-ERK1/2 pathways [319]. Activation of the TRPV1 channels in the skeletal muscle stimulates mitochondrial biogenesis and hypertrophy [321,322]. However, there is no evidence that eCBs are involved in these TRPV1-mediated processes in the skeletal muscle.

A study by Crespillo et al. demonstrated that the activity of the skeletal muscle ECS depends on the consumed diet. Treatment with an inverse CB1 agonist restores HFD-induced alterations in skeletal muscle cells [316], highlighting the importance of the ECS in muscle cells for metabolic health and body weight control.

3.8. Adipose Tissue

Besides WAT, the ECS is also present in brown adipose tissue (BAT), where it contributes to the thermogenic function of fat cells and regulates body weight by directly affecting energy expenditure [237]. In WAT, eCBs and leptin are negatively correlated [323]. In times the ECS is stimulated in adipose tissue, cascades for energy storage are activated, leading to increased de novo production of lipids and glucose uptake. As a consequence, the expression of the hormone adiponectin, a cytokine with anti-inflammatory features, is downregulated, which has an impact on the insulin sensitivity at distant tissues like the skeletal muscle and the adipose tissue itself, and, on top of that, causes a local inflammatory process in the adipose tissue [324,325].

Obesity and its comorbidities are often accompanied by inflammation of the adipose tissue, which is suggested to accelerate the onset of metabolic syndrome [326]. Therefore, many groups aim at the identification of new pharmaceutical targets to influence this adipose tissue inflammation [327,328]. While specific targets are upregulated in the course of DIO-associated inflammation of WAT, such as the transcription factor E2F1 [329], it is overall accepted that inflammation in metabolically active organs links the development of insulin resistance and liver diseases to pathways of the immune system [330,331]. In DIO, the treatment with Rimonabant reverses the downregulation of adiponectin, causing anti-inflammatory effects [324]. Analysis of human subcutaneous adipose tissue of obese participants, when compared to lean controls, revealed a decrease in FAAH activity, increased eCB levels but a decreased expression level of the CB1 receptor [238]. The authors suggest that CB1 may be regulated by a negative feedback loop and that its downregulation is a secondary effect of the increased eCB levels. In this regard, the same study showed an upregulation of CB1 and FAAH in mature human adipocytes in contrast to pre-adipocytes, highlighting the physiological relevance of the ECS in mature human adipocytes [238]. As previously mentioned, CB1 activation results in adipogenesis and lipogenesis, which leads to an impaired mitochondrial function in DIO [231,332,333]. Upon CB1 activation, there is a downregulation of PPARγ coactivator 1a (Ppargc1a), triggering a decrease of mitochondrial mass and function in WAT. In contrast, a blockade of CB1 the expression of Ppargc1a is increased leading to an elevated mitochondrial biogenesis [320,333].

Activated CB1 favors WAT and inhibits thermogenesis in BAT and beige adipose tissue [334]. The effect on BAT is presumably mediated by CB1-induced inhibition of the sympathetic tone. Accordingly, the pharmacological blockade of CB1 results in differentiation of white into beige adipocytes [335]. Similar to brown adipocytes, beige adipocytes have an enriched number of mitochondria and a higher activity of the enzyme AMPK and uncoupling protein 1 (UCP1). In addition to their common task in thermogenesis, beige and brown adipocytes show many distinguished characteristics, as beige adipocytes are derived from another embryonic precursor cell [336]. Within subcutaneous WAT, clusters of beige adipocytes, can develop due to different stimuli [337].

Normally, the BAT protects our body against cold environments using high-caloric nutrients for the required energy [338]. A cold environment leads to noradrenaline release from sympathetic neurons which activates lipolysis in BAT and WAT through activation of β3-adrenoceptors [237,339]. In BAT, the released fatty acids are transferred to mitochondria for β-oxidation and heat production, depending on the presence of UCP1. UCP1 enables the exothermic production of ATP, resulting in heat production, required for stabilization of the body temperature [339]. In BAT, the ECS represents an autocrine negative feedback mechanism: after cold exposure, β3-adrenoceptor activation increases eCB levels in BAT, which in turn attenuate the sympathetic tone and thereby decrease browning [237]. Overall, specific targeting of adipocyte CB1 represents an interesting interventional approach in order to treat obesity and metabolic syndrome [340], since a recent study clearly indicated that adipocyte CB1 plays a key regulatory role in the crosstalk among adipocytes, immune cells, and the sympathetic nervous system [341].

3.9. The ECS in Neuroendocrine Circuitries Being Relevant for Body Weight Control

The pituitary gland is an important endocrine interface between the hypothalamus and the peripheral endocrine glands. With regard to body weight control, the hypothalamic-pituitary-adrenal (HPA) and hypothalamic-pituitary-thyroid (HPT) axes represent the most significant functional systems and will be addressed here.

3.10. Hypothalamic-Pituitary-Adrenal Axis (HPA) and the ECS

The activation of the HPA axis due to stress is necessary for survival. This axis is regulated by different brain structures and is adjusted by eCB signaling [168,342]. In this regard, there clearly exist site-specific roles of the ECS within the HPA, and divergent functions of AEA and 2-AG in the HPA were observed [343]. While a few studies report on acute activation of the HPA triggered by cannabis consumption or by the use of CB1 agonists, numerous studies revealed that the ECS is involved in stabilization of the HPA axis under physiological, basal conditions, while upon stressful mediators, the ECS is thought to dampen the stress response finally allowing for the recovery of homeostasis [344].

Indeed, CB1 was detected in both the pituitary and adrenal gland [345,346]. The authors showed that CB1 is located in human adrenal cortex cells and that peripheral steroidogenesis and cortisol release are inhibited by synthetic cannabinoids [347]. Further studies demonstrated that inhibition of the ECS results in an increase of circulating corticosterone concentrations in animal models of stress, like forced swimming and tail suspension [348,349]. Injection of CB1 and CB2 inverse agonists into the third ventricle acutely increased serum corticosterone levels in stressed rats [344]. In accordance to these results, previous studies demonstrated that i.p. AM251 treatment raised both, the basal control and stress-induced levels of HPA-axis activity [350–352]. In line with this, elevation of eCBs, as induced by treatment with FAAH inhibitor, decreased the stress-induced corticosterone serum levels [344]. However, another study showed that acute central application of AEA induced secretion of adrenocorticotropin (ACTH) hormone [353]. The release of ACTH is not influenced by the genetic deletion of CB1 or the pharmacological treatment with CB1 blockers [354]. The authors suggested that there is another interaction between the ECS and the HPA axis besides the pituitary. Indeed, the adrenal gland expresses CB1 but not CB2 in the cortex [347]. ACTH, as a main regulator of steroid biosynthesis and -secretion, promotes corticosterone secretion, which is inhibited by AEA. Interestingly, this effect was only partially reversed by CB1 blockers, but completely reversed by the blockade of TRPV1 [344]. These findings link AEA, as a full agonist of TRPV1 channels, with peripheral effects of ACTH on adrenal cortex, since ACTH induces expression of the TRPV1 channel [355].

3.11. The ECS in Hypothalamic-Pituitary-Thyroid (HPT) and Growth Hormone (GH) Axes

Besides important developmental functions such as control of CNS maturation and longitudinal body growth, the thyroid hormones thyroxine (T4) and triiodothyronine (T3) represent indispensible regulators of thermogenesis and energy metabolism and therefore contribute to body weight regulation [356]. In this, hypothalamic thyrotropin-releasing hormone (TRH) stimulates the synthesis and secretion of pituitary thyrotropin (TSH) in the anterior lobe, which finally activates biosynthesis and secretion of T4 and T3 in the thyroid gland. Moreover, a close functional interrelation exists between the HPT and GH axes [357]. In the anterior pituitary, GH release is stimulated by the hypothalamic GHRH (growth hormone-releasing hormone) [358]. The application of CB1 agonists let to decreased GH levels [359]. This effect was presumably mediated indirectly by cannabinoid-dependent inhibition of GHRH release in the hypothalamus [358]. Thyroid hormones and GH interact in regulation of insulin-like growth factor-1 (IGF-1) levels [360]. IGF-1 represents an important metabolic molecule, which induces cell growth and differentiation. In this regard, the ECS is suggested to be involved in growth control by regulation of the GH/IGF-1 axis [361].

Administration of AEA led to an acute decrease in TSH and T4, but not T3 levels in rat serum, while application of CB1 inverse agonists acutely raised TSH levels [362]. These findings are overall in line with previous reports showing that THC reduces serum TSH, T4 and T3 [363], while the synthetic CB1/CB2 agonist WIN 55212-2 reduced T4 and T3, but did not alter TSH levels [364]. In this regard, central CB1 in the hypothalamus are thought to mediate the acute effects of cannabinoids on the HPT axis. Basically, glutamatergic synapses that contain CB1 and contact with TRH neurons in the PVN were identified [365]. Accordingly, studies showed that THC application reduced TRH amounts [366], and eCBs directly affected activity of TRH positive parvocellular neurons in the PVN, potentially by eCBs driven DSE at glutamatergic input synapses [367]. Thus, a general negative modulation of the HPT axis by the ECS is postulated. Besides these central effects, eCBs might also be able to directly modulate TSH and T4/T3 secretion since CB1 was detected in pituitary and thyroid gland as well [368].

4. Therapeutic Targeting of the ECS in Body Weight Regulation—Clinical Implications and Pharmacological Perspectives

4.1. The Medical Potential of the ECS in Treatment of Pathological Weight Loss

Historically, both, the recreational consumption of marihuana and the controlled administration of THC promoted appetite and resulted in increased food intake in sated humans [369]. However, a hyperphagic response to THC was not observed in all human individuals [370]. Specifically, THC consumption led to favored intake of caloric dense palatable foods, accompanied with moderate weight gain upon chronic application within a few weeks [371,372]. It was also observed in these studies that by smoking marihuana, the orexigenic effect of THC was more pronounced at lower when compared to higher doses, assuming a biphasic feeding response upon THC treatment [369]. In mice, when cannabinoids were applied in a sub-psychotropic dose range, lower doses of e.g., THC increased while higher (still sub-psychotropic) doses decreased feeding [369,373]. Besides stimulation of food intake, CB1-driven decrease of energy expenditure may also account for treatment of body weight loss. Indeed, CB1 activation at postganglionic sympathetic neurons induced sympatholytic effects finally resulting in reduced energy expenditure [227]. Together, pharmacological activation of CB1 induces appetite, promotes food consumption and reduces energy expenditure and thus might be helpful for patients suffering from chronic loss of appetite and severe reduction in body weight.

Thus, numerous indications exist that pharmacological promotion of CB1 signaling will potentially result in body weight regain in patients suffering from anorexia. Anorectic patients suffering from psychiatric disorders such as anorexia nervosa or bulimia, or patients affected by the cancer anorexia-cachexia syndrome could potentially benefit from CB1-activation [9]. Unfortunately, it is still controversially discussed whether treating anorexia with CB1 agonists represents a promising therapeutic option or not. Many clinicians are worried about the acute and chronic psychotropic effects of CB1 agonists, and the state of scientific knowledge on use of cannabinoids in the clinics in order to treat anorexia is still enigmatic [374,375]. While the overall possibility of decreasing body weight by pharmacological blockade of CB1 signaling is evident, a fully established and well-accepted pharmacotherapy which increases food intake and results in body weight gain by promoting CB1 signaling is still lacking.

One reason might be the fact that the orexigenic effect of CB1 agonists strongly depend on the individual's metabolic state, since the orexigenic effect was most pronounced in sated persons when compared to fasted individuals [370]. As reviewed above, this orexigenic effect of cannabinoids is primarily associated with central CB1 signaling leading to increased food seeking, amplified sensory detection of food, consumption of caloric dense palatable food and downregulation of energy expenditure. Notably, chronic consumption of marihuana, e.g., for recreational purposes, does not necessarily lead to development of severe obesity or metabolic syndrome, potentially due to pharmacological habituation. Another assumption in this regard was that chronic consumption of THC might lead to shifts in the gut microbiome upon prolonged treatment, which finally also may account for limitations in cannabinoid-driven weight gain [293].

In the group of patients suffering from the cancer anorexia-cachexia syndrome, tumor by-products and/or host cytokine release combined with metabolic abnormalities might lead to an imbalanced ECS in both, central and peripheral circuitries [376,377]. While THC safely and effectively induced caloric intake, mood and sleep in anorectic HIV patients [378,379], orexigenic effects of THC were not detected in a phase III study on patients with cancer anorexia-cachexia [380]. This still equivocal set of clinical studies might be due to the lack of resilient data obtained in phase I/II studies carefully eliciting pharmacokinetic, dose-concentration and concentration-response data in cancer patients suffering from anorexia [381]. Principally, it is suggested that a chronically underactive ECS exists under anorectic conditions [186,377]. In patients suffering from anorexia or bulimia nervosa, an upregulation of CB1 was observed in cortical and subcortical areas of the brain [186]. It is supposed that under anorectic conditions, eCB-driven pathways contribute to abnormal hedonic input into brain areas managing sensory, interoceptive and motivational signals. Major differences for CB1 density in anorexia and bulimia nervosa patients were observed in the insular cortex, an area that not only codes for sensory detection of taste, flavor and oral texture of food, but also for rewarding properties of food [382,383]. Alongside altered CB1 density was detected in frontal and temporal areas of the cortex, regions well known for their interoceptive abilities required for integration of a variety of different sensations [384]. However, the main question remaining open here still is whether the variations observed for CB1 in anorexia reflect a cause or consequence of the disease. Nevertheless, only a few clinical trials have already taken place which have shown that the treatment with dronabinol, a dual CB1/CB2 agonist, leads to a little but significant weight gain in anorexia rodent models and humans with anorexia nervosa, potentially due to a reduction in the urge to be physically active [376,377]. In line with these findings, dronabinol reduced activity and attenuated weight loss in a rat model for activity-based anorexia [375]. Many cancer patients are suffering from nausea and vomiting in the course or after chemotherapy. In this, CB1 agonists displayed a well-tolerated anti-emetic drug, reducing nausea and vomiting, however, besides these acute beneficial effects, only some short-term improvement in appetite was detected, with no or some long-term improvements in body weight were documented in these patients [376].

In conclusion, much more research is needed to clarify the pathological role of the ECS in anorexia. Moreover, the pharmacokinetics of selective CB1 and CB2 agonists or of dual CB1/CB2 agonists have to be tested more systematically in clinical trials aiming at therapy of anorexia [381]. Alongside, another pharmacological approach in order to induce CB1/CB2 signaling could be based on inhibitors blocking specific enzymes responsible for degradation of eCBs [385]. In mouse models for anxiety or pain, pharmacological or genetic blockade of eCB degrading enzymes such as FAAH or MAGL led to increased levels of AEA and 2-AG, respectively, which finally resulted in analgesic and anxiolytic effects [386–388]. However, the pain-reducing effects observed in mouse and rat models have not yet been successfully transferred into humans [389]. In order to treat depression (anxiety)-like behaviors, in which FAAH blockade was described as a successful therapeutic option in mouse models [390], it recently occurred that participants in a phase 1 study of a compound known as BIA 10-2474, a presumed selective FAAH inhibitor, were hospitalized with severe neurological symptoms, presumably due to off-target proteins [391]. Overall, this tragedy finally indicates that ongoing further research on the ECS is still required and that much more critical considerations are needed for the performance of clinical trials that are based on interspecies translational approaches when regarding the ECS. Fortunately, a collaborative effort between multiple academic and industry laboratories revealed that HU910, HU308 and JWH133 represent the most selective CB2 agonists and thus being the most recommendable candidates to test for CB2 selective effects in pathophysiology of anorexia [392]. Basically, neuroinflammatory alterations are associated with neuropsychiatric disorders and polymorphisms in the CB2 gene have been reported not only in depression and schizophrenia but also in eating disorders [393]. Thus, besides CB1, the selective targeting of CB2 might be also relevant for the pharmacological treatment of eating disorders. Indeed, a polymorphism of the CB2 gene could be associated with anorexia nervosa and bulimia [394]. In mouse models, CB2 blockade by AM630 decreased food intake under non-fasting conditions while the same drug (AM630), when administered following food deprivation, increased food intake [395,396]. Thus, while antagonism of the CB1 receptor induces anorexia irrespective of fed or fasted states, the effects of CB2 receptor agonists on food intake appear to depend on the current metabolic state. This finally indicates that both CB1 and CB2 affect food intake in rodents, although the underlying mechanisms remain to be determined [393].

4.2. The Medical Potential of the ECS in Treatment of Overeating and Obesity

As highlighted above, chronic activation of the ECS is strongly linked with obesity and its co-morbidities. For example; plasma eCBs are not only elevated in obese patients but also in patients with type-2 diabetes [397]. In this disease the dietary intake of fatty acids plays an important role in determining tissue eCB levels [287,288]. Thus, CB1 blockade was thought to represent a useful tool for the treatment of obesity. In 2006 the first generation of CB1 inverse agonists represented by rimonabant and other "nabant" drugs was discovered in Europe [398]. Rimonabant, marketed as Acomplia (in Europe) and trademarked as Zimulti (USPTO, Washington, DC, USA) was the first clinical approved CB1-dependent drug. Its main properties represent restoring insulin sensitivity in DIO, normalizing fat cell size, preventing visceral fat accumulation and decreasing subcutaneous fat [399–401]. Acomplia also improved cardiovascular risk factors such as low adiponectin, high HDL and high triglyceride levels [402]. The underlying mechanisms, however, were largely unknown. In this regard, the first attention has focused on adiponectin [403]. Plasma adiponectin as well as the adiponectin gene expression in visceral fat was increased during rimonabant treatment. Also expression of adiponectin receptor 1 and 2 was enhanced; hence it is proposed that the increase of the adiponectin gene expression elevated the adiponectin delivery into the liver [404]. Furthermore, rimonabant plays a liver-protecting role in obesity by reducing inflammatory reactions and increasing fat oxidation, resulting in a decreased accumulation of lipids in the liver [405]. Additional studies showed that peripheral but not central injection of rimonabant elicited decreased triglycerides in WAT, illustrating that fat reduction induced by rimonabant is independent on its central effects on food intake [406]. In this, rimonabant further induced activation of the sympathetic nervous system highlighting that bidirectional circuits between the periphery and the brain are involved in CB1-dependent regulation of feeding [407]. Unfortunately, rimonabant not just reduced body weight independently of reduction in food intake but also resulted in high levels of psychiatric side effects [408]. Due to this devastating effect, Acomplia was pulled from markets in Europe, never received a FDA approval in the US and research focus has shifted to sole peripheral CB1 inverse agonists to eliminate the CNS side effects. Today, rimonabant is thus considered as an unacceptable treatment of obesity and its co-morbidities [398], and one of the most relevant pitfalls for research associated with the relevance of body weight control was the clinical failure of rimonabant [409].

4.3. Omitting Central CB1—Is It Sufficient to Medicate Morbid Body Weight Solely by Selective Targeting of Peripheral CB1?

Several other first generation "nabant" like inverse agonists have failed phase 2 or 3 clinical trials due to the aforementioned undesirable CNS effects described for rimonabant [244]. Thus, aiming at avoidance of undesired psychotropic side effects, blood-brain-barrier impermeable CB1 inverse agonists, such as JD5037 or TM38837 and global neutral antagonists that are brain penetrant, such as AM4113 were developed as second generation CB1-dependent pharmaceuticals, and so far have been successfully tested in rodent models of obesity and metabolic syndrome [403]. Since several studies suggested that the central side effects of Rimonabant were due to its structure as an inverse agonist, brain penetrant neutral CB1 antagonists might avoid these detrimental CNS effects. Indeed, this assumption holds true for the anti-obesity effects of AM4113, a drug, which although reaching the brain did not show typical central side effects as induced by "nabant" like inverse agonists before [410]. Moreover, the use of the neutral antagonists at putative lower doses will account for less central side effects as well [403]. Overall, second generation CB1 blocker showed the same beneficial metabolic effects when compared to rimonabant, but instead did not show detrimental central side effects in animal models. Administration of global or peripheral neutral antagonists, as well as of peripherally restricted inverse agonists showed great beneficial potential for the treatment of obesity and metabolic disease. Here the peripherally restricted CB1 inverse agonist JD5037 and the neutral antagonist AM6545 have to be mentioned. Both of them reduced obesity, reversed leptin resistance and improved hepatic steatosis, dyslipidemia and insulin resistance [403,411]. Moreover, peripheral blockade of CB1 led to the recovery of central leptin sensitivity [110,412]. There are still ongoing studies designing and testing for other new generation CB1 blockers, such as "Compound 2p" and "Compound 10q" which peripherally target the ECS, and look very promising as an alternative treatment of metabolic diseases [403]. In this regard, putative milestones for targeted drug discovery presumably will be the discovery and description of the crystal structure of human CB1, as revealed in complex with AM6538 and taranabant as stabilizing antagonists, respectively [413,414]. Moreover, crystal structure of agonist-bound human CB1 showed important conformational changes in the overall structure in relation to the aforementioned antagonist-bound state [415]. Altogether, the recent discovery of the CB1 crystal structure should lead to the design of chemically diverse ligands with distinct pharmacological properties [415].

As discussed before for anorexia, pharmacological targeting of CB2 might also have therapeutic implications to treat overeating and obesity. While CB1 is increased in obese rodents, CB2 is decreased in peripheral tissues, arguing that CB2 possibly opposes the pro-obesity effects of CB1 signaling [416]. Indeed, CB2 is present in metabolically active tissues, such as liver, pancreatic islets, adipose tissue and skeletal muscle [417]. Besides its localization, the inhibition and/or deletion of CB2 led to an increased food intake in non-obese rodents as well as increased body weight and adipose tissue hypertrophy [417]. Thus, recent studies discuss the possibility of CB2 stimulation in order to reduce food intake and body weight gain without having an impact on mood [416,417]. Chronic treatment of DIO mice with the CB2 agonist JWH015 reduced food intake and fat mass of retroperitoneal and inguinal WAT as well as adipocyte cell size [417]. In more detail, body weight loss was accompanied by increased markers of lipolysis, elevated expression of the anti-inflammatory cytokine IL-10 and by reduction of the pro-inflammatory marker TNF-alpha [417]. Thus it appears that by silencing the activated immune system, which has a key role in worsening obesity and metabolic diseases, CB2 signaling might obtain anti-obesity effect. This assumption is further supported by the findings that age-associated obesity was pronounced in CB2-deficient mice fed a normal laboratory chow [416].

4.4. Positive and Negative Allosteric CB1 Ligands: New Therapeutic Avenues for Treating Eating Disorders and Restoration of Morbid Body Weight?

In silico mapping of allosteric binding sites at human CB1 supports the idea that body weight regulating effects being transduced by orthosteric CB1 ligands could potentially be affected by allosteric ligands [418]. Numerous synthetic and natural allosteric CB1 modulators with negative or positive effects on orthosteric ligand (cannabinoid) binding efficacy were described so far in vitro [419]. Several endogenous small molecules such as lipoxin A4, pregnenolone and PEPCAN-12 were identified as intrinsic allosteric CB1 ligands [419,420]. Being part of the Hpa (a-hemoglobin-derived peptide hemopressin: PVNFKLSH) neuropeptide family, PEPCAN (peptide endocannabinoid)-12, also known as RVD-hemopressin, was first described in 2012 as a negative allosteric modulator of CB1 [421]. Interestingly PEPCAN-12 is a non-lipid molecule being released from noradrenergic neurons in the CNS, and was shown to decrease food intake in obese mice [420,422]. Another structurally similar peptide called hemopressin is also considered as an allosteric CB1 inhibitor. When compared to CB1 inverse agonists, hemopressin also shows a dose-dependent hypotensive effect in mice [423,424]. It further decreased food intake in normal and obese rodents without any adverse side effects [424]. However, many allosteric ligands so far being described and tested in vitro have not yet shown a sustained effect on CB1 signaling in vivo [425]. Thus, research still has to put a lot of effort into the successful establishment of allosteric CB1 ligands as potential future pharmacological tools in the clinics. Before, much more insight into mechanistic properties of allosteric CB1 ligands is required. For example, it was shown that ORG27569, PSNCBAM-1, and PEPCAN-12 decreased eCB-driven DSE in autoptic hippocampal neurons [422]. Using the same experimental setup, positive allosteric modulators of eCB-driven effects in neurons were identified as well [426]. Finally, another natural allosteric CB1 inhibitor is represented by the neurosteroid pregnenolone. It was shown that pregnenolone binds to CB1 without affecting binding of orthosteric agonists. Downstream effects of pregnenolone are thought to be independent of adenylyl cyclase/cAMP-driven pathways, but should occur via inhibition of the MAPK pathway. Chronic administration of pregnenolone does not cause anxiety in DIO mice [422].

In conclusion, research on allosteric mechanisms at CB1 and other target sites for eCBs is of great interest and high relevance in basic research. Here, the overall goal should be the generation of mechanistic insights in order to develop safe and reliable drugs being able to treat morbid body weight regulation in underweight, overweight and obese patients worldwide.

Overall, the knowledge about the involvement of the ECS in body weight control increased significantly in the last years and is still growing. Recent mechanistic insights into eCB-driven pathways participating in body weight control, and the design of novel pharmacological tools might lead to a major breakthrough in the development of cannabinoid medicines for treatment of adverse body weight development.

Author Contributions: M.K. conceptualized, supervised and edited the manuscript. H.H., B.B., L.D. and M.K. wrote the manuscript and designed the figures.

Acknowledgments: This work was supported by the Deutsche Forschungsgemeinschaft CRC obesity mechanisms (1052/A7).

Conflicts of Interest: The authors declare no conflict of interest.

References

1. Gao, Q.; Horvath, T.L. Neurobiology of feeding and energy expenditure. *Annu. Rev. Neurosci.* **2007**, *30*, 367–398. [CrossRef] [PubMed]

2. Adair, L.S.; Fall, C.H.; Osmond, C.; Stein, A.D.; Martorell, R.; Ramirez-Zea, M.; Sachdev, H.S.; Dahly, D.L.; Bas, I.; Norris, S.A.; et al. Associations of linear growth and relative weight gain during early life with adult health and human capital in countries of low and middle income: Findings from five birth cohort studies. *Lancet* **2013**, *382*, 525–534. [CrossRef]

3. Smolen, J.S.; Burmester, G.R.; Combeet, B. NCD Risk Factor Collaboration (NCD-RisC) Worldwide trends in body-mass index, underweight, overweight, and obesity from 1975 to 2016: A pooled analysis of 2416 population-based measurement studies in 128.9 million children, adolescents, and adults. *Lancet* **2017**, *390*, 2627–2642.

4. Galgani, J.; Ravussin, E. Energy metabolism, fuel selection and body weight regulation. *Int. J. Obes. (Lond.)* **2008**, *32* (Suppl. 7), S109–S119. [CrossRef] [PubMed]

5. Koch, M.; Horvath, T.L. Molecular and cellular regulation of hypothalamic melanocortin neurons controlling food intake and energy metabolism. *Mol. Psychiatry* **2014**, *19*, 752–761. [CrossRef] [PubMed]

6. Wells, J.C. The evolution of human adiposity and obesity: Where did it all go wrong? *Dis. Models Mech.* **2012**, *5*, 595–607. [CrossRef] [PubMed]

7. Dietrich, M.O.; Horvath, T.L. Hypothalamic control of energy balance: Insights into the role of synaptic plasticity. *Trends Neurosci.* **2013**, *36*, 65–73. [CrossRef] [PubMed]

8. Speakman, J.R. The evolution of body fatness: Trading off disease and predation risk. *J. Exp. Biol.* **2018**, *221*, jeb167254. [CrossRef] [PubMed]

9. Koch, M. Cannabinoid receptor signaling in central regulation of feeding behavior: A mini-review. *Front. Neurosci.* **2017**, *11*, 293. [CrossRef] [PubMed]

10. Li, H.-L. An archaeological and historical account of cannabis in China. *Econ. Bot.* **1973**, *28*, 437–448. [CrossRef]

11. Fleming, M.P.; Clarke, R.C. Physical evidence for the antiquity of *Cannabis sativa* L. *J. Int. Hemp Assoc.* **1998**, *5*, 80–93.

12. Brand, E.J.; Zhao, Z. Cannabis in Chinese medicine: Are some traditional indications referenced in ancient literature related to cannabinoids? *Front. Pharmacol.* **2017**, *8*, 108. [CrossRef] [PubMed]

13. Mechoulam, R.; Shvo, Y. Hashish—I. The structure of cannabidiol. *Tetrahedron* **1963**, *19*, 2073–2078. [CrossRef]

14. Gaoni, Y.; Mechoulam, R. Isolation, structure, and partial synthesis of an active constituent of hashish. *J. Am. Chem. Soc.* **1964**, *86*, 1646–1647. [CrossRef]

15. Mechoulam, R.; Gaoni, Y. Hashish—IV. The isolation and structure of cannabinolic cannabidiolic and cannabigerolic acids. *Tetrahedron* **1965**, *21*, 1223–1229. [CrossRef]

16. Mechoulam, R.; Hanuš, L.O.; Pertwee, R.; Howlett, A.C. Early phytocannabinoid chemistry to endocannabinoids and beyond. *Nat. Rev. Neurosci.* **2014**, *15*, 757–764. [CrossRef] [PubMed]

17. Mechoulam, R. Conversation with raphael mechoulam. *Addiction* **2007**, *102*, 887–893. [PubMed]

18. Devane, W.A.; Dysarz, F.A., III; Johnson, M.R.; Melvin, L.S.; Howlett, A.C. Determination and characterization of a cannabinoid receptor in rat brain. *Mol. Pharmacol.* **1988**, *34*, 605–613. [PubMed]

19. Munro, S.; Thomas, K.L.; Abu-Shaar, M. Molecular characterization of a peripheral receptor for cannabinoids. *Nature* **1993**, *365*, 61–65. [CrossRef] [PubMed]

20. Galiegue, S.; Mary, S.; Marchand, J.; Dussossoy, D.; Carriere, D.; Carayon, P.; Bouaboula, M.; Shire, D.; Le Fur, G.; Casellas, P. Expression of central and peripheral cannabinoid receptors in human immune tissues and leukocyte subpopulations. *Eur. J. Biochem.* **1995**, *232*, 54–61. [CrossRef] [PubMed]

21. Devane, W.A.; Hanus, L.; Breuer, A.; Pertwee, R.G.; Stevenson, L.A.; Griffin, G.; Gibson, D.; Mandelbaum, A.; Etinger, A.; Mechoulam, R. Isolation and structure of a brain constituent that binds to the cannabinoid receptor. *Science (N.Y.)* **1992**, *258*, 1946–1949. [CrossRef]

22. Mechoulam, R.; Ben-Shabat, S.; Hanus, L.; Ligumsky, M.; Kaminski, N.E.; Schatz, A.R.; Gopher, A.; Almog, S.; Martin, B.R.; Compton, D.R.; et al. Identification of an endogenous 2-monoglyceride, present in canine gut, that binds to cannabinoid receptors. *Biochem. Pharmacol.* **1995**, *50*, 83–90. [CrossRef]

23. Maccarrone, M.; Bab, I.; Bíró, T.; Cabral, G.A.; Dey, S.K.; Di Marzo, V.; Konje, J.C.; Kunos, G.; Mechoulam, R.; Pacher, P.; et al. Endocannabinoid signaling at the periphery: 50 years after thc. *Trends Pharmacol. Sci.* **2015**, *36*, 277–296. [CrossRef] [PubMed]

24. Pertwee, R.G. The therapeutic potential of drugs that target cannabinoid receptors or modulate the tissue levels or actions of endocannabinoids. *AAPS J.* **2005**, *7*, E625–E654. [CrossRef] [PubMed]

25. Blankman, J.L.; Cravatt, B.F. Chemical probes of endocannabinoid metabolism. *Pharmacol. Rev.* **2013**, *65*, 849–871. [CrossRef] [PubMed]

26. Alger, B.E.; Kim, J. Supply and demand for endocannabinoids. *Trends Neurosci.* **2011**, *34*, 304–315. [CrossRef] [PubMed]

27. Gyombolai, P.; Pap, D.; Turu, G.; Catt, K.J.; Bagdy, G.; Hunyady, L. Regulation of endocannabinoid release by G proteins: A paracrine mechanism of G protein-coupled receptor action. *Mol. Cell. Endocrinol.* **2012**, *353*, 29–36. [CrossRef] [PubMed]

28. Liu, J.; Wang, L.; Harvey-White, J.; Huang, B.X.; Kim, H.Y.; Luquet, S.; Palmiter, R.D.; Krystal, G.; Rai, R.; Mahadevan, A.; et al. Multiple pathways involved in the biosynthesis of anandamide. *Neuropharmacology* **2008**, *54*, 1–7. [CrossRef] [PubMed]

29. Leishman, E.; Mackie, K.; Luquet, S.; Bradshaw, H.B. Lipidomics profile of a NAPE-PLD KO mouse provides evidence of a broader role of this enzyme in lipid metabolism in the brain. *Biochim. Biophys. Acta (BBA)-Mol. Cell Biol. Lipids* **2016**, *1861*, 491–500. [CrossRef] [PubMed]

30. Glaser, S.T.; Abumrad, N.A.; Fatade, F.; Kaczocha, M.; Studholme, K.M.; Deutsch, D.G. Evidence against the presence of an anandamide transporter. *Proc. Natl. Acad. Sci. USA* **2003**, *100*, 4269–4274. [CrossRef] [PubMed]

31. Chicca, A.; Marazzi, J.; Nicolussi, S.; Gertsch, J.G. Evidence for bidirectional endocannabinoid transport across cell membranes. *J. Biol. Chem.* **2012**, *287*, 34660–34682. [CrossRef] [PubMed]

32. Seillier, A.; Giuffrida, A. The cannabinoid transporter inhibitor omdm-2 reduces social interaction: Further evidence for transporter-mediated endocannabinoid release. *Neuropharmacology* **2018**, *130*, 1–9. [CrossRef] [PubMed]

33. Fowler, C.J. Transport of endocannabinoids across the plasma membrane and within the cell. *FEBS J.* **2013**, *280*, 1895–1904. [CrossRef] [PubMed]

34. Bojesen, I.N.; Hansen, H.S. Binding of anandamide to bovine serum albumin. *J. Lipid Res.* **2003**, *44*, 1790–1794. [CrossRef] [PubMed]

35. Kano, M. Endocannabinoid-mediated control of synaptic transmission. *Phys. Rev.* **2009**, *89*, 309–380. [CrossRef] [PubMed]

36. Turu, G.; Hunyady, L. Signal transduction of the CB1 cannabinoid receptor. *J. Mol. Endocrinol.* **2010**, *44*, 75–85. [CrossRef] [PubMed]

37. Morello, G.; Imperatore, R.; Palomba, L.; Finelli, C.; Labruna, G.; Pasanisi, F.; Sacchetti, L.; Buono, L.; Piscitelli, F.; Orlando, P.; et al. Orexin-a represses satiety-inducing pomc neurons and contributes to obesity via stimulation of endocannabinoid signaling. *Proc. Natl. Acad. Sci. USA* **2016**, *113*, 4759–4764. [CrossRef] [PubMed]

38. Busquets-Garcia, A.; Bains, J.; Marsicano, G. CB1 receptor signaling in the brain: Extracting specificity from ubiquity. *Neuropsychopharmacology* **2018**, *43*, 4–20. [CrossRef] [PubMed]

39. Bacci, A.; Huguenard, J.R.; Prince, D.A. Long-lasting self-inhibition of neocortical interneurons mediated by endocannabinoids. *Nature* **2004**, *431*, 312–316. [CrossRef] [PubMed]

40. Pertwee, R.G.; Howlett, A.C.; Abood, M.E.; Alexander, S.P.H.; Marzo, V.D.; Elphick, M.R.; Greasley, P.J.; Hansen, H.S.; Kunos, G. International union of basic and clinical pharmacology. LXXIX. Cannabinoid receptors and their ligands: Beyond CB1 and CB2. *Pharmacol. Rev.* **2010**, *62*, 588–631. [CrossRef] [PubMed]

41. Benard, G.; Massa, F.; Puente, N.; Lourenco, J.; Bellocchio, L.; Soria-Gomez, E.; Matias, I.; Delamarre, A.; Metna-Laurent, M.; Cannich, A.; et al. Mitochondrial CB(1) receptors regulate neuronal energy metabolism. *Nat. Neurosci.* **2012**, *15*, 558–564. [CrossRef] [PubMed]

42. Viader, A.; Blankman, J.L.; Zhong, P.; Liu, X.; Schlosburg, J.E.; Joslyn, C.M.; Liu, Q.S.; Tomarchio, A.J.; Lichtman, A.H.; Selley, D.E.; et al. Metabolic interplay between astrocytes and neurons regulates endocannabinoid action. *Cell Rep.* **2015**, *12*, 798–808. [CrossRef] [PubMed]

43. Navarrete, M.; Araque, A. Endocannabinoids mediate neuron-astrocyte communication. *Neuron* **2008**, *57*, 883–893. [CrossRef] [PubMed]

44. Scheller, A.; Kirchhoff, F. Endocannabinoids and heterogeneity of glial cells in brain function. *Front. Integr. Neurosci.* **2016**, *10*, 24. [CrossRef] [PubMed]

45. Mecha, M.; Feliú, A.; Carrillo-Salinas, F.J.; Rueda-Zubiaurre, A.; Ortega-Gutiérrez, S.; de Sola, R.G.; Guaza, C. Endocannabinoids drive the acquisition of an alternative phenotype in microglia. *Brain Behav. Immun.* **2015**, *49*, 233–245. [CrossRef] [PubMed]

46. Gómez-Gonzalo, M.; Navarrete, M.; Perea, G.; Covelo, A.; Martín-Fernández, M.; Shigemoto, R.; Luján, R.; Araque, A. Endocannabinoids induce lateral long-term potentiation of transmitter release by stimulation of gliotransmission. *Cereb. Cortex* **2015**, *25*, 3699–3712. [CrossRef] [PubMed]

47. Araque, A.; Castillo, P.E.; Manzoni, O.J.; Tonini, R. Synaptic functions of endocannabinoid signaling in health and disease. *Neuropharmacology* **2017**, *124*, 13–24. [CrossRef] [PubMed]

48. Koch, M.; Varela, L.; Kim, J.G.; Kim, J.D.; Hernández-Nuño, F.; Simonds, S.E.; Castorena, C.M.; Vianna, C.R.; Elmquist, J.K.; Morozov, Y.M.; et al. Hypothalamic pomc neurons promote cannabinoid-induced feeding. *Nature* **2015**, *519*, 45–50. [CrossRef] [PubMed]

49. Garfield, A.S.; Shah, B.P.; Burgess, C.R.; Li, M.M.; Li, C.; Steger, J.S.; Madara, J.C.; Campbell, J.N.; Kroeger, D.; Scammell, T.E.; et al. Dynamic GABAergic afferent modulation of AgRP neurons. *Nat. Neurosci.* **2016**, *19*, 1628–1635. [CrossRef] [PubMed]

50. Rossi, M.A.; Stuber, G.D. Overlapping brain circuits for homeostatic and hedonic feeding. *Cell Metab.* **2018**, *27*, 42–56. [CrossRef] [PubMed]

51. Novelle, M.G.; Dieguez, C. Food addiction and binge eating: Lessons learned from animal models. *Nutrients* **2018**, *10*, 71. [CrossRef] [PubMed]

52. Jager, G.; Witkamp, R.F. The endocannabinoid system and appetite: Relevance for food reward. *Nutr. Res. Rev.* **2014**, *27*, 172–185. [CrossRef] [PubMed]

53. Mechoulam, R.; Berry, E.M.; Avraham, Y.; Di Marzo, V.; Fride, E. Endocannabinoids, feeding and suckling—From our perspective. *Int. J. Obes.* **2006**, *30*, 24–28. [CrossRef] [PubMed]

54. Fride, E.; Ginzburg, Y.; Breuer, A.; Bisogno, T.; Di Marzo, V.; Mechoulam, R. Critical role of the endogenous cannabinoid system in mouse pup suckling and growth. *Eur. J. Pharmacol.* **2001**, *419*, 207–214. [CrossRef]

55. Fride, E.; Foox, A.; Rosenberg, E.; Faigenboim, M.; Cohen, V.; Barda, L.; Blau, H.; Mechoulam, R. Milk intake and survival in newborn cannabinoid CB1 receptor knockout mice: Evidence for a "CB3" receptor. *Eur. J. Pharmacol.* **2003**, *461*, 27–34. [CrossRef]

56. Aguirre, C.A.; Castillo, V.A.; Llanos, M.N. Excess of the endocannabinoid anandamide during lactation induces overweight, fat accumulation and insulin resistance in adult mice. *Diabetol. Metab. Syndr.* **2012**, *4*, 35. [CrossRef] [PubMed]

57. Aguirre, C.A.; Castillo, V.A.; Llanos, M.N. The endocannabinoid anandamide during lactation increases body fat content and CB1 receptor levels in mice adipose tissue. *Nutr. Diabetes* **2015**, *5*, e167. [CrossRef] [PubMed]

58. Aguirre, C.; Castillo, V.; Llanos, M. Oral administration of the endocannabinoid anandamide during lactation: Effects on hypothalamic cannabinoid type 1 receptor and food intake in adult mice. *J. Nutr. Metab.* **2017**, *2017*, 2945010. [CrossRef] [PubMed]

59. Garry, A.; Rigourd, V.; Amirouche, A.; Fauroux, V.; Aubry, S.; Serreau, R. Cannabis and breastfeeding. *J. Toxicol.* **2009**, *2009*, 596149. [CrossRef] [PubMed]

60. Ravinet Trillou, C.; Delgorge, C.; Menet, C.; Arnone, M.; Soubrie, P. CB1 cannabinoid receptor knockout in mice leads to leanness, resistance to diet-induced obesity and enhanced leptin sensitivity. *Int. J. Obes. Relat. Metab. Disord.* **2004**, *28*, 640–648. [CrossRef] [PubMed]

61. Massa, F.; Mancini, G.; Schmidt, H.; Steindel, F.; Mackie, K.; Angioni, C.; Oliet, S.H.R.; Geisslinger, G.; Lutz, B. Alterations in the hippocampal endocannabinoid system in diet-induced obese mice. *J. Neurosci.* **2010**, *30*, 6273–6281. [CrossRef] [PubMed]

62. Zimmer, A.; Zimmer, A.M.; Hohmann, A.G.; Herkenham, M.; Bonner, T.I. Increased mortality, hypoactivity, and hypoalgesia in cannabinoid CB1 receptor knockout mice. *Proc. Natl. Acad. Sci. USA* **1999**, *96*, 5780–5785. [CrossRef] [PubMed]

63. Busquets-Garcia, A.; Desprez, T.; Metna-Laurent, M.; Bellocchio, L.; Marsicano, G.; Soria-Gomez, E. Dissecting the cannabinergic control of behavior: The where matters. *BioEssays News Rev. Mol. Cell. Dev. Biol.* **2015**, *37*, 1215–1225. [CrossRef] [PubMed]

64. Saper, C.B.; Lowell, B.B. The hypothalamus. *Curr. Biol.* **2014**, *24*, R1111–R1116. [CrossRef] [PubMed]

65. Wu, Q.; Lemus, M.B.; Stark, R.; Bayliss, J.A.; Reichenbach, A.; Lockie, S.H.; Andrews, Z.B. The temporal pattern of cfos activation in hypothalamic, cortical, and brainstem nuclei in response to fasting and refeeding in male mice. *Endocrinology* **2014**, *155*, 840–853. [CrossRef] [PubMed]

66. Date, Y.; Shimbara, T.; Koda, S.; Toshinai, K.; Ida, T.; Murakami, N.; Miyazato, M.; Kokame, K.; Ishizuka, Y.; Ishida, Y.; et al. Peripheral ghrelin transmits orexigenic signals through the noradrenergic pathway from the hindbrain to the hypothalamus. *Cell Metab.* **2006**, *4*, 323–331. [CrossRef] [PubMed]

67. Cowley, M.A.; Smart, J.L.; Rubinstein, M.; Cerdán, M.G.; Diano, S.; Horvath, T.L.; Cone, R.D.; Low, M.J. Leptin activates anorexigenic pomc neurons through a neural network in the arcuate nucleus. *Nature* **2001**, *411*, 480–484. [CrossRef] [PubMed]

68. Andermann, M.L.; Lowell, B.B. Toward a wiring diagram understanding of appetite control. *Neuron* **2017**, *95*, 757–778. [CrossRef] [PubMed]

69. Morozov, Y.M.; Koch, M.; Rakic, P.; Horvath, T.L. Cannabinoid type 1 receptor-containing axons innervate NPY/AgRP neurons in the mouse arcuate nucleus. *Mol. Metab.* **2017**, *6*, 374–381. [CrossRef] [PubMed]

70. Zhang, X.; van den Pol, A.N. Hypothalamic arcuate nucleus tyrosine hydroxylase neurons play orexigenic role in energy homeostasis. *Nat. Neurosci.* **2016**, *19*, 1341–1347. [CrossRef] [PubMed]

71. Campbell, J.N.; Macosko, E.Z.; Fenselau, H.; Pers, T.H.; Lyubetskaya, A.; Tenen, D.; Goldman, M.; Verstegen, A.M.; Resch, J.M.; McCarroll, S.A.; et al. A molecular census of arcuate hypothalamus and median eminence cell types. *Nat. Neurosci.* **2017**, *20*, 484–496. [CrossRef] [PubMed]

72. Kim, J.G.; Sun, B.H.; Dietrich, M.O.; Koch, M.; Yao, G.Q.; Diano, S.; Insogna, K.; Horvath, T.L. Agrp neurons regulate bone mass. *Cell Rep.* **2015**, *13*, 8–14. [CrossRef] [PubMed]

73. Matarese, G.; Procaccini, C.; Menale, C.; Kim, J.G.; Kim, J.D.; Diano, S.; Diano, N.; De Rosa, V.; Dietrich, M.O.; Horvath, T.L. Hunger-promoting hypothalamic neurons modulate effector and regulatory t-cell responses. *Proc. Natl. Acad. Sci. USA* **2013**, *110*, 6193–6198. [CrossRef] [PubMed]

74. Sims, J.S.; Lorden, J.F. Effect of paraventricular nucleus lesions on body weight, food intake and insulin levels. *Behav. Brain Res.* **1986**, *22*, 265–281. [CrossRef]

75. Rinaman, L. Oxytocinergic inputs to the nucleus of the solitary tract and dorsal motor nucleus of the vagus in neonatal rats. *J. Comp. Neurol.* **1998**, *399*, 101–109. [CrossRef]

76. Arletti, R.; Benelli, A.; Bertolini, A. Oxytocin inhibits food and fluid intake in rats. *Physiol. Behav.* **1990**, *48*, 825–830. [CrossRef]

77. Spetter, M.S.; Hallschmid, M. Current findings on the role of oxytocin in the regulation of food intake. *Physiol. Behav.* **2017**, *176*, 31–39. [CrossRef] [PubMed]

78. Romano, A.; Tempesta, B.; Provensi, G.; Passani, M.B.; Gaetani, S. Central mechanisms mediating the hypophagic effects of oleoylethanolamide and *N*-acylphosphatidylethanolamines: Different lipid signals? *Front. Pharmacol.* **2015**, *6*, 137. [CrossRef] [PubMed]

79. Romano, A.; Potes, C.S.; Tempesta, B.; Cassano, T.; Cuomo, V.; Lutz, T.; Gaetani, S. Hindbrain noradrenergic input to the hypothalamic PVN mediates the activation of oxytocinergic neurons induced by the satiety factor oleoylethanolamide. *Am. J. Physiol. Endocrinol. Metab.* **2013**, *305*, E1266–E1273. [CrossRef] [PubMed]

80. Gaetani, S.; Fu, J.; Cassano, T.; Dipasquale, P.; Romano, A.; Righetti, L.; Cianci, S.; Laconca, L.; Giannini, E.; Scaccianoce, S.; et al. The fat-induced satiety factor oleoylethanolamide suppresses feeding through central release of oxytocin. *J. Neurosci.* **2010**, *30*, 8096–8101. [CrossRef] [PubMed]

81. Bonnavion, P.; Mickelsen, L.E.; Fujita, A.; de Lecea, L.; Jackson, A.C. Hubs and spokes of the lateral hypothalamus: Cell types, circuits and behaviour. *J. Physiol.* **2016**, *594*, 6443–6462. [CrossRef] [PubMed]

82. Qu, D.; Ludwig, D.S.; Gammeltoft, S.; Piper, M.; Pelleymounter, M.A.; Cullen, M.J.; Mathes, W.F.; Przypek, R.; Kanarek, R.; Maratos-Flier, E. A role for melanin-concentrating hormone in the central regulation of feeding behaviour. *Nature* **1996**, *380*, 243–247. [CrossRef] [PubMed]

83. Shaimada, M.; Tritos, N.A.; Lowell, B.B.; Flier, J.S.; Maratos-Flier, E. Mice lacking melanin-concentrating hormone are hypophagic and lean. *Nature* **1998**, *396*, 670–674. [CrossRef] [PubMed]

84. Sakurai, T.; Amemiya, A.; Ishii, M.; Matsuzaki, I.; Chemelli, R.M.; Tanaka, H.; Williams, S.C.; Richardson, J.A.; Kozlowski, G.P.; Wilson, S.; et al. Orexins and orexin receptors: A family of hypothalamic neuropeptides and G protein-coupled receptors that regulate feeding behavior. *Cell* **1998**, *92*, 573–585. [CrossRef]

85. Aston-Jones, G.; Smith, R.J.; Sartor, G.C.; Moorman, D.E.; Massi, L.; Tahsili-Fahadan, P.; Richardson, K.A. Lateral hypothalamic orexin/hypocretin neurons: A role in reward-seeking and addiction. *Brain Res.* **2010**, *1314*, 74–90. [CrossRef] [PubMed]

86. Chemelli, R.M.; Willie, J.T.; Sinton, C.M.; Elmquist, J.K.; Scammell, T.; Lee, C.; Richardson, J.A.; Williams, S.C.; Xiong, Y.; Kisanuki, Y.; et al. Narcolepsy in orexin knockout mice: Molecular genetics of sleep regulation. *Cell* **1999**, *98*, 437–451. [CrossRef]

87. Huang, H.; Acuna-Goycolea, C.; Li, Y.; Cheng, H.M.; Obrietan, K.; van den Pol, A.N. Cannabinoids excite hypothalamic melanin-concentrating hormone but inhibit hypocretin/orexin neurons: Implications for cannabinoid actions on food intake and cognitive arousal. *J. Neurosci.* **2007**, *27*, 4870–4881. [CrossRef] [PubMed]

88. Horvath, T.L.; Gao, X.B. Input organization and plasticity of hypocretin neurons: Possible clues to obesity's association with insomnia. *Cell Metab.* **2005**, *1*, 279–286. [CrossRef] [PubMed]

89. Cristino, L.; Busetto, G.; Imperatore, R.; Ferrandino, I.; Palomba, L.; Silvestri, C.; Petrosino, S.; Orlando, P.; Bentivoglio, M.; Mackie, K.; et al. Obesity-driven synaptic remodeling affects endocannabinoid control of orexinergic neurons. *Proc. Natl. Acad. Sci. USA* **2013**, *110*, E2229–E2238. [CrossRef] [PubMed]

90. Alpar, A.; Harkany, T. Orexin neurons use endocannabinoids to break obesity-induced inhibition. *Proc. Natl. Acad. Sci. USA* **2013**, *110*, 9625–9626. [CrossRef] [PubMed]

91. Becker, T.M.; Favero, M.; Di Marzo, V.; Cristino, L.; Busetto, G. Endocannabinoid-dependent disinhibition of orexinergic neurons: Electrophysiological evidence in leptin-knockout obese mice. *Mol. Metab.* **2017**, *6*, 594–601. [CrossRef] [PubMed]

92. Moreno, E.; Chiarlone, A.; Medrano, M.; Puigdellívol, M.; Bibic, L.; Howell, L.A.; Resel, E.; Puente, N.; Casarejos, M.J.; Perucho, J.; et al. Singular location and signaling profile of adenosine A2A-cannabinoid CB1receptor heteromers in the dorsal striatum. *Neuropsychopharmacology* **2017**, *43*, 964–977. [CrossRef] [PubMed]

93. Jo, Y.H.; Chen, Y.J.; Chua, S.C., Jr.; Talmage, D.A.; Role, L.W. Integration of endocannabinoid and leptin signaling in an appetite-related neural circuit. *Neuron* **2005**, *48*, 1055–1066. [CrossRef] [PubMed]

94. Harris, G.C.; Wimmer, M.; Aston-Jones, G. A role for lateral hypothalamic orexin neurons in reward seeking. *Nature* **2005**, *437*, 556–559. [CrossRef] [PubMed]

95. Ch'ng, S.S.; Lawrence, A.J. Distribution of the orexin-1 receptor (OX1R) in the mouse forebrain and rostral brainstem: A characterisation of OX1R-eGFP mice. *J. Chem. Neuroanat.* **2015**, *66–67*, 1–9. [CrossRef] [PubMed]

96. Parise, E.M.; Lilly, N.; Kay, K.; Dossat, A.M.; Seth, R.; Overton, J.M.; Williams, D.L. Evidence for the role of hindbrain orexin-1 receptors in the control of meal size. *Am. J. Physiol. Regul. Integr. Comp. Physiol.* **2011**, *301*, R1692–R1699. [CrossRef] [PubMed]

97. Tung, L.W.; Lu, G.L.; Lee, Y.H.; Yu, L.; Lee, H.J.; Leishman, E.; Bradshaw, H.; Hwang, L.L.; Hung, M.S.; Mackie, K.; et al. Orexins contribute to restraint stress-induced cocaine relapse by endocannabinoid-mediated disinhibition of dopaminergic neurons. *Nat. Commun.* **2016**, *7*, 12199. [CrossRef] [PubMed]

98. Date, Y.; Kojima, M.; Hosoda, H.; Sawaguchi, A.; Mondal, M.S.; Suganuma, T.; Matsukura, S.; Kangawa, K.; Nakazato, M. Ghrelin, a novel growth hormone-releasing acylated peptide, is synthesized in a distinct endocrine cell type in the gastrointestinal tracts of rats and humans. *Endocrinology* **2000**, *141*, 4255–4261. [CrossRef] [PubMed]

99. Alen, F.; Crespo, I.; Ramirez-Lopez, M.T.; Jagerovic, N.; Goya, P.; de Fonseca, F.R.; de Heras, R.G.; Orio, L. Ghrelin-induced orexigenic effect in rats depends on the metabolic status and is counteracted by peripheral cb1 receptor antagonism. *PLoS ONE* **2013**, *8*, e60918. [CrossRef] [PubMed]

100. Hashiguchi, H.; Sheng, Z.; Routh, V.; Gerzanich, V.; Simard, J.M.; Bryan, J. Direct versus indirect actions of ghrelin on hypothalamic NPY neurons. *PLoS ONE* **2017**, *12*, e0184261. [CrossRef] [PubMed]

101. Kola, B.; Farkas, I.; Christ-Crain, M.; Wittmann, G.; Lolli, F.; Amin, F.; Harvey-White, J.; Liposits, Z.; Kunos, G.; Grossman, A.B.; et al. The orexigenic effect of ghrelin is mediated through central activation of the endogenous cannabinoid system. *PLoS ONE* **2008**, *3*, e1797. [CrossRef] [PubMed]

102. Kalafateli, A.L.; Vallöf, D.; Jörnulf, J.W.; Heilig, M.; Jerlhag, E. A cannabinoid receptor antagonist attenuates ghrelin-induced activation of the mesolimbic dopamine system in mice. *Physiol. Behav.* **2018**, *184*, 211–219. [CrossRef] [PubMed]

103. Myers, M.G., Jr.; Leibel, R.L.; Seeley, R.J.; Schwartz, M.W. Obesity and leptin resistance: Distinguishing cause from effect. *Trends Endocrinol. Metab.* **2010**, *21*, 643–651. [CrossRef] [PubMed]

104. Mitchell, S.E.; Nogueiras, R.; Morris, A.; Tovar, S.; Grant, C.; Cruickshank, M.; Rayner, D.V.; Dieguez, C.; Williams, L.M. Leptin receptor gene expression and number in the brain are regulated by leptin level and nutritional status. *J. Physiol.* **2009**, *587*, 3573–3585. [CrossRef] [PubMed]

105. Krugel, U.; Schraft, T.; Kittner, H.; Kiess, W.; Illes, P. Basal and feeding-evoked dopamine release in the rat nucleus accumbens is depressed by leptin. *Eur. J. Pharmacol.* **2003**, *482*, 185–187. [CrossRef] [PubMed]

106. Matheny, M.; Strehler, K.Y.; King, M.; Tumer, N.; Scarpace, P.J. Targeted leptin receptor blockade: Role of ventral tegmental area and nucleus of the solitary tract leptin receptors in body weight homeostasis. *J. Endocrinol.* **2014**, *222*, 27–41. [CrossRef] [PubMed]

107. Banks, W.A.; Farr, S.A.; Salameh, T.S.; Niehoff, M.L.; Rhea, E.M.; Morley, J.E.; Hanson, A.J.; Hansen, K.M.; Craft, S. Triglycerides cross the blood-brain barrier and induce central leptin and insulin receptor resistance. *Int. J. Obes. (Lond.)* **2018**, *42*, 391–397. [CrossRef] [PubMed]

108. Di Marzo, V.; Goparaju, S.K.; Wang, L.; Liu, J.; Batkai, S.; Jarai, Z.; Fezza, F.; Miura, G.I.; Palmiter, R.D.; Sugiura, T.; et al. Leptin-regulated endocannabinoids are involved in maintaining food intake. *Nature* **2001**, *410*, 822–825. [CrossRef] [PubMed]

109. Wierucka-Rybak, M.; Wolak, M.; Juszczak, M.; Drobnik, J.; Bojanowska, E. The inhibitory effect of combination treatment with leptin and cannabinoid cb1 receptor agonist on food intake and body weight gain is mediated by serotonin 1b and 2c receptors. *J. Physiol. Pharmacol. Off. J. Pol. Physiol. Soc.* **2016**, *67*, 457–463.

110. Tam, J.; Szanda, G.; Drori, A.; Liu, Z.; Cinar, R.; Kashiwaya, Y.; Reitman, M.L.; Kunos, G. Peripheral cannabinoid-1 receptor blockade restores hypothalamic leptin signaling. *Mol. Metab.* **2017**, *6*, 1113–1125. [CrossRef] [PubMed]

111. Rehfeld, J.F. Cholecystokinin-from local gut hormone to ubiquitous messenger. *Front. Endocrinol.* **2017**, *8*, 47. [CrossRef] [PubMed]

112. Antin, J.; Gibbs, J.; Holt, J.; Young, R.C.; Smith, G.P. Cholecystokinin elicits the complete behavioral sequence of satiety in rats. *J. Comp. Physiol. Psychol.* **1975**, *89*, 784–790. [CrossRef] [PubMed]

113. Crawley, J.N.; Kiss, J.Z.; Mezey, E. Bilateral midbrain transections block the behavioral effects of cholecystokinin on feeding and exploration in rats. *Brain Res.* **1984**, *322*, 316–321. [CrossRef]

114. Roman, C.W.; Derkach, V.A.; Palmiter, R.D. Genetically and functionally defined NTS to PBN brain circuits mediating anorexia. *Nat. Commun.* **2016**, *7*, 11905. [CrossRef] [PubMed]

115. Chhatwal, J.P.; Gutman, A.R.; Maguschak, K.A.; Bowser, M.E.; Yang, Y.; Davis, M.; Ressler, K.J. Functional interactions between endocannabinoid and CCK neurotransmitter systems may be critical for extinction learning. *Neuropsychopharmacology* **2009**, *34*, 509–521. [CrossRef] [PubMed]

116. Mitchell, V.A.; Jeong, H.J.; Drew, G.M.; Vaughan, C.W. Cholecystokinin exerts an effect via the endocannabinoid system to inhibit gabaergic transmission in midbrain periaqueductal gray. *Neuropsychopharmacology* **2011**, *36*, 1801–1810. [CrossRef] [PubMed]

117. Khlaifia, A.; Matias, I.; Cota, D.; Tell, F. Nutritional status-dependent endocannabinoid signalling regulates the integration of rat visceral information. *J. Physiol.* **2017**, *595*, 3267–3285. [CrossRef] [PubMed]

118. Van Houten, M.; Posner, B.I.; Kopriwa, B.M.; Brawer, J.R. Insulin binding sites localized to nerve terminals in rat median eminence and arcuate nucleus. *Science* **1980**, *207*, 1081–1083. [CrossRef] [PubMed]

119. Sipols, A.J.; Baskin, D.G.; Schwartz, M.W. Effect of intracerebroventricular insulin infusion on diabetic hyperphagia and hypothalamic neuropeptide gene expression. *Diabetes* **1995**, *44*, 147–151. [CrossRef] [PubMed]

120. Williams, K.W.; Margatho, L.O.; Lee, C.E.; Choi, M.; Lee, S.; Scott, M.M.; Elias, C.F.; Elmquist, J.K. Segregation of acute leptin and insulin effects in distinct populations of arcuate proopiomelanocortin neurons. *J. Neurosci.* **2010**, *30*, 2472–2479. [CrossRef] [PubMed]

121. Loh, K.; Zhang, L.; Brandon, A.; Wang, Q.; Begg, D.; Qi, Y.; Fu, M.; Kulkarni, R.; Teo, J.; Baldock, P.; et al. Insulin controls food intake and energy balance via npy neurons. *Mol. Metab.* **2017**, *6*, 574–584. [CrossRef] [PubMed]

122. Larsen, P.J.; Tang-Christensen, M.; Holst, J.J.; Ørskov, C. Distribution of glucagon-like peptide-1 and other preproglucagon-derived peptides in the rat hypothalamus and brainstem. *Neuroscience* **1997**, *77*, 257–270. [CrossRef]

123. Cork, S.C.; Richards, J.E.; Holt, M.K.; Gribble, F.M.; Reimann, F.; Trapp, S. Distribution and characterisation of glucagon-like peptide-1 receptor expressing cells in the mouse brain. *Mol. Metab.* **2015**, *4*, 718–731. [CrossRef] [PubMed]

124. Trapp, S.; Richards, J.E. The gut hormone glucagon-like peptide-1 produced in brain: Is this physiologically relevant? *Curr. Opin. Pharmacol.* **2013**, *13*, 964–969. [CrossRef] [PubMed]

125. McMahon, L.R.; Wellman, P.J. Pvn infusion of GLP-1-(7—36) amide suppresses feeding but does not induce aversion or alter locomotion in rats. *Am. J. Physiol.-Regul. Integr. Comp. Physiol.* **1998**, *274*, R23–R29. [CrossRef]

126. Liu, J.; Conde, K.; Zhang, P.; Lilascharoen, V.; Xu, Z.; Lim, B.K.; Seeley, R.J.; Zhu, J.J.; Scott, M.M.; Pang, Z.P. Enhanced AMPA receptor trafficking mediates the anorexigenic effect of endogenous glucagon-like peptide-1 in the paraventricular hypothalamus. *Neuron* **2017**, *96*, 897.e895–909.e895. [CrossRef] [PubMed]

127. Cheng, Y.H.; Ho, M.S.; Huang, W.T.; Chou, Y.T.; King, K. Modulation of glucagon-like peptide-1 (GLP-1) potency by endocannabinoid-like lipids represents a novel mode of regulating GLP-1 receptor signaling. *J. Biol. Chem.* **2015**, *290*, 14302–14313. [CrossRef] [PubMed]

128. Witkamp, R.F. The role of fatty acids and their endocannabinoid-like derivatives in the molecular regulation of appetite. *Mol. Asp. Med.* **2018**, in press. [CrossRef] [PubMed]

129. Khan, M.Z.; He, L. The role of polyunsaturated fatty acids and GPR40 receptor in brain. *Neuropharmacology* **2017**, *113*, 639–651. [CrossRef] [PubMed]

130. Lafourcade, M.; Larrieu, T.; Mato, S.; Duffaud, A.; Sepers, M.; Matias, I.; De Smedt-Peyrusse, V.; Labrousse, V.F.; Bretillon, L.; Matute, C.; et al. Nutritional omega-3 deficiency abolishes endocannabinoid-mediated neuronal functions. *Nat. Neurosci.* **2011**, *14*, 345–350. [CrossRef] [PubMed]

131. Hawkins, R.A.; O'Kane, R.L.; Simpson, I.A.; Vina, J.R. Structure of the blood-brain barrier and its role in the transport of amino acids. *J. Nutr.* **2006**, *136*, 218s–226s. [CrossRef] [PubMed]

132. Gietzen, D.W.; Hao, S.; Anthony, T.G. Mechanisms of food intake repression in indispensable amino acid deficiency. *Annu. Rev. Nutr.* **2007**, *27*, 63–78. [CrossRef] [PubMed]

133. Heeley, N.; Blouet, C. Central amino acid sensing in the control of feeding behavior. *Front. Endocrinol. (Lausanne)* **2016**, *7*, 148. [CrossRef] [PubMed]

134. Thorens, B. Sensing of glucose in the brain. *Handb. Exp. Pharmacol.* **2012**, *209*, 277–294.

135. Grabauskas, G.; Song, I.; Zhou, S.; Owyang, C. Electrophysiological identification of glucose-sensing neurons in rat nodose ganglia. *J. Physiol.* **2010**, *588*, 617–632. [CrossRef] [PubMed]

136. Karnani, M.; Burdakov, D. Multiple hypothalamic circuits sense and regulate glucose levels. *Am. J. Physiol. Regul. Integr. Comp. Physiol.* **2011**, *300*, R47–R55. [CrossRef] [PubMed]

137. Parton, L.E.; Ye, C.P.; Coppari, R.; Enriori, P.J.; Choi, B.; Zhang, C.Y.; Xu, C.; Vianna, C.R.; Balthasar, N.; Lee, C.E.; et al. Glucose sensing by pomc neurons regulates glucose homeostasis and is impaired in obesity. *Nature* **2007**, *449*, 228–232. [CrossRef] [PubMed]

138. Murphy, B.A.; Fioramonti, X.; Jochnowitz, N.; Fakira, K.; Gagen, K.; Contie, S.; Lorsignol, A.; Penicaud, L.; Martin, W.J.; Routh, V.H. Fasting enhances the response of arcuate neuropeptide Y-glucose-inhibited neurons to decreased extracellular glucose. *Am. J. Physiol. Cell Physiol.* **2009**, *296*, C746–C756. [CrossRef] [PubMed]

139. Abraham, M.A.; Rasti, M.; Bauer, P.V.; Lam, T.K.T. Leptin enhances hypothalamic lactate dehydrogenase A (LDHA)-dependent glucose sensing to lower glucose production in high-fat-fed rats. *J. Biol. Chem.* **2018**, *293*, 4159–4166. [CrossRef] [PubMed]

140. Chari, M.; Yang, C.S.; Lam, C.K.; Lee, K.; Mighiu, P.; Kokorovic, A.; Cheung, G.W.; Lai, T.Y.; Wang, P.Y.; Lam, T.K. Glucose transporter-1 in the hypothalamic glial cells mediates glucose sensing to regulate glucose production in vivo. *Diabetes* **2011**, *60*, 1901–1906. [CrossRef] [PubMed]

141. Allard, C.; Carneiro, L.; Grall, S.; Cline, B.H.; Fioramonti, X.; Chretien, C.; Baba-Aissa, F.; Giaume, C.; Penicaud, L.; Leloup, C. Hypothalamic astroglial connexins are required for brain glucose sensing-induced insulin secretion. *J. Cereb. Blood Flow Metab.* **2014**, *34*, 339–346. [CrossRef] [PubMed]

142. Fuente-Martin, E.; Garcia-Caceres, C.; Granado, M.; de Ceballos, M.L.; Sanchez-Garrido, M.A.; Sarman, B.; Liu, Z.W.; Dietrich, M.O.; Tena-Sempere, M.; Argente-Arizon, P.; et al. Leptin regulates glutamate and glucose transporters in hypothalamic astrocytes. *J. Clin. Investig.* **2012**, *122*, 3900–3913. [CrossRef] [PubMed]

143. Bosier, B.; Bellocchio, L.; Metna-Laurent, M.; Soria-Gomez, E.; Matias, I.; Hebert-Chatelain, E.; Cannich, A.; Maitre, M.; Leste-Lasserre, T.; Cardinal, P.; et al. Astroglial cb1 cannabinoid receptors regulate leptin signaling in mouse brain astrocytes. *Mol. Metab.* **2013**, *2*, 393–404. [CrossRef] [PubMed]

144. Frayling, C.; Britton, R.; Dale, N. Atp-mediated glucosensing by hypothalamic tanycytes. *J. Physiol.* **2011**, *589*, 2275–2286. [CrossRef] [PubMed]

145. Elizondo-Vega, R.; Cortes-Campos, C.; Barahona, M.J.; Oyarce, K.A.; Carril, C.A.; Garcia-Robles, M.A. The role of tanycytes in hypothalamic glucosensing. *J. Cell. Mol. Med.* **2015**, *19*, 1471–1482. [CrossRef] [PubMed]

146. Schultz, W. Neuronal reward and decision signals: From theories to data. *Physiol. Rev.* **2015**, *95*, 853–951. [CrossRef] [PubMed]

147. Leonard, W.R.; Snodgrass, J.J.; Robertson, M.L. Evolutionary perspectives on fat ingestion and metabolism in humans. In *Fat Detection: Taste, Texture, and Post Ingestive Effects*; Montmayeur, J.P., le Coutre, J., Eds.; CRC Press: Boca Raton, FL, USA, 2010.

148. Berridge, K.C. Food reward: Brain substrates of wanting and liking. *Neurosci. Biobehav. Rev.* **1996**, *20*, 1–25. [CrossRef]

149. Rogers, P.J. Why a palatability construct is needed. *Appetite* **1990**, *14*, 167–170. [CrossRef]

150. Covey, D.P.; Mateo, Y.; Sulzer, D.; Cheer, J.F.; Lovinger, D.M. Endocannabinoid modulation of dopamine neurotransmission. *Neuropharmacology* **2017**, *124*, 52–61. [CrossRef] [PubMed]

151. Gardner, E.L. Endocannabinoid signaling system and brain reward: Emphasis on dopamine. *Pharmacol. Biochem. Behav.* **2005**, *81*, 263–284. [CrossRef] [PubMed]

152. Julian, M.D.; Martin, A.B.; Cuellar, B.; Rodriguez De Fonseca, F.; Navarro, M.; Moratalla, R.; Garcia-Segura, L.M. Neuroanatomical relationship between type 1 cannabinoid receptors and dopaminergic systems in the rat basal ganglia. *Neuroscience* **2003**, *119*, 309–318. [CrossRef]

153. Cheer, J.F.; Kendall, D.A.; Mason, R.; Marsden, C.A. Differential cannabinoid-induced electrophysiological effects in rat ventral tegmentum. *Neuropharmacology* **2003**, *44*, 633–641. [CrossRef]

154. Turner, B.D.; Kashima, D.T.; Manz, K.M.; Grueter, C.A.; Grueter, B.A. Synaptic plasticity in the nucleus accumbens: Lessons learned from experience. *ACS Chem. Neurosci.* **2018**. [CrossRef] [PubMed]

155. Mogenson, G.J.; Jones, D.L.; Yim, C.Y. From motivation to action: Functional interface between the limbic system and the motor system. *Prog. Neurobiol.* **1980**, *14*, 69–97. [CrossRef]

156. Kirkham, T.C.; Williams, C.M.; Fezza, F.; Marzo, V.D. Endocannabinoid levels in rat limbic forebrain and hypothalamus in relation to fasting, feeding and satiation: Stimulation of eating by 2-arachidonoyl glycerol. *Br. J. Pharmacol.* **2002**, *136*, 550–557. [CrossRef] [PubMed]

157. Robbe, D.; Kopf, M.; Remaury, A.; Bockaert, J.; Manzoni, O.J. Endogenous cannabinoids mediate long-term synaptic depression in the nucleus accumbens. *Proc. Natl. Acad. Sci. USA* **2002**, *99*, 8384–8388. [CrossRef] [PubMed]

158. Anselme, P.; Robinson, M.J. "Wanting," "liking," and their relation to consciousness. *J. Exp. Psychol. Anim. Learn. Cogn.* **2016**, *42*, 123–140. [CrossRef] [PubMed]

159. Howard, J.D.; Gottfried, J.A.; Tobler, P.N.; Kahnt, T. Identity-specific coding of future rewards in the human orbitofrontal cortex. *Proc. Natl. Acad. Sci. USA* **2015**, *112*, 5195–5200. [CrossRef] [PubMed]

160. Suzuki, S.; Cross, L.; O'Doherty, J.P. Elucidating the underlying components of food valuation in the human orbitofrontal cortex. *Nat. Neurosci.* **2017**, *20*, 1780–1786. [CrossRef] [PubMed]

161. Stalnaker, T.A.; Cooch, N.K.; McDannald, M.A.; Liu, T.L.; Wied, H.; Schoenbaum, G. Orbitofrontal neurons infer the value and identity of predicted outcomes. *Nat. Commun.* **2014**, *5*, 3926. [CrossRef] [PubMed]

162. Foerde, K.; Steinglass, J.E.; Shohamy, D.; Walsh, B.T. Neural mechanisms supporting maladaptive food choices in anorexia nervosa. *Nat. Neurosci.* **2015**, *18*, 1571–1573. [CrossRef] [PubMed]

163. Satta, V.; Scherma, M.; Piscitelli, F.; Usai, P.; Castelli, M.P.; Bisogno, T.; Fratta, W.; Fadda, P. Limited access to a high fat diet alters endocannabinoid tone in female rats. *Front. Neurosci.* **2018**, *12*, 40. [CrossRef] [PubMed]

164. Arnone, M.; Maruani, J.; Chaperon, F.; Thiebot, M.H.; Poncelet, M.; Soubrie, P.; Le Fur, G. Selective inhibition of sucrose and ethanol intake by SR 141716, an antagonist of central cannabinoid (CB1) receptors. *Psychopharmacology (Berl.)* **1997**, *132*, 104–106. [CrossRef] [PubMed]

165. Abel, E.L. Effects of marihuana on the solution of anagrams, memory and appetite. *Nature* **1971**, *231*, 260–261. [CrossRef] [PubMed]

166. Williams, C.M.; Rogers, P.J.; Kirkham, T.C. Hyperphagia in pre-fed rats following oral delta9-THC. *Phys. Behav.* **1998**, *65*, 343–346. [CrossRef]

167. Sofia, R.D.; Knobloch, L.C. Comparative effects of various naturally occurring cannabinoids on food, sucrose and water consumption by rats. *Pharmacol. Biochem. Behav.* **1976**, *4*, 591–599. [CrossRef]

168. Tasker, J.G.; Chen, C.; Fisher, M.O.; Fu, X.; Rainville, J.R.; Weiss, G.L. Endocannabinoid regulation of neuroendocrine systems. *Int. Rev. Neurobiol.* **2015**, *125*, 163–201. [PubMed]

169. Glick, S.D.; Milloy, S. Increased and decreased eating following THC administration. *Psychon. Sci.* **1972**, *29*, 6. [CrossRef]

170. Hao, S.; Avraham, Y.; Mechoulam, R.; Berry, E.M. Low dose anandamide affects food intake, cognitive function, neurotransmitter and corticosterone levels in diet-restricted mice. *Eur. J. Pharmacol.* **2000**, *392*, 147–156. [CrossRef]

171. Williams, C.M.; Kirkham, T.C. Anandamide induces overeating: Mediation by central cannabinoid (CB1) receptors. *Psychopharmacology* **1999**, *143*, 315–317. [CrossRef] [PubMed]

172. De Luca, M.A.; Solinas, M.; Bimpisidis, Z.; Goldberg, S.R.; Di Chiara, G. Cannabinoid facilitation of behavioral and biochemical hedonic taste responses. *Neuropharmacology* **2012**, *63*, 161–168. [CrossRef] [PubMed]

173. Soria-Gomez, E.; Bellocchio, L.; Reguero, L.; Lepousez, G.; Martin, C.; Bendahmane, M.; Ruehle, S.; Remmers, F.; Desprez, T.; Matias, I.; et al. The endocannabinoid system controls food intake via olfactory processes. *Nat. Neurosci.* **2014**, *17*, 407–415. [CrossRef] [PubMed]

174. Tarragon, E.; Moreno, J.J. Role of endocannabinoids on sweet taste perception, food preference, and obesity-related disorders. *Chem. Senses* **2017**, *43*, 3–16. [CrossRef] [PubMed]

175. Livneh, Y.; Andermann, M.L. Yummy or yucky? Ask your central amygdala. *Nat. Neurosci.* **2017**, *20*, 1321–1322. [CrossRef] [PubMed]

176. Saper, C.B.; Loewy, A.D. Efferent connections of the parabrachial nucleus in the rat. *Brain Res.* **1980**, *197*, 291–317. [CrossRef]

177. DiPatrizio, N.V.; Simansky, K.J. Activating parabrachial cannabinoid cb1 receptors selectively stimulates feeding of palatable foods in rats. *J. Neurosci.* **2008**, *28*, 9702–9709. [CrossRef] [PubMed]

178. Norgren, R.; Hajnal, A.; Mungarndee, S.S. Gustatory reward and the nucleus accumbens. *Physiol. Behav.* **2006**, *89*, 531–535. [CrossRef] [PubMed]

179. Befort, K. Interactions of the opioid and cannabinoid systems in reward: Insights from knockout studies. *Front. Pharmacol.* **2015**, *6*, 6. [PubMed]

180. Caref, K.; Nicola, S.M. Endogenous opioids in the nucleus accumbens promote approach to high-fat food in the absense of caloric need. *eLife* **2018**, *7*, e34955. [CrossRef] [PubMed]

181. Marsicano, G.; Lutz, B. Expression of the cannabinoid receptor CB1 in distinct neuronal subpopulations in the adult mouse forebrain. *Eur. J. Neurosci.* **1999**, *11*, 4213–4225. [CrossRef] [PubMed]

182. Winters, B.D.; Kruger, J.M.; Huang, X.; Gallaher, Z.R.; Ishikawa, M.; Czaja, K.; Krueger, J.M.; Huang, Y.H.; Schluter, O.M.; Dong, Y. Cannabinoid receptor 1-expressing neurons in the nucleus accumbens. *Proc. Natl Acad. Sci. USA* **2012**, *109*, E2717–E2725. [CrossRef] [PubMed]

183. Finlayson, G. Food addiction and obesity: Unnecessary medicalization of hedonic overeating. *Nat. Rev. Endocrinol.* **2017**, *13*, 493–498. [CrossRef] [PubMed]

184. Rolls, E.T. Taste, olfactory, and food reward value processing in the brain. *Prog. Neurobiol.* **2015**, *127–128*, 64–90. [CrossRef] [PubMed]

185. Livneh, Y.; Ramesh, R.N.; Burgess, C.R.; Levandowski, K.M.; Madara, J.C.; Fenselau, H.; Goldey, G.J.; Diaz, V.E.; Jikomes, N.; Resch, J.M.; et al. Homeostatic circuits selectively gate food cue responses in insular cortex. *Nature* **2017**, *546*, 611–616. [CrossRef] [PubMed]

186. Gerard, N.; Pieters, G.; Goffin, K.; Bormans, G.; Van Laere, K. Brain type 1 cannabinoid receptor availability in patients with anorexia and bulimia nervosa. *Biol. Psychiatry* **2011**, *70*, 777–784. [CrossRef] [PubMed]

187. Khlaifia, A.; Farah, H.; Gackiere, F.; Tell, F. Anandamide, cannabinoid type 1 receptor, and nmda receptor activation mediate non-hebbian presynaptically expressed long-term depression at the first central synapse for visceral afferent fibers. *J. Neurosci.* **2013**, *33*, 12627–12637. [CrossRef] [PubMed]

188. Ueno, H.; Nakazato, M. Mechanistic relationship between the vagal afferent pathway, central nervous system and peripheral organs in appetite regulation. *J. Diabetes Investig.* **2016**, *7*, 812–818. [CrossRef] [PubMed]

189. Schwartz, G.J.; Salorio, C.F.; Skoglund, C.; Moran, T.H. Gut vagal afferent lesions increase meal size but do not block gastric preload-induced feeding suppression. *Am. J. Physiol.-Regul. Integr. Comp. Physiol.* **1999**, *276*, R1623–R1629. [CrossRef]

190. Davidson, T.L.; Kanoski, S.E.; Schier, L.A.; Clegg, D.J.; Benoit, S.C. A potential role for the hippocampus in energy intake and body weight regulation. *Curr. Opin. Pharmacol.* **2007**, *7*, 613–616. [CrossRef] [PubMed]

191. Sharkey, K.A.; Darmani, N.A.; Parker, L.A. Regulation of nausea and vomiting by cannabinoids and the endocannabinoid system. *Eur. J. Pharmacol.* **2014**, *722*, 134–146. [CrossRef] [PubMed]

192. Singh, P.; Yoon, S.S.; Kuo, B. Nausea: A review of pathophysiology and therapeutics. *Ther. Adv. Gastroenterol.* **2016**, *9*, 98–112. [CrossRef] [PubMed]

193. Vincent, B.J.; McQuiston, D.J.; Einhorn, L.H.; Nagy, C.M.; Brames, M.J. Review of cannabinoids and their antiemetic effectiveness. *Drugs* **1983**, *25* (Suppl. 1), 52–62. [CrossRef] [PubMed]

194. Allen, J.H.; de Moore, G.M.; Heddle, R.; Twartz, J.C. Cannabinoid hyperemesis: Cyclical hyperemesis in association with chronic cannabis abuse. *Gut* **2004**, *53*, 1566–1570. [CrossRef] [PubMed]

195. Emsley, J.G.; Macklis, J.D. Astroglial heterogeneity closely reflects the neuronal-defined anatomy of the adult murine CNS. *Neuron Glia Biol.* **2006**, *2*, 175–186. [CrossRef] [PubMed]

196. Matyash, V.; Kettenmann, H. Heterogeneity in astrocyte morphology and physiology. *Brain Res. Rev.* **2010**, *63*, 2–10. [CrossRef] [PubMed]

197. Oberheim, N.A.; Goldman, S.A.; Nedergaard, M. Heterogeneity of astrocytic form and function. *Methods Mol. Biol.* **2012**, *814*, 23–45. [PubMed]

198. Panatier, A.; Vallee, J.; Haber, M.; Murai, K.K.; Lacaille, J.C.; Robitaille, R. Astrocytes are endogenous regulators of basal transmission at central synapses. *Cell* **2011**, *146*, 785–798. [CrossRef] [PubMed]

199. Benedetti, B.; Matyash, V.; Kettenmann, H. Astrocytes control gabaergic inhibition of neurons in the mouse barrel cortex. *J. Physiol.* **2011**, *589*, 1159–1172. [CrossRef] [PubMed]

200. Kang, J.; Jiang, L.; Goldman, S.A.; Nedergaard, M. Astrocyte-mediated potentiation of inhibitory synaptic transmission. *Nat. Neurosci.* **1998**, *1*, 683–692. [CrossRef] [PubMed]

201. Araque, A.; Parpura, V.; Sanzgiri, R.P.; Haydon, P.G. Tripartite synapses: Glia, the unacknowledged partner. *Trends Neurosci.* **1999**, *22*, 208–215. [CrossRef]

202. Henneberger, C.; Papouin, T.; Oliet, S.H.; Rusakov, D.A. Long-term potentiation depends on release of D-serine from astrocytes. *Nature* **2010**, *463*, 232–236. [CrossRef] [PubMed]

203. Araque, A.; Carmignoto, G.; Haydon, P.G.; Oliet, S.H.; Robitaille, R.; Volterra, A. Gliotransmitters travel in time and space. *Neuron* **2014**, *81*, 728–739. [CrossRef] [PubMed]

204. Carriba, P.; Ortiz, O.; Patkar, K.; Justinova, Z.; Stroik, J.; Themann, A.; Muller, C.; Woods, A.S.; Hope, B.T.; Ciruela, F.; et al. Striatal adenosine A2a and cannabinoid CB1 receptors form functional heteromeric complexes that mediate the motor effects of cannabinoids. *Neuropsychopharmacology* **2007**, *32*, 2249–2259. [CrossRef] [PubMed]

205. Yang, L.; Qi, Y.; Yang, Y. Astrocytes control food intake by inhibiting agrp neuron activity via adenosine a1 receptors. *Cell Rep.* **2015**, *11*, 798–807. [CrossRef] [PubMed]

206. Garcia-Caceres, C.; Quarta, C.; Varela, L.; Gao, Y.; Gruber, T.; Legutko, B.; Jastroch, M.; Johansson, P.; Ninkovic, J.; Yi, C.X.; et al. Astrocytic insulin signaling couples brain glucose uptake with nutrient availability. *Cell* **2016**, *166*, 867–880. [CrossRef] [PubMed]

207. Leloup, C.; Allard, C.; Carneiro, L.; Fioramonti, X.; Collins, S.; Penicaud, L. Glucose and hypothalamic astrocytes: More than a fueling role? *Neuroscience* **2016**, *323*, 110–120. [CrossRef] [PubMed]

208. Rottkamp, D.M.; Rudenko, I.A.; Maier, M.T.; Roshanbin, S.; Yulyaningsih, E.; Perez, L.; Valdearcos, M.; Chua, S.; Koliwad, S.K.; Xu, A.W. Leptin potentiates astrogenesis in the developing hypothalamus. *Mol. Metab.* **2015**, *4*, 881–889. [CrossRef] [PubMed]

209. Kim, J.G.; Suyama, S.; Koch, M.; Jin, S.; Argente-Arizon, P.; Argente, J.; Liu, Z.W.; Zimmer, M.R.; Jeong, J.K.; Szigeti-Buck, K.; et al. Leptin signaling in astrocytes regulates hypothalamic neuronal circuits and feeding. *Nat. Neurosci.* **2014**, *17*, 908–910. [CrossRef] [PubMed]

210. Chowen, J.A.; Argente-Arizon, P.; Freire-Regatillo, A.; Frago, L.M.; Horvath, T.L.; Argente, J. The role of astrocytes in the hypothalamic response and adaptation to metabolic signals. *Prog. Neurobiol.* **2016**, *144*, 68–87. [CrossRef] [PubMed]

211. Rodriguez, E.M.; Blazquez, J.L.; Pastor, F.E.; Pelaez, B.; Pena, P.; Peruzzo, B.; Amat, P. Hypothalamic tanycytes: A key component of brain-endocrine interaction. *Int. Rev. Cytol.* **2005**, *247*, 89–164. [CrossRef]

212. Lazutkaite, G.; Solda, A.; Lossow, K.; Meyerhof, W.; Dale, N. Amino acid sensing in hypothalamic tanycytes via umami taste receptors. *Mol. Metab.* **2017**, *6*, 1480–1492. [CrossRef] [PubMed]

213. Balland, E.; Dam, J.; Langlet, F.; Caron, E.; Steculorum, S.; Messina, A.; Rasika, S.; Falluel-Morel, A.; Anouar, Y.; Dehouck, B.; et al. Hypothalamic tanycytes are an erk-gated conduit for leptin into the brain. *Cell Metab.* **2014**, *19*, 293–301. [CrossRef] [PubMed]

214. Suarez, J.; Romero-Zerbo, S.Y.; Rivera, P.; Bermudez-Silva, F.J.; Perez, J.; De Fonseca, F.R.; Fernandez-Llebrez, P. Endocannabinoid system in the adult rat circumventricular areas: An immunohistochemical study. *J. Comp. Neurol.* **2010**, *518*, 3065–3085. [CrossRef] [PubMed]

215. Goodman, T.; Hajihosseini, M.K. Hypothalamic tanycytes-masters and servants of metabolic, neuroendocrine, and neurogenic functions. *Front. Neurosci.* **2015**, *9*, 387. [CrossRef] [PubMed]

216. De Souza, C.T.; Araujo, E.P.; Bordin, S.; Ashimine, R.; Zollner, R.L.; Boschero, A.C.; Saad, M.J.; Velloso, L.A. Consumption of a fat-rich diet activates a proinflammatory response and induces insulin resistance in the hypothalamus. *Endocrinology* **2005**, *146*, 4192–4199. [CrossRef] [PubMed]

217. Andre, C.; Guzman-Quevedo, O.; Rey, C.; Remus-Borel, J.; Clark, S.; Castellanos-Jankiewicz, A.; Ladeveze, E.; Leste-Lasserre, T.; Nadjar, A.; Abrous, D.N.; et al. Inhibiting microglia expansion prevents diet-induced hypothalamic and peripheral inflammation. *Diabetes* **2017**, *66*, 908–919. [CrossRef] [PubMed]

218. Jin, S.; Kim, J.G.; Park, J.W.; Koch, M.; Horvath, T.L.; Lee, B.J. Hypothalamic TLR2 triggers sickness behavior via a microglia-neuronal axis. *Sci. Rep.* **2016**, *6*, 29424. [CrossRef] [PubMed]

219. Buckley, N.E.; McCoy, K.L.; Mezey, E.; Bonner, T.; Zimmer, A.; Felder, C.C.; Glass, M.; Zimmer, A. Immunomodulation by cannabinoids is absent in mice deficient for the cannabinoid CB(2) receptor. *Eur. J. Pharmacol.* **2000**, *396*, 141–149. [CrossRef]

220. Nunez, E.; Benito, C.; Pazos, M.R.; Barbachano, A.; Fajardo, O.; Gonzalez, S.; Tolon, R.M.; Romero, J. Cannabinoid CB2 receptors are expressed by perivascular microglial cells in the human brain: An immunohistochemical study. *Synapse* **2004**, *53*, 208–213. [CrossRef] [PubMed]

221. Carlisle, S.J.; Marciano-Cabral, F.; Staab, A.; Ludwick, C.; Cabral, G.A. Differential expression of the CB2 cannabinoid receptor by rodent macrophages and macrophage-like cells in relation to cell activation. *Int. Immunopharmacol.* **2002**, *2*, 69–82. [CrossRef]

222. Carrier, E.J.; Kearn, C.S.; Barkmeier, A.J.; Breese, N.M.; Yang, W.; Nithipatikom, K.; Pfister, S.L.; Campbell, W.B.; Hillard, C.J. Cultured rat microglial cells synthesize the endocannabinoid 2-arachidonylglycerol, which increases proliferation via a CB2 receptor-dependent mechanism. *Mol. Pharmacol.* **2004**, *65*, 999–1007. [CrossRef] [PubMed]

223. Li, Y.; Kim, J. Distinct roles of neuronal and microglial CB2 cannabinoid receptors in the mouse hippocampus. *Neuroscience* **2017**, *363*, 11–25. [CrossRef] [PubMed]

224. Palazuelos, J.; Aguado, T.; Pazos, M.R.; Julien, B.; Carrasco, C.; Resel, E.; Sagredo, O.; Benito, C.; Romero, J.; Azcoitia, I.; et al. Microglial CB2 cannabinoid receptors are neuroprotective in huntington's disease excitotoxicity. *Brain J. Neurol.* **2009**, *132*, 3152–3164. [CrossRef] [PubMed]

225. Maresz, K.; Carrier, E.J.; Ponomarev, E.D.; Hillard, C.J.; Dittel, B.N. Modulation of the cannabinoid CB2 receptor in microglial cells in response to inflammatory stimuli. *J. Neurochem.* **2005**, *95*, 437–445. [CrossRef] [PubMed]

226. Li, Y.; Kim, J. Neuronal expression of CB2 cannabinoid receptor mrnas in the mouse hippocampus. *Neuroscience* **2015**, *311*, 253–267. [CrossRef] [PubMed]

227. Quarta, C.; Bellocchio, L.; Mancini, G.; Mazza, R.; Cervino, C.; Braulke, L.J.; Fekete, C.; Latorre, R.; Nanni, C.; Bucci, M.; et al. CB(1) signaling in forebrain and sympathetic neurons is a key determinant of endocannabinoid actions on energy balance. *Cell Metab.* **2010**, *11*, 273–285. [CrossRef] [PubMed]

228. Deveaux, V.; Cadoudal, T.; Ichigotani, Y.; Teixeira-Clerc, F.; Louvet, A.; Manin, S.; Nhieu, J.T.; Belot, M.P.; Zimmer, A.; Even, P.; et al. Cannabinoid CB2 receptor potentiates obesity-associated inflammation, insulin resistance and hepatic steatosis. *PLoS ONE* **2009**, *4*, e5844. [CrossRef] [PubMed]

229. Barutta, F.; Piscitelli, F.; Pinach, S.; Bruno, G.; Gambino, R.; Rastaldi, M.P.; Salvidio, G.; Di Marzo, V.; Cavallo Perin, P.; Gruden, G. Protective role of cannabinoid receptor type 2 in a mouse model of diabetic nephropathy. *Diabetes* **2011**, *60*, 2386–2396. [CrossRef] [PubMed]

230. Gruden, G.; Barutta, F.; Kunos, G.; Pacher, P. Role of the endocannabinoid system in diabetes and diabetic complications. *Br. J. Pharmacol.* **2016**, *173*, 1116–1127. [CrossRef] [PubMed]

231. Cota, D.; Marsicano, G.; Tschop, M.; Grubler, Y.; Flachskamm, C.; Schubert, M.; Auer, D.; Yassouridis, A.; Thone-Reineke, C.; Ortmann, S.; et al. The endogenous cannabinoid system affects energy balance via central orexigenic drive and peripheral lipogenesis. *J. Clin. Investig.* **2003**, *112*, 423–431. [CrossRef] [PubMed]

232. Osei-Hyiaman, D.; DePetrillo, M.; Pacher, P.; Liu, J.; Radaeva, S.; Batkai, S.; Harvey-White, J.; Mackie, K.; Offertaler, L.; Wang, L.; et al. Endocannabinoid activation at hepatic CB1 receptors stimulates fatty acid synthesis and contributes to diet-induced obesity. *J. Clin. Investig.* **2005**, *115*, 1298–1305. [CrossRef] [PubMed]

233. Jourdan, T.; Djaouti, L.; Demizieux, L.; Gresti, J.; Verges, B.; Degrace, P. CB1 antagonism exerts specific molecular effects on visceral and subcutaneous fat and reverses liver steatosis in diet-induced obese mice. *Diabetes* **2010**, *59*, 926–934. [CrossRef] [PubMed]

234. Osei-Hyiaman, D.; Liu, J.; Zhou, L.; Godlewski, G.; Harvey-White, J.; Jeong, W.I.; Batkai, S.; Marsicano, G.; Lutz, B.; Buettner, C.; et al. Hepatic CB1 receptor is required for development of diet-induced steatosis, dyslipidemia, and insulin and leptin resistance in mice. *J. Clin. Investig.* **2008**, *118*, 3160–3169. [CrossRef] [PubMed]

235. Dinh, T.P.; Carpenter, D.; Leslie, F.M.; Freund, T.F.; Katona, I.; Sensi, S.L.; Kathuria, S.; Piomelli, D. Brain monoglyceride lipase participating in endocannabinoid inactivation. *Proc. Natl. Acad. Sci. USA* **2002**, *99*, 10819–10824. [CrossRef] [PubMed]

236. Karlsson, M.; Contreras, J.A.; Hellman, U.; Tornqvist, H.; Holm, C. Cdna cloning, tissue distribution, and identification of the catalytic triad of monoglyceride lipase. Evolutionary relationship to esterases, lysophospholipases, and haloperoxidases. *J. Biol. Chem.* **1997**, *272*, 27218–27223. [CrossRef] [PubMed]

237. Krott, L.M.; Piscitelli, F.; Heine, M.; Borrino, S.; Scheja, L.; Silvestri, C.; Heeren, J.; Di Marzo, V. Endocannabinoid regulation in white and brown adipose tissue following thermogenic activation. *J. Lipid Res.* **2016**, *57*, 464–473. [CrossRef] [PubMed]

238. Engeli, S.; Bohnke, J.; Feldpausch, M.; Gorzelniak, K.; Janke, J.; Batkai, S.; Pacher, P.; Harvey-White, J.; Luft, F.C.; Sharma, A.M.; et al. Activation of the peripheral endocannabinoid system in human obesity. *Diabetes* **2005**, *54*, 2838–2843. [CrossRef] [PubMed]

239. Jourdan, T.; Godlewski, G.; Kunos, G. Endocannabinoid regulation of beta-cell functions: Implications for glycaemic control and diabetes. *Diabetes Obes. Metab.* **2016**, *18*, 549–557. [CrossRef] [PubMed]

240. Kunos, G.; Osei-Hyiaman, D.; Liu, J.; Godlewski, G.; Batkai, S. Endocannabinoids and the control of energy homeostasis. *J. Biol. Chem.* **2008**, *283*, 33021–33025. [CrossRef] [PubMed]

241. Chambers, A.P.; Vemuri, V.K.; Peng, Y.; Wood, J.T.; Olszewska, T.; Pittman, Q.J.; Makriyannis, A.; Sharkey, K.A. A neutral CB1 receptor antagonist reduces weight gain in rat. *Am. J. Physiol. Regul. Integr. Comp. Physiol.* **2007**, *293*, R2185–R2193. [CrossRef] [PubMed]

242. Fernandez, J.R.; Allison, D.B. Rimonabant sanofi-synthelabo. *Curr. Opin. Investig. Drugs* **2004**, *5*, 430–435. [PubMed]

243. Sam, A.H.; Salem, V.; Ghatei, M.A. Rimonabant: From rio to ban. *J. Obes.* **2011**, *2011*, 432607. [CrossRef] [PubMed]

244. Ward, S.J.; Raffa, R.B. Rimonabant redux and strategies to improve the future outlook of CB1 receptor neutral-antagonist/inverse-agonist therapies. *Obesity (Silver Spring)* **2011**, *19*, 1325–1334. [CrossRef] [PubMed]

245. Yoshida, R.; Ohkuri, T.; Jyotaki, M.; Yasuo, T.; Horio, N.; Yasumatsu, K.; Sanematsu, K.; Shigemura, N.; Yamamoto, T.; Margolskee, R.F.; et al. Endocannabinoids selectively enhance sweet taste. *Proc. Natl. Acad. Sci. USA* **2010**, *107*, 935–939. [CrossRef] [PubMed]

246. Laugerette, F.; Passilly-Degrace, P.; Patris, B.; Niot, I.; Febbraio, M.; Montmayeur, J.P.; Besnard, P. Cd36 involvement in orosensory detection of dietary lipids, spontaneous fat preference, and digestive secretions. *J. Clin. Investig.* **2005**, *115*, 3177–3184. [CrossRef] [PubMed]

247. Sclafani, A.; Ackroff, K.; Abumrad, N.A. CD36 gene deletion reduces fat preference and intake but not post-oral fat conditioning in mice. *Am. J. Physiol. Regul. Integr. Comp. Physiol.* **2007**, *293*, R1823–R1832. [CrossRef] [PubMed]

248. Niki, M.; Jyotaki, M.; Yoshida, R.; Yasumatsu, K.; Shigemura, N.; DiPatrizio, N.V.; Piomelli, D.; Ninomiya, Y. Modulation of sweet taste sensitivities by endogenous leptin and endocannabinoids in mice. *J. Physiol.* **2015**, *593*, 2527–2545. [CrossRef] [PubMed]

249. Matias, I.; Gatta-Cherifi, B.; Tabarin, A.; Clark, S.; Leste-Lasserre, T.; Marsicano, G.; Piazza, P.V.; Cota, D. Endocannabinoids measurement in human saliva as potential biomarker of obesity. *PLoS ONE* **2012**, *7*, e42399. [CrossRef] [PubMed]

250. Choromanska, K.; Choromanska, B.; Dabrowska, E.; Baczek, W.; Mysliwiec, P.; Dadan, J.; Zalewska, A. Saliva of obese patients—Is it different? *Postepy Hig. Med. Dosw. (Online)* **2015**, *69*, 1190–1195. [CrossRef] [PubMed]

251. DiPatrizio, N.V.; Joslin, A.; Jung, K.M.; Piomelli, D. Endocannabinoid signaling in the gut mediates preference for dietary unsaturated fats. *FASEB J.* **2013**, *27*, 2513–2520. [CrossRef] [PubMed]

252. Passilly-Degrace, P.; Chevrot, M.; Bernard, A.; Ancel, D.; Martin, C.; Besnard, P. Is the taste of fat regulated? *Biochimie* **2014**, *96*, 3–7. [CrossRef] [PubMed]

253. Mattes, R.D. Oral fatty acid signaling and intestinal lipid processing: Support and supposition. *Physiol. Behav.* **2011**, *105*, 27–35. [CrossRef] [PubMed]

254. Stewart, J.E.; Feinle-Bisset, C.; Keast, R.S. Fatty acid detection during food consumption and digestion: Associations with ingestive behavior and obesity. *Prog. Lipid Res.* **2011**, *50*, 225–233. [CrossRef] [PubMed]

255. Simopoulos, A.P. An increase in the omega-6/omega-3 fatty acid ratio increases the risk for obesity. *Nutrients* **2016**, *8*, 128. [CrossRef] [PubMed]

256. Artmann, A.; Petersen, G.; Hellgren, L.I.; Boberg, J.; Skonberg, C.; Nellemann, C.; Hansen, S.H.; Hansen, H.S. Influence of dietary fatty acids on endocannabinoid and *N*-acylethanolamine levels in rat brain, liver and small intestine. *Biochim. Biophys. Acta* **2008**, *1781*, 200–212. [CrossRef] [PubMed]

257. Higgs, S.; Williams, C.M.; Kirkham, T.C. Cannabinoid influences on palatability: Microstructural analysis of sucrose drinking after delta(9)-tetrahydrocannabinol, anandamide, 2-arachidonoyl glycerol and sr141716. *Psychopharmacology (Berl.)* **2003**, *165*, 370–377. [CrossRef] [PubMed]

258. Kim, U.K.; Wooding, S.; Riaz, N.; Jorde, L.B.; Drayna, D. Variation in the human tas1r taste receptor genes. *Chem. Senses* **2006**, *31*, 599–611. [CrossRef] [PubMed]

259. Loper, H.B.; La Sala, M.; Dotson, C.; Steinle, N. Taste perception, associated hormonal modulation, and nutrient intake. *Nutr. Rev.* **2015**, *73*, 83–91. [CrossRef] [PubMed]

260. Yoshida, R.; Niki, M.; Jyotaki, M.; Sanematsu, K.; Shigemura, N.; Ninomiya, Y. Modulation of sweet responses of taste receptor cells. *Semin. Cell Dev. Biol.* **2013**, *24*, 226–231. [CrossRef] [PubMed]

261. Kopach, O.; Vats, J.; Netsyk, O.; Voitenko, N.; Irving, A.; Fedirko, N. Cannabinoid receptors in submandibular acinar cells: Functional coupling between saliva fluid and electrolytes secretion and Ca^{2+} signalling. *J. Cell Sci.* **2012**, *125*, 1884–1895. [CrossRef] [PubMed]

262. Prestifilippo, J.P.; Fernandez-Solari, J.; de la Cal, C.; Iribarne, M.; Suburo, A.M.; Rettori, V.; McCann, S.M.; Elverdin, J.C. Inhibition of salivary secretion by activation of cannabinoid receptors. *Exp. Biol. Med. (Maywood)* **2006**, *231*, 1421–1429. [CrossRef] [PubMed]

263. Izzo, A.A.; Sharkey, K.A. Cannabinoids and the gut: New developments and emerging concepts. *Pharmacol. Ther.* **2010**, *126*, 21–38. [CrossRef] [PubMed]

264. Fichna, J.; Bawa, M.; Thakur, G.A.; Tichkule, R.; Makriyannis, A.; McCafferty, D.M.; Sharkey, K.A.; Storr, M. Cannabinoids alleviate experimentally induced intestinal inflammation by acting at central and peripheral receptors. *PLoS ONE* **2014**, *9*, e109115. [CrossRef] [PubMed]

265. Kinsey, S.G.; Nomura, D.K.; O'Neal, S.T.; Long, J.Z.; Mahadevan, A.; Cravatt, B.F.; Grider, J.R.; Lichtman, A.H. Inhibition of monoacylglycerol lipase attenuates nonsteroidal anti-inflammatory drug-induced gastric hemorrhages in mice. *J. Pharmacol. Exp. Ther.* **2011**, *338*, 795–802. [CrossRef] [PubMed]

266. Massa, F.; Sibaev, A.; Marsicano, G.; Blaudzun, H.; Storr, M.; Lutz, B. Vanilloid receptor (TRPV1)-deficient mice show increased susceptibility to dinitrobenzene sulfonic acid induced colitis. *J. Mol. Med. (Berl.)* **2006**, *84*, 142–146. [CrossRef] [PubMed]

267. O'Sullivan, S.E. Cannabinoids go nuclear: Evidence for activation of peroxisome proliferator-activated receptors. *Br. J. Pharmacol.* **2007**, *152*, 576–582. [CrossRef] [PubMed]

268. Fredriksson, R.; Hoglund, P.J.; Gloriam, D.E.; Lagerstrom, M.C.; Schioth, H.B. Seven evolutionarily conserved human rhodopsin G protein-coupled receptors lacking close relatives. *FEBS Lett.* **2003**, *554*, 381–388. [CrossRef]

269. Ryberg, E.; Larsson, N.; Sjogren, S.; Hjorth, S.; Hermansson, N.O.; Leonova, J.; Elebring, T.; Nilsson, K.; Drmota, T.; Greasley, P.J. The orphan receptor GPR55 is a novel cannabinoid receptor. *Br. J. Pharmacol.* **2007**, *152*, 1092–1101. [CrossRef] [PubMed]

270. Fu, J.; Gaetani, S.; Oveisi, F.; Lo Verme, J.; Serrano, A.; Rodriguez De Fonseca, F.; Rosengarth, A.; Luecke, H.; Di Giacomo, B.; Tarzia, G.; et al. Oleylethanolamide regulates feeding and body weight through activation of the nuclear receptor ppar-alpha. *Nature* **2003**, *425*, 90–93. [CrossRef] [PubMed]

271. Ahern, G.P. Activation of trpv1 by the satiety factor oleoylethanolamide. *J. Biol. Chem.* **2003**, *278*, 30429–30434. [CrossRef] [PubMed]

272. Borrelli, F.; Izzo, A.A. Role of acylethanolamides in the gastrointestinal tract with special reference to food intake and energy balance. *Best Pract. Res. Clin. Endocrinol. Metab.* **2009**, *23*, 33–49. [CrossRef] [PubMed]

273. Piomelli, D.; Beltramo, M.; Giuffrida, A.; Stella, N. Endogenous cannabinoid signaling. *Neurobiol. Dis.* **1998**, *5*, 462–473. [CrossRef] [PubMed]

274. Astarita, G.; Rourke, B.C.; Andersen, J.B.; Fu, J.; Kim, J.H.; Bennett, A.F.; Hicks, J.W.; Piomelli, D. Postprandial increase of oleoylethanolamide mobilization in small intestine of the burmese python (python molurus). *Am. J. Physiol. Regul. Integr. Comp. Physiol.* **2006**, *290*, R1407–R1412. [CrossRef] [PubMed]

275. Izzo, A.A.; Piscitelli, F.; Capasso, R.; Marini, P.; Cristino, L.; Petrosino, S.; Di Marzo, V. Basal and fasting/refeeding-regulated tissue levels of endogenous ppar-alpha ligands in zucker rats. *Obesity (Silver Spring)* **2010**, *18*, 55–62. [CrossRef] [PubMed]

276. Lo Verme, J.; Gaetani, S.; Fu, J.; Oveisi, F.; Burton, K.; Piomelli, D. Regulation of food intake by oleoylethanolamide. *Cell. Mol. Life Sci.* **2005**, *62*, 708–716. [CrossRef] [PubMed]

277. Rodriguez de Fonseca, F.; Navarro, M.; Gomez, R.; Escuredo, L.; Nava, F.; Fu, J.; Murillo-Rodriguez, E.; Giuffrida, A.; LoVerme, J.; Gaetani, S.; et al. An anorexic lipid mediator regulated by feeding. *Nature* **2001**, *414*, 209–212. [CrossRef] [PubMed]

278. Karwad, M.A.; Macpherson, T.; Wang, B.; Theophilidou, E.; Sarmad, S.; Barrett, D.A.; Larvin, M.; Wright, K.L.; Lund, J.N.; O'Sullivan, S.E. Oleoylethanolamine and palmitoylethanolamine modulate intestinal permeability in vitro via TRPV1 and PPARalpha. *FASEB J.* **2017**, *31*, 469–481. [CrossRef] [PubMed]

279. Lauffer, L.M.; Iakoubov, R.; Brubaker, P.L. GPR119 is essential for oleoylethanolamide-induced glucagon-like peptide-1 secretion from the intestinal enteroendocrine L-cell. *Diabetes* **2009**, *58*, 1058–1066. [CrossRef] [PubMed]

280. Cani, P.D.; Plovier, H.; Van Hul, M.; Geurts, L.; Delzenne, N.M.; Druart, C.; Everard, A. Endocannabinoids—At the crossroads between the gut microbiota and host metabolism. *Nat. Rev. Endocrinol.* **2016**, *12*, 133–143. [CrossRef] [PubMed]

281. Di Marzo, V.; Matias, I. Endocannabinoid control of food intake and energy balance. *Nat. Neurosci.* **2005**, *8*, 585–589. [CrossRef] [PubMed]

282. Massa, F.; Storr, M.; Lutz, B. The endocannabinoid system in the physiology and pathophysiology of the gastrointestinal tract. *J. Mol. Med. (Berl.)* **2005**, *83*, 944–954. [CrossRef] [PubMed]

283. Tellez, L.A.; Medina, S.; Han, W.; Ferreira, J.G.; Licona-Limon, P.; Ren, X.; Lam, T.T.; Schwartz, G.J.; de Araujo, I.E. A gut lipid messenger links excess dietary fat to dopamine deficiency. *Science* **2013**, *341*, 800–802. [CrossRef] [PubMed]

284. Monteleone, P.; Matias, I.; Martiadis, V.; De Petrocellis, L.; Maj, M.; Di Marzo, V. Blood levels of the endocannabinoid anandamide are increased in anorexia nervosa and in binge-eating disorder, but not in bulimia nervosa. *Neuropsychopharmacology* **2005**, *30*, 1216–1221. [CrossRef] [PubMed]

285. Argueta, D.A.; DiPatrizio, N.V. Peripheral endocannabinoid signaling controls hyperphagia in western diet-induced obesity. *Physiol. Behav.* **2017**, *171*, 32–39. [CrossRef] [PubMed]

286. Berge, K.; Piscitelli, F.; Hoem, N.; Silvestri, C.; Meyer, I.; Banni, S.; Di Marzo, V. Chronic treatment with krill powder reduces plasma triglyceride and anandamide levels in mildly obese men. *Lipids Health Dis.* **2013**, *12*, 78. [CrossRef] [PubMed]

287. Berger, A.; Crozier, G.; Bisogno, T.; Cavaliere, P.; Innis, S.; Di Marzo, V. Anandamide and diet: Inclusion of dietary arachidonate and docosahexaenoate leads to increased brain levels of the corresponding *N*-acylethanolamines in piglets. *Proc. Natl. Acad. Sci. USA* **2001**, *98*, 6402–6406. [CrossRef] [PubMed]

288. Watanabe, S.; Doshi, M.; Hamazaki, T. N-3 polyunsaturated fatty acid (PUFA) deficiency elevates and n-3 pufa enrichment reduces brain 2-arachidonoylglycerol level in mice. *Prostaglandins Leukot. Essent. Fatty Acids* **2003**, *69*, 51–59. [CrossRef]

289. Nieves, D.; Moreno, J.J. Effect of arachidonic and eicosapentaenoic acid metabolism on raw 264.7 macrophage proliferation. *J. Cell. Physiol.* **2006**, *208*, 428–434. [CrossRef] [PubMed]

290. Petersen, G.; Sorensen, C.; Schmid, P.C.; Artmann, A.; Tang-Christensen, M.; Hansen, S.H.; Larsen, P.J.; Schmid, H.H.; Hansen, H.S. Intestinal levels of anandamide and oleoylethanolamide in food-deprived rats are regulated through their precursors. *Biochim. Biophys. Acta* **2006**, *1761*, 143–150. [CrossRef] [PubMed]

291. Sykaras, A.G.; Demenis, C.; Case, R.M.; McLaughlin, J.T.; Smith, C.P. Duodenal enteroendocrine i-cells contain mRNA transcripts encoding key endocannabinoid and fatty acid receptors. *PLoS ONE* **2012**, *7*, e42373. [CrossRef] [PubMed]

292. Rousseaux, C.; Thuru, X.; Gelot, A.; Barnich, N.; Neut, C.; Dubuquoy, L.; Dubuquoy, C.; Merour, E.; Geboes, K.; Chamaillard, M.; et al. Lactobacillus acidophilus modulates intestinal pain and induces opioid and cannabinoid receptors. *Nat. Med.* **2007**, *13*, 35–37. [CrossRef] [PubMed]

293. Cluny, N.L.; Keenan, C.M.; Reimer, R.A.; Le Foll, B.; Sharkey, K.A. Prevention of diet-induced obesity effects on body weight and gut microbiota in mice treated chronically with delta9-tetrahydrocannabinol. *PLoS ONE* **2015**, *10*, e0144270. [CrossRef] [PubMed]

294. DiPatrizio, N.V.; Astarita, G.; Schwartz, G.; Li, X.; Piomelli, D. Endocannabinoid signal in the gut controls dietary fat intake. *Proc. Natl. Acad. Sci. USA* **2011**, *108*, 12904–12908. [CrossRef] [PubMed]

295. Cooper, M.E.; Regnell, S.E. The hepatic cannabinoid 1 receptor as a modulator of hepatic energy state and food intake. *Br. J. Clin. Pharmacol.* **2014**, *77*, 21–30. [CrossRef] [PubMed]

296. Jeong, W.I.; Osei-Hyiaman, D.; Park, O.; Liu, J.; Batkai, S.; Mukhopadhyay, P.; Horiguchi, N.; Harvey-White, J.; Marsicano, G.; Lutz, B.; et al. Paracrine activation of hepatic CB1 receptors by stellate cell-derived endocannabinoids mediates alcoholic fatty liver. *Cell Metab.* **2008**, *7*, 227–235. [CrossRef] [PubMed]

297. Liu, J.; Cinar, R.; Xiong, K.; Godlewski, G.; Jourdan, T.; Lin, Y.; Ntambi, J.M.; Kunos, G. Monounsaturated fatty acids generated via stearoyl coa desaturase-1 are endogenous inhibitors of fatty acid amide hydrolase. *Proc. Natl. Acad. Sci. USA* **2013**, *110*, 18832–18837. [CrossRef] [PubMed]

298. Chanda, D.; Kim, Y.H.; Li, T.; Misra, J.; Kim, D.K.; Kim, J.R.; Kwon, J.; Jeong, W.I.; Ahn, S.H.; Park, T.S.; et al. Hepatic cannabinoid receptor type 1 mediates alcohol-induced regulation of bile acid enzyme genes expression via crebh. *PLoS ONE* **2013**, *8*, e68845. [CrossRef] [PubMed]

299. Magotti, P.; Bauer, I.; Igarashi, M.; Babagoli, M.; Marotta, R.; Piomelli, D.; Garau, G. Structure of human *N*-acylphosphatidylethanolamine-hydrolyzing phospholipase D: Regulation of fatty acid ethanolamide biosynthesis by bile acids. *Structure* **2015**, *23*, 598–604. [CrossRef] [PubMed]

300. Margheritis, E.; Castellani, B.; Magotti, P.; Peruzzi, S.; Romeo, E.; Natali, F.; Mostarda, S.; Gioiello, A.; Piomelli, D.; Garau, G. Bile acid recognition by nape-pld. *ACS Chem. Biol.* **2016**, *11*, 2908–2914. [CrossRef] [PubMed]

301. Linari, G.; Agostini, S.; Amadoro, G.; Ciotti, M.T.; Florenzano, F.; Improta, G.; Petrella, C.; Severini, C.; Broccardo, M. Involvement of cannabinoid CB1- and CB2-receptors in the modulation of exocrine pancreatic secretion. *Pharmacol. Res.* **2009**, *59*, 207–214. [CrossRef] [PubMed]

302. Michler, T.; Storr, M.; Kramer, J.; Ochs, S.; Malo, A.; Reu, S.; Goke, B.; Schafer, C. Activation of cannabinoid receptor 2 reduces inflammation in acute experimental pancreatitis via intra-acinar activation of p38 and MK2-dependent mechanisms. *Am. J. Physiol. Gastrointest. Liver Physiol.* **2013**, *304*, G181–G192. [CrossRef] [PubMed]

303. Doyle, M.E. The role of the endocannabinoid system in islet biology. *Curr. Opin. Endocrinol. Diabetes Obes.* **2011**, *18*, 153–158. [CrossRef] [PubMed]

304. Rohrbach, K.; Thomas, M.A.; Glick, S.; Fung, E.N.; Wang, V.; Watson, L.; Gregory, P.; Antel, J.; Pelleymounter, M.A. Ibipinabant attenuates beta-cell loss in male zucker diabetic fatty rats independently of its effects on body weight. *Diabetes Obes. Metab.* **2012**, *14*, 555–564. [CrossRef] [PubMed]

305. Jourdan, T.; Godlewski, G.; Cinar, R.; Bertola, A.; Szanda, G.; Liu, J.; Tam, J.; Han, T.; Mukhopadhyay, B.; Skarulis, M.C.; et al. Activation of the Nlrp3 inflammasome in infiltrating macrophages by endocannabinoids mediates beta cell loss in type 2 diabetes. *Nat. Med.* **2013**, *19*, 1132–1140. [CrossRef] [PubMed]

306. Juan-Pico, P.; Fuentes, E.; Bermudez-Silva, F.J.; Javier Diaz-Molina, F.; Ripoll, C.; Rodriguez de Fonseca, F.; Nadal, A. Cannabinoid receptors regulate Ca(2+) signals and insulin secretion in pancreatic beta-cell. *Cell Calcium* **2006**, *39*, 155–162. [CrossRef] [PubMed]

307. Starowicz, K.M.; Cristino, L.; Matias, I.; Capasso, R.; Racioppi, A.; Izzo, A.A.; Di Marzo, V. Endocannabinoid dysregulation in the pancreas and adipose tissue of mice fed with a high-fat diet. *Obesity (Silver Spring)* **2008**, *16*, 553–565. [CrossRef] [PubMed]

308. Horvath, B.; Mukhopadhyay, P.; Hasko, G.; Pacher, P. The endocannabinoid system and plant-derived cannabinoids in diabetes and diabetic complications. *Am. J. Pathol.* **2012**, *180*, 432–442. [CrossRef] [PubMed]

309. Malenczyk, K.; Jazurek, M.; Keimpema, E.; Silvestri, C.; Janikiewicz, J.; Mackie, K.; Di Marzo, V.; Redowicz, M.J.; Harkany, T.; Dobrzyn, A. CB1 cannabinoid receptors couple to focal adhesion kinase to control insulin release. *J. Biol. Chem.* **2013**, *288*, 32685–32699. [CrossRef] [PubMed]

310. Kim, W.; Lao, Q.; Shin, Y.K.; Carlson, O.D.; Lee, E.K.; Gorospe, M.; Kulkarni, R.N.; Egan, J.M. Cannabinoids induce pancreatic beta-cell death by directly inhibiting insulin receptor activation. *Sci. Signal.* **2012**, *5*, ra23. [CrossRef] [PubMed]

311. Malenczyk, K.; Keimpema, E.; Piscitelli, F.; Calvigioni, D.; Bjorklund, P.; Mackie, K.; Di Marzo, V.; Hokfelt, T.G.; Dobrzyn, A.; Harkany, T. Fetal endocannabinoids orchestrate the organization of pancreatic islet microarchitecture. *Proc. Natl. Acad. Sci. USA* **2015**, *112*, E6185–E6194. [CrossRef] [PubMed]

312. Bermudez-Silva, F.J.; Sanchez-Vera, I.; Suarez, J.; Serrano, A.; Fuentes, E.; Juan-Pico, P.; Nadal, A.; Rodriguez de Fonseca, F. Role of cannabinoid CB2 receptors in glucose homeostasis in rats. *Eur. J. Pharmacol.* **2007**, *565*, 207–211. [CrossRef] [PubMed]

313. Pacher, P.; Mechoulam, R. Is lipid signaling through cannabinoid 2 receptors part of a protective system? *Prog. Lipid Res.* **2011**, *50*, 193–211. [CrossRef] [PubMed]

314. Cavuoto, P.; McAinch, A.J.; Hatzinikolas, G.; Cameron-Smith, D.; Wittert, G.A. Effects of cannabinoid receptors on skeletal muscle oxidative pathways. *Mol. Cell. Endocrinol.* **2007**, *267*, 63–69. [CrossRef] [PubMed]

315. Cavuoto, P.; McAinch, A.J.; Hatzinikolas, G.; Janovska, A.; Game, P.; Wittert, G.A. The expression of receptors for endocannabinoids in human and rodent skeletal muscle. *Biochem. Biophys. Res. Commun.* **2007**, *364*, 105–110. [CrossRef] [PubMed]

316. Crespillo, A.; Suarez, J.; Bermudez-Silva, F.J.; Rivera, P.; Vida, M.; Alonso, M.; Palomino, A.; Lucena, M.A.; Serrano, A.; Perez-Martin, M.; et al. Expression of the cannabinoid system in muscle: Effects of a high-fat diet and CB1 receptor blockade. *Biochem. J.* **2011**, *433*, 175–185. [CrossRef] [PubMed]

317. Eckardt, K.; Sell, H.; Taube, A.; Koenen, M.; Platzbecker, B.; Cramer, A.; Horrighs, A.; Lehtonen, M.; Tennagels, N.; Eckel, J. Cannabinoid type 1 receptors in human skeletal muscle cells participate in the negative crosstalk between fat and muscle. *Diabetologia* **2009**, *52*, 664–674. [CrossRef] [PubMed]

318. Esposito, I.; Proto, M.C.; Gazzerro, P.; Laezza, C.; Miele, C.; Alberobello, A.T.; D'Esposito, V.; Beguinot, F.; Formisano, P.; Bifulco, M. The cannabinoid cb1 receptor antagonist rimonabant stimulates 2-deoxyglucose uptake in skeletal muscle cells by regulating the expression of phosphatidylinositol-3-kinase. *Mol. Pharmacol.* **2008**, *74*, 1678–1686. [CrossRef] [PubMed]

319. Lipina, C.; Stretton, C.; Hastings, S.; Hundal, J.S.; Mackie, K.; Irving, A.J.; Hundal, H.S. Regulation of MAP kinase-directed mitogenic and protein kinase B-mediated signaling by cannabinoid receptor type 1 in skeletal muscle cells. *Diabetes* **2010**, *59*, 375–385. [CrossRef] [PubMed]

320. Tedesco, L.; Valerio, A.; Dossena, M.; Cardile, A.; Ragni, M.; Pagano, C.; Pagotto, U.; Carruba, M.O.; Vettor, R.; Nisoli, E. Cannabinoid receptor stimulation impairs mitochondrial biogenesis in mouse white adipose tissue, muscle, and liver: The role of enos, p38 mapk, and ampk pathways. *Diabetes* **2010**, *59*, 2826–2836. [CrossRef] [PubMed]

321. Luo, Z.; Ma, L.; Zhao, Z.; He, H.; Yang, D.; Feng, X.; Ma, S.; Chen, X.; Zhu, T.; Cao, T.; et al. Trpv1 activation improves exercise endurance and energy metabolism through PGC-1alpha upregulation in mice. *Cell Res.* **2012**, *22*, 551–564. [CrossRef] [PubMed]

322. Ito, N.; Ruegg, U.T.; Kudo, A.; Miyagoe-Suzuki, Y.; Takeda, S. Capsaicin mimics mechanical load-induced intracellular signaling events: Involvement of TRPV1-mediated calcium signaling in induction of skeletal muscle hypertrophy. *Channels (Austin)* **2013**, *7*, 221–224. [CrossRef] [PubMed]

323. Buettner, C.; Muse, E.D.; Cheng, A.; Chen, L.; Scherer, T.; Pocai, A.; Su, K.; Cheng, B.; Li, X.; Harvey-White, J.; et al. Leptin controls adipose tissue lipogenesis via central, STAT3-independent mechanisms. *Nat. Med.* **2008**, *14*, 667–675. [CrossRef] [PubMed]

324. Ge, Q.; Maury, E.; Rycken, L.; Gerard, J.; Noel, L.; Detry, R.; Navez, B.; Brichard, S.M. Endocannabinoids regulate adipokine production and the immune balance of omental adipose tissue in human obesity. *Int. J. Obes. (Lond.)* **2013**, *37*, 874–880. [CrossRef] [PubMed]

325. Murumalla, R.; Bencharif, K.; Gence, L.; Bhattacharya, A.; Tallet, F.; Gonthier, M.P.; Petrosino, S.; di Marzo, V.; Cesari, M.; Hoareau, L.; et al. Effect of the cannabinoid receptor-1 antagonist SR141716A on human adipocyte inflammatory profile and differentiation. *J. Inflamm. (Lond.)* **2011**, *8*, 33. [CrossRef] [PubMed]

326. Barazzoni, R.; Gortan Cappellari, G.; Ragni, M.; Nisoli, E. Insulin resistance in obesity: An overview of fundamental alterations. *Eat. Weight Disord.* **2018**, *23*, 149–157. [CrossRef] [PubMed]

327. Braune, J.; Weyer, U.; Hobusch, C.; Mauer, J.; Bruning, J.C.; Bechmann, I.; Gericke, M. Il-6 regulates m2 polarization and local proliferation of adipose tissue macrophages in obesity. *J. Immunol.* **2017**, *198*, 2927–2934. [CrossRef] [PubMed]

328. Braune, J.; Weyer, U.; Matz-Soja, M.; Hobusch, C.; Kern, M.; Kunath, A.; Kloting, N.; Kralisch, S.; Bluher, M.; Gebhardt, R.; et al. Hedgehog signalling in myeloid cells impacts on body weight, adipose tissue inflammation and glucose metabolism. *Diabetologia* **2017**, *60*, 889–899. [CrossRef] [PubMed]

329. Haim, Y.; Bluher, M.; Konrad, D.; Goldstein, N.; Kloting, N.; Harman-Boehm, I.; Kirshtein, B.; Ginsberg, D.; Tarnovscki, T.; Gepner, Y.; et al. ASK1 (MAP3K5) is transcriptionally upregulated by E2F1 in adipose tissue in obesity, molecularly defining a human dys-metabolic obese phenotype. *Mol. Metab.* **2017**, *6*, 725–736. [CrossRef] [PubMed]

330. Chatzigeorgiou, A.; Chavakis, T. Immune cells and metabolism. *Handb Exp. Pharmacol.* **2016**, *233*, 221–249. [PubMed]

331. Seijkens, T.; Kusters, P.; Chatzigeorgiou, A.; Chavakis, T.; Lutgens, E. Immune cell crosstalk in obesity: A key role for costimulation? *Diabetes* **2014**, *63*, 3982–3991. [CrossRef] [PubMed]

332. Bensaid, M.; Gary-Bobo, M.; Esclangon, A.; Maffrand, J.P.; Le Fur, G.; Oury-Donat, F.; Soubrie, P. The cannabinoid CB1 receptor antagonist SR141716 increases Acrp30 mRNA expression in adipose tissue of obese fa/fa rats and in cultured adipocyte cells. *Mol. Pharmacol.* **2003**, *63*, 908–914. [CrossRef] [PubMed]

333. Tedesco, L.; Valerio, A.; Cervino, C.; Cardile, A.; Pagano, C.; Vettor, R.; Pasquali, R.; Carruba, M.O.; Marsicano, G.; Lutz, B.; et al. Cannabinoid type 1 receptor blockade promotes mitochondrial biogenesis through endothelial nitric oxide synthase expression in white adipocytes. *Diabetes* **2008**, *57*, 2028–2036. [CrossRef] [PubMed]

334. Silvestri, C.; Di Marzo, V. The endocannabinoid system in energy homeostasis and the etiopathology of metabolic disorders. *Cell Metab.* **2013**, *17*, 475–490. [CrossRef] [PubMed]

335. Perwitz, N.; Wenzel, J.; Wagner, I.; Buning, J.; Drenckhan, M.; Zarse, K.; Ristow, M.; Lilienthal, W.; Lehnert, H.; Klein, J. Cannabinoid type 1 receptor blockade induces transdifferentiation towards a brown fat phenotype in white adipocytes. *Diabetes Obes. Metab.* **2010**, *12*, 158–166. [CrossRef] [PubMed]

336. Seale, P.; Bjork, B.; Yang, W.; Kajimura, S.; Chin, S.; Kuang, S.; Scime, A.; Devarakonda, S.; Conroe, H.M.; Erdjument-Bromage, H.; et al. Prdm16 controls a brown fat/skeletal muscle switch. *Nature* **2008**, *454*, 961–967. [CrossRef] [PubMed]

337. Vitali, A.; Murano, I.; Zingaretti, M.C.; Frontini, A.; Ricquier, D.; Cinti, S. The adipose organ of obesity-prone C57BL/6J mice is composed of mixed white and brown adipocytes. *J. Lipid Res.* **2012**, *53*, 619–629. [CrossRef] [PubMed]

338. Bartelt, A.; Heeren, J. The holy grail of metabolic disease: Brown adipose tissue. *Curr. Opin. Lipidol.* **2012**, *23*, 190–195. [CrossRef] [PubMed]

339. Cannon, B.; Nedergaard, J. Brown adipose tissue: Function and physiological significance. *Physiol. Rev.* **2004**, *84*, 277–359. [CrossRef] [PubMed]

340. Hawkins, M.N.; Horvath, T.L. Cannabis in fat: High hopes to treat obesity. *J. Clin. Investig.* **2017**, *127*, 3918–3920. [CrossRef] [PubMed]

341. Ruiz de Azua, I.; Mancini, G.; Srivastava, R.K.; Rey, A.A.; Cardinal, P.; Tedesco, L.; Zingaretti, C.M.; Sassmann, A.; Quarta, C.; Schwitter, C.; et al. Adipocyte cannabinoid receptor CB1 regulates energy homeostasis and alternatively activated macrophages. *J. Clin. Investig.* **2017**, *127*, 4148–4162. [CrossRef] [PubMed]

342. Crowe, M.S.; Nass, S.R.; Gabella, K.M.; Kinsey, S.G. The endocannabinoid system modulates stress, emotionality, and inflammation. *Brain Behav. Immun.* **2014**, *42*, 1–5. [CrossRef] [PubMed]

343. Hill, M.N.; Tasker, J.G. Endocannabinoid signaling, glucocorticoid-mediated negative feedback, and regulation of the hypothalamic-pituitary-adrenal axis. *Neuroscience* **2012**, *204*, 5–16. [CrossRef] [PubMed]

344. Surkin, P.N.; Gallino, S.L.; Luce, V.; Correa, F.; Fernandez-Solari, J.; De Laurentiis, A. Pharmacological augmentation of endocannabinoid signaling reduces the neuroendocrine response to stress. *Psychoneuroendocrinology* **2018**, *87*, 131–140. [CrossRef] [PubMed]

345. Howlett, A.C.; Barth, F.; Bonner, T.I.; Cabral, G.; Casellas, P.; Devane, W.A.; Felder, C.C.; Herkenham, M.; Mackie, K.; Martin, B.R.; et al. International union of pharmacology. XXVII. Classification of cannabinoid receptors. *Pharmacol. Rev.* **2002**, *54*, 161–202. [CrossRef] [PubMed]

346. Mechoulam, R.; Parker, L.A. The endocannabinoid system and the brain. *Annu. Rev. Psychol.* **2013**, *64*, 21–47. [CrossRef] [PubMed]

347. Ziegler, C.G.; Mohn, C.; Lamounier-Zepter, V.; Rettori, V.; Bornstein, S.R.; Krug, A.W.; Ehrhart-Bornstein, M. Expression and function of endocannabinoid receptors in the human adrenal cortex. *Horm. Metab. Res.* **2010**, *42*, 88–92. [CrossRef] [PubMed]

348. Evanson, N.K.; Tasker, J.G.; Hill, M.N.; Hillard, C.J.; Herman, J.P. Fast feedback inhibition of the HPA axis by glucocorticoids is mediated by endocannabinoid signaling. *Endocrinology* **2010**, *151*, 4811–4819. [CrossRef] [PubMed]

349. Pertwee, R.G. Endocannabinoids and their pharmacological actions. *Handb. Exp. Pharmacol.* **2015**, *231*, 1–37. [PubMed]

350. Hill, M.N.; McEwen, B.S. Involvement of the endocannabinoid system in the neurobehavioural effects of stress and glucocorticoids. *Prog. Neuropsychopharmacol. Biol. Psychiatry* **2010**, *34*, 791–797. [CrossRef] [PubMed]

351. Newsom, R.J.; Osterlund, C.; Masini, C.V.; Day, H.E.; Spencer, R.L.; Campeau, S. Cannabinoid receptor type 1 antagonism significantly modulates basal and loud noise induced neural and hypothalamic-pituitary-adrenal axis responses in male sprague-dawley rats. *Neuroscience* **2012**, *204*, 64–73. [CrossRef] [PubMed]

352. Patel, S.; Roelke, C.T.; Rademacher, D.J.; Cullinan, W.E.; Hillard, C.J. Endocannabinoid signaling negatively modulates stress-induced activation of the hypothalamic-pituitary-adrenal axis. *Endocrinology* **2004**, *145*, 5431–5438. [CrossRef] [PubMed]

353. Feldman, S.; Weidenfeld, J. Involvement of endogeneous glutamate in the stimulatory effect of norepinephrine and serotonin on the hypothalamo-pituitary-adrenocortical axis. *Neuroendocrinology* **2004**, *79*, 43–53. [CrossRef] [PubMed]

354. Rabasa, C.; Pastor-Ciurana, J.; Delgado-Morales, R.; Gomez-Roman, A.; Carrasco, J.; Gagliano, H.; Garcia-Gutierrez, M.S.; Manzanares, J.; Armario, A. Evidence against a critical role of CB1 receptors in adaptation of the hypothalamic-pituitary-adrenal axis and other consequences of daily repeated stress. *Eur. Neuropsychopharmacol.* **2015**, *25*, 1248–1259. [CrossRef] [PubMed]

355. Ross, R.A. Anandamide and vanilloid TRPV1 receptors. *Br. J. Pharmacol.* **2003**, *140*, 790–801. [CrossRef] [PubMed]

356. Ortiga-Carvalho, T.M.; Chiamolera, M.I.; Pazos-Moura, C.C.; Wondisford, F.E. Hypothalamus-pituitary-thyroid axis. *Comp. Physiol.* **2016**, *6*, 1387–1428.

357. Behan, L.A.; Monson, J.P.; Agha, A. The interaction between growth hormone and the thyroid axis in hypopituitary patients. *Clin. Endocrinol. (Oxf.)* **2011**, *74*, 281–288. [CrossRef] [PubMed]

358. Pagotto, U.; Marsicano, G.; Cota, D.; Lutz, B.; Pasquali, R. The emerging role of the endocannabinoid system in endocrine regulation and energy balance. *Endocr. Rev.* **2006**, *27*, 73–100. [CrossRef] [PubMed]

359. Kokka, N.; Garcia, J.F. Effects of delta 9-THC on growth hormone and ACTH secretion in rats. *Life Sci.* **1974**, *15*, 329–338. [CrossRef]

360. Wolf, M.; Ingbar, S.H.; Moses, A.C. Thyroid hormone and growth hormone interact to regulate insulin-like growth factor-i messenger ribonucleic acid and circulating levels in the rat. *Endocrinology* **1989**, *125*, 2905–2914. [CrossRef] [PubMed]

361. Li, Z.; Schmidt, S.F.; Friedman, J.M. Developmental role for endocannabinoid signaling in regulating glucose metabolism and growth. *Diabetes* **2013**, *62*, 2359–2367. [CrossRef] [PubMed]

362. Da Veiga, M.A.; Fonseca Bloise, F.; Costa, E.S.R.H.; Souza, L.L.; Almeida, N.A.; Oliveira, K.J.; Pazos-Moura, C.C. Acute effects of endocannabinoid anandamide and CB1 receptor antagonist, AM251 in the regulation of thyrotropin secretion. *J. Endocrinol.* **2008**, *199*, 235–242. [CrossRef] [PubMed]

363. Hillard, C.J.; Farber, N.E.; Hagen, T.C.; Bloom, A.S. The effects of delta 9-tetrahydrocannabinol on serum thyrotropin levels in the rat. *Pharmacol. Biochem. Behav.* **1984**, *20*, 547–550. [CrossRef]

364. Porcella, A.; Marchese, G.; Casu, M.A.; Rocchitta, A.; Lai, M.L.; Gessa, G.L.; Pani, L. Evidence for functional cb1 cannabinoid receptor expressed in the rat thyroid. *Eur. J. Endocrinol.* **2002**, *147*, 255–261. [CrossRef] [PubMed]

365. Deli, L.; Wittmann, G.; Kallo, I.; Lechan, R.M.; Watanabe, M.; Liposits, Z.; Fekete, C. Type 1 cannabinoid receptor-containing axons innervate hypophysiotropic thyrotropin-releasing hormone-synthesizing neurons. *Endocrinology* **2009**, *150*, 98–103. [CrossRef] [PubMed]

366. Lomax, P. The effect of marihuana on pituitary-thyroid activity in the rat. *Agents Actions* **1970**, *1*, 252–257. [CrossRef] [PubMed]

367. Di, S.; Malcher-Lopes, R.; Halmos, K.C.; Tasker, J.G. Nongenomic glucocorticoid inhibition via endocannabinoid release in the hypothalamus: A fast feedback mechanism. *J. Neurosci.* **2003**, *23*, 4850–4857. [CrossRef] [PubMed]

368. Pagotto, U.; Marsicano, G.; Fezza, F.; Theodoropoulou, M.; Grubler, Y.; Stalla, J.; Arzberger, T.; Milone, A.; Losa, M.; Di Marzo, V.; et al. Normal human pituitary gland and pituitary adenomas express cannabinoid receptor type 1 and synthesize endogenous cannabinoids: First evidence for a direct role of cannabinoids on hormone modulation at the human pituitary level. *J. Clin. Endocrinol. Metab.* **2001**, *86*, 2687–2696. [PubMed]

369. Simon, V.; Cota, D. Mechanisms in endocrinology: Endocannabinoids and metabolism: Past, present and future. *Eur. J. Endocrinol.* **2017**, *176*, R309–R324. [CrossRef] [PubMed]

370. Hollister, L.E. Hunger and appetite after single doses of marihuana, alcohol, and dextroamphetamine. *Clin. Pharmacol. Ther.* **1971**, *12*, 44–49. [CrossRef] [PubMed]

371. Foltin, R.W.; Fischman, M.W.; Byrne, M.F. Effects of smoked marijuana on food intake and body weight of humans living in a residential laboratory. *Appetite* **1988**, *11*, 1–14. [CrossRef]

372. Greenberg, I.; Kuehnle, J.; Mendelson, J.H.; Bernstein, J.G. Effects of marihuana use on body weight and caloric intake in humans. *Psychopharmacology (Berl.)* **1976**, *49*, 79–84. [PubMed]

373. Bellocchio, L.; Lafenetre, P.; Cannich, A.; Cota, D.; Puente, N.; Grandes, P.; Chaouloff, F.; Piazza, P.V.; Marsicano, G. Bimodal control of stimulated food intake by the endocannabinoid system. *Nat. Neurosci.* **2010**, *13*, 281–283. [CrossRef] [PubMed]

374. Graap, H.; Erim, Y.; Paslakis, G. The effect of dronabinol in a male patient with anorexia nervosa suffering from severe acute urge to be physically active. *Int. J. Eat. Disord.* **2018**, *51*, 180–183. [CrossRef] [PubMed]

375. Scherma, M.; Satta, V.; Collu, R.; Boi, M.F.; Usai, P.; Fratta, W.; Fadda, P. Cannabinoid CB1/CB2 receptor agonists attenuate hyperactivity and body weight loss in a rat model of activity-based anorexia. *Br. J. Pharmacol.* **2017**, *174*, 2682–2695. [CrossRef] [PubMed]

376. Inui, A. Cancer anorexia-cachexia syndrome: Current issues in research and management. *CA Cancer J. Clin.* **2002**, *52*, 72–91. [CrossRef] [PubMed]

377. Osei-Hyiaman, D. Endocannabinoid system in cancer cachexia. *Curr. Opin. Clin. Nutr. Metab. Care* **2007**, *10*, 443–448. [CrossRef] [PubMed]

378. Bedi, G.; Foltin, R.W.; Gunderson, E.W.; Rabkin, J.; Hart, C.L.; Comer, S.D.; Vosburg, S.K.; Haney, M. Efficacy and tolerability of high-dose dronabinol maintenance in hiv-positive marijuana smokers: A controlled laboratory study. *Psychopharmacology (Berl.)* **2010**, *212*, 675–686. [CrossRef] [PubMed]

379. Haney, M.; Gunderson, E.W.; Rabkin, J.; Hart, C.L.; Vosburg, S.K.; Comer, S.D.; Foltin, R.W. Dronabinol and marijuana in HIV-positive marijuana smokers. Caloric intake, mood, and sleep. *J. Acquir. Immune Defic. Syndr.* **2007**, *45*, 545–554. [CrossRef] [PubMed]

380. Cannabis In-Cachexia-Study-Group; Strasser, F.; Luftner, D.; Possinger, K.; Ernst, G.; Ruhstaller, T.; Meissner, W.; Ko, Y.D.; Schnelle, M.; Reif, M.; et al. Comparison of orally administered cannabis extract and delta-9-tetrahydrocannabinol in treating patients with cancer-related anorexia-cachexia syndrome: A multicenter, phase III, randomized, double-blind, placebo-controlled clinical trial from the cannabis-in-cachexia-study-group. *J. Clin. Oncol.* **2006**, *24*, 3394–3400. [PubMed]

381. Reuter, S.E.; Martin, J.H. Pharmacokinetics of cannabis in cancer cachexia-anorexia syndrome. *Clin. Pharmacokinet.* **2016**, *55*, 807–812. [CrossRef] [PubMed]

382. Wagner, A.; Aizenstein, H.; Mazurkewicz, L.; Fudge, J.; Frank, G.K.; Putnam, K.; Bailer, U.F.; Fischer, L.; Kaye, W.H. Altered insula response to taste stimuli in individuals recovered from restricting-type anorexia nervosa. *Neuropsychopharmacology* **2008**, *33*, 513–523. [CrossRef] [PubMed]

383. Kaye, W.H.; Bailer, U.F. Understanding the neural circuitry of appetitive regulation in eating disorders. *Biol. Psychiatry* **2011**, *70*, 704–705. [CrossRef] [PubMed]

384. Haase, L.; Cerf-Ducastel, B.; Murphy, C. Cortical activation in response to pure taste stimuli during the physiological states of hunger and satiety. *Neuroimage* **2009**, *44*, 1008–1021. [CrossRef] [PubMed]

385. Petrosino, S.; Di Marzo, V. Faah and magl inhibitors: Therapeutic opportunities from regulating endocannabinoid levels. *Curr. Opin. Investig. Drugs* **2010**, *11*, 51–62. [PubMed]

386. Kwilasz, A.J.; Abdullah, R.A.; Poklis, J.L.; Lichtman, A.H.; Negus, S.S. Effects of the fatty acid amide hydrolase inhibitor URB597 on pain-stimulated and pain-depressed behavior in rats. *Behav. Pharmacol.* **2014**, *25*, 119–129. [CrossRef] [PubMed]

387. Nozaki, C.; Markert, A.; Zimmer, A. Inhibition of faah reduces nitroglycerin-induced migraine-like pain and trigeminal neuronal hyperactivity in mice. *Eur. Neuropsychopharmacol.* **2015**, *25*, 1388–1396. [CrossRef] [PubMed]

388. Mulvihill, M.M.; Nomura, D.K. Therapeutic potential of monoacylglycerol lipase inhibitors. *Life Sci.* **2013**, *92*, 492–497. [CrossRef] [PubMed]

389. Huggins, J.P.; Smart, T.S.; Langman, S.; Taylor, L.; Young, T. An efficient randomised, placebo-controlled clinical trial with the irreversible fatty acid amide hydrolase-1 inhibitor PF-04457845, which modulates endocannabinoids but fails to induce effective analgesia in patients with pain due to osteoarthritis of the knee. *Pain* **2012**, *153*, 1837–1846. [PubMed]

390. Marco, E.M.; Rapino, C.; Caprioli, A.; Borsini, F.; Laviola, G.; Maccarrone, M. Potential therapeutic value of a novel faah inhibitor for the treatment of anxiety. *PLoS ONE* **2015**, *10*, e0137034. [CrossRef] [PubMed]

391. Van Esbroeck, A.C.M.; Janssen, A.P.A.; Cognetta, A.B., 3rd; Ogasawara, D.; Shpak, G.; van der Kroeg, M.; Kantae, V.; Baggelaar, M.P.; de Vrij, F.M.S.; Deng, H.; et al. Activity-based protein profiling reveals off-target proteins of the faah inhibitor bia 10-2474. *Science* **2017**, *356*, 1084–1087. [CrossRef] [PubMed]

392. Soethoudt, M.; Grether, U.; Fingerle, J.; Grim, T.W.; Fezza, F.; de Petrocellis, L.; Ullmer, C.; Rothenhausler, B.; Perret, C.; van Gils, N.; et al. Cannabinoid CB2 receptor ligand profiling reveals biased signalling and off-target activity. *Nat. Commun.* **2017**, *8*, 13958. [CrossRef] [PubMed]

393. Roche, M.; Finn, D.P. Brain CB(2) receptors: Implications for neuropsychiatric disorders. *Pharmaceuticals (Basel)* **2010**, *3*, 2517–2553. [CrossRef] [PubMed]

394. Ishiguro, H.; Carpio, O.; Horiuchi, Y.; Shu, A.; Higuchi, S.; Schanz, N.; Benno, R.; Arinami, T.; Onaivi, E.S. A nonsynonymous polymorphism in cannabinoid CB2 receptor gene is associated with eating disorders in humans and food intake is modified in mice by its ligands. *Synapse* **2010**, *64*, 92–96. [CrossRef] [PubMed]

395. Onaivi, E.S.; Carpio, O.; Ishiguro, H.; Schanz, N.; Uhl, G.R.; Benno, R. Behavioral effects of CB2 cannabinoid receptor activation and its influence on food and alcohol consumption. *Ann. N. Y. Acad. Sci.* **2008**, *1139*, 426–433. [CrossRef] [PubMed]

396. Werner, N.A.; Koch, J.E. Effects of the cannabinoid antagonists AM281 and AM630 on deprivation-induced intake in lewis rats. *Brain Res.* **2003**, *967*, 290–292. [CrossRef]

397. Engeli, S. Dysregulation of the endocannabinoid system in obesity. *J. Neuroendocrinol.* **2008**, *20* (Suppl. 1), 110–115. [CrossRef] [PubMed]

398. Chen, W.; Xu, C.; Liu, H.Y.; Long, L.; Zhang, W.; Zheng, Z.B.; Xie, Y.D.; Wang, L.L.; Li, S. Novel selective cannabinoid CB(1) receptor antagonist MJ08 with potent in vivo bioactivity and inverse agonistic effects. *Acta Pharmacol. Sin.* **2011**, *32*, 1148–1158. [CrossRef] [PubMed]

399. Chen, B.; Hu, N. Rimonabant improves metabolic parameters partially attributed to restoration of high voltage-activated Ca^{2+} channels in skeletal muscle in hfd-fed mice. *Braz. J. Med. Biol. Res.* **2017**, *50*, e6141. [CrossRef] [PubMed]

400. Lipina, C.; Vaanholt, L.M.; Davidova, A.; Mitchell, S.E.; Storey-Gordon, E.; Hambly, C.; Irving, A.J.; Speakman, J.R.; Hundal, H.S. CB1 receptor blockade counters age-induced insulin resistance and metabolic dysfunction. *Aging Cell* **2016**, *15*, 325–335. [CrossRef] [PubMed]

401. Shrestha, N.; Cuffe, J.S.M.; Hutchinson, D.S.; Headrick, J.P.; Perkins, A.V.; McAinch, A.J.; Hryciw, D.H. Peripheral modulation of the endocannabinoid system in metabolic disease. *Drug Discov. Today* **2018**, *23*, 592–604. [CrossRef] [PubMed]

402. Pacher, P.; Steffens, S.; Hasko, G.; Schindler, T.H.; Kunos, G. Cardiovascular effects of marijuana and synthetic cannabinoids: The good, the bad, and the ugly. *Nat. Rev. Cardiol.* **2018**, *15*, 151–166. [CrossRef] [PubMed]

403. Richey, J.M.; Woolcott, O. Re-visiting the endocannabinoid system and its therapeutic potential in obesity and associated diseases. *Curr. Diabetes Rep.* **2017**, *17*, 99. [CrossRef] [PubMed]

404. Kabir, M.; Iyer, M.S.; Richey, J.M.; Woolcott, O.O.; Asare Bediako, I.; Wu, Q.; Kim, S.P.; Stefanovski, D.; Kolka, C.M.; Hsu, I.R.; et al. Cb1r antagonist increases hepatic insulin clearance in fat-fed dogs likely via upregulation of liver adiponectin receptors. *Am. J. Physiol. Endocrinol. Metab.* **2015**, *309*, E747–E758. [CrossRef] [PubMed]

405. Tam, J.; Liu, J.; Mukhopadhyay, B.; Cinar, R.; Godlewski, G.; Kunos, G. Endocannabinoids in liver disease. *Hepatology* **2011**, *53*, 346–355. [CrossRef] [PubMed]

406. Nogueiras, R.; Veyrat-Durebex, C.; Suchanek, P.M.; Klein, M.; Tschop, J.; Caldwell, C.; Woods, S.C.; Wittmann, G.; Watanabe, M.; Liposits, Z.; et al. Peripheral, but not central, CB1 antagonism provides food intake-independent metabolic benefits in diet-induced obese rats. *Diabetes* **2008**, *57*, 2977–2991. [CrossRef] [PubMed]

407. Bellocchio, L.; Soria-Gomez, E.; Quarta, C.; Metna-Laurent, M.; Cardinal, P.; Binder, E.; Cannich, A.; Delamarre, A.; Haring, M.; Martin-Fontecha, M.; et al. Activation of the sympathetic nervous system mediates hypophagic and anxiety-like effects of CB(1) receptor blockade. *Proc. Natl. Acad. Sci. USA* **2013**, *110*, 4786–4791. [CrossRef] [PubMed]

408. Padwal, R.S.; Majumdar, S.R. Drug treatments for obesity: Orlistat, sibutramine, and rimonabant. *Lancet* **2007**, *369*, 71–77. [CrossRef]

409. Christensen, R.; Kristensen, P.K.; Bartels, E.M.; Bliddal, H.; Astrup, A. Efficacy and safety of the weight-loss drug rimonabant: A meta-analysis of randomised trials. *Lancet* **2007**, *370*, 1706–1713. [CrossRef]

410. Gueye, A.B.; Pryslawsky, Y.; Trigo, J.M.; Poulia, N.; Delis, F.; Antoniou, K.; Loureiro, M.; Laviolette, S.R.; Vemuri, K.; Makriyannis, A.; et al. The CB1 neutral antagonist AM4113 retains the therapeutic efficacy of the inverse agonist rimonabant for nicotine dependence and weight loss with better psychiatric tolerability. *Int. J. Neuropsychopharmacol.* **2016**, *19*, pyw068. [CrossRef] [PubMed]

411. Randall, P.A.; Vemuri, V.K.; Segovia, K.N.; Torres, E.F.; Hosmer, S.; Nunes, E.J.; Santerre, J.L.; Makriyannis, A.; Salamone, J.D. The novel cannabinoid CB1 antagonist AM6545 suppresses food intake and food-reinforced behavior. *Pharmacol. Biochem. Behav.* **2010**, *97*, 179–184. [CrossRef] [PubMed]

412. Cota, D. The brain strikes back: Hypothalamic targets for peripheral CB1 receptor inverse agonism. *Mol. Metab.* **2017**, *6*, 1077–1078. [CrossRef] [PubMed]

413. Hua, T.; Vemuri, K.; Pu, M.; Qu, L.; Han, G.W.; Wu, Y.; Zhao, S.; Shui, W.; Li, S.; Korde, A.; et al. Crystal structure of the human cannabinoid receptor CB1. *Cell* **2016**, *167*, 750–762.e714. [CrossRef] [PubMed]

414. Shao, Z.; Yin, J.; Chapman, K.; Grzemska, M.; Clark, L.; Wang, J.; Rosenbaum, D.M. High-resolution crystal structure of the human CB1 cannabinoid receptor. *Nature* **2016**, *540*, 602–606. [CrossRef] [PubMed]

415. Hua, T.; Vemuri, K.; Nikas, S.P.; Laprairie, R.B.; Wu, Y.; Qu, L.; Pu, M.; Korde, A.; Jiang, S.; Ho, J.H.; et al. Crystal structures of agonist-bound human cannabinoid receptor CB1. *Nature* **2017**, *547*, 468–471. [CrossRef] [PubMed]

416. Schmitz, K.; Mangels, N.; Haussler, A.; Ferreiros, N.; Fleming, I.; Tegeder, I. Pro-inflammatory obesity in aged cannabinoid-2 receptor-deficient mice. *Int. J. Obes. (Lond.)* **2016**, *40*, 366–379. [CrossRef] [PubMed]

417. Verty, A.N.; Stefanidis, A.; McAinch, A.J.; Hryciw, D.H.; Oldfield, B. Anti-obesity effect of the CB2 receptor agonist JWH-015 in diet-induced obese mice. *PLoS ONE* **2015**, *10*, e0140592. [CrossRef] [PubMed]

418. Sabatucci, A.; Tortolani, D.; Dainese, E.; Maccarrone, M. In silico mapping of allosteric ligand binding sites in type-1 cannabinoid receptor. *Biotechnol. Appl. Biochem.* **2018**, *65*, 21–28. [CrossRef] [PubMed]

419. Alaverdashvili, M.; Laprairie, R.B. The future of type 1 cannabinoid receptor allosteric ligands. *Drug Metab. Rev.* **2018**, *50*, 14–25. [CrossRef] [PubMed]

420. Bauer, M.; Chicca, A.; Tamborrini, M.; Eisen, D.; Lerner, R.; Lutz, B.; Poetz, O.; Pluschke, G.; Gertsch, J. Identification and quantification of a new family of peptide endocannabinoids (pepcans) showing negative allosteric modulation at CB1 receptors. *J. Biol. Chem.* **2012**, *287*, 36944–36967. [CrossRef] [PubMed]

421. Lewis, R.A.; Austen, K.F.; Drazen, J.M.; Soter, N.A.; Figueiredo, J.C.; Corey, E.J. Structure, function, and metabolism of leukotriene constituents of SRS-A. *Adv. Prostaglandin Thromboxane Leukot. Res.* **1982**, *9*, 137–151. [PubMed]

422. Straiker, A.; Mitjavila, J.; Yin, D.; Gibson, A.; Mackie, K. Aiming for allosterism: Evaluation of allosteric modulators of CB1 in a neuronal model. *Pharmacol. Res.* **2015**, *99*, 370–376. [CrossRef] [PubMed]

423. Heimann, A.S.; Gomes, I.; Dale, C.S.; Pagano, R.L.; Gupta, A.; de Souza, L.L.; Luchessi, A.D.; Castro, L.M.; Giorgi, R.; Rioli, V.; et al. Hemopressin is an inverse agonist of CB1 cannabinoid receptors. *Proc. Natl. Acad. Sci. USA* **2007**, *104*, 20588–20593. [CrossRef] [PubMed]

424. Macedonio, G.; Stefanucci, A.; Maccallini, C.; Mirzaie, S.; Novellino, E.; Mollica, A. Hemopressin peptides as modulators of the endocannabinoid system and their potential applications as therapeutic tools. *Protein Pept. Lett.* **2016**, *23*, 1045–1051. [CrossRef] [PubMed]

425. Gamage, T.F.; Farquhar, C.E.; Lefever, T.W.; Thomas, B.F.; Nguyen, T.; Zhang, Y.; Wiley, J.L. The great divide: Separation between in vitro and in vivo effects of psncbam-based CB1 receptor allosteric modulators. *Neuropharmacology* **2017**, *125*, 365–375. [CrossRef] [PubMed]

426. Mitjavila, J.; Yin, D.; Kulkarni, P.M.; Zanato, C.; Thakur, G.A.; Ross, R.; Greig, I.; Mackie, K.; Straiker, A. Enantiomer-specific positive allosteric modulation of CB1 signaling in autaptic hippocampal neurons. *Pharmacol. Res.* **2018**, *129*, 475–481. [CrossRef] [PubMed]

Permissions

All chapters in this book were first published in PHARMACEUTICALS, by MDPI; hereby published with permission under the Creative Commons Attribution License or equivalent. Every chapter published in this book has been scrutinized by our experts. Their significance has been extensively debated. The topics covered herein carry significant findings which will fuel the growth of the discipline. They may even be implemented as practical applications or may be referred to as a beginning point for another development.

The contributors of this book come from diverse backgrounds, making this book a truly international effort. This book will bring forth new frontiers with its revolutionizing research information and detailed analysis of the nascent developments around the world.

We would like to thank all the contributing authors for lending their expertise to make the book truly unique. They have played a crucial role in the development of this book. Without their invaluable contributions this book wouldn't have been possible. They have made vital efforts to compile up to date information on the varied aspects of this subject to make this book a valuable addition to the collection of many professionals and students.

This book was conceptualized with the vision of imparting up-to-date information and advanced data in this field. To ensure the same, a matchless editorial board was set up. Every individual on the board went through rigorous rounds of assessment to prove their worth. After which they invested a large part of their time researching and compiling the most relevant data for our readers.

The editorial board has been involved in producing this book since its inception. They have spent rigorous hours researching and exploring the diverse topics which have resulted in the successful publishing of this book. They have passed on their knowledge of decades through this book. To expedite this challenging task, the publisher supported the team at every step. A small team of assistant editors was also appointed to further simplify the editing procedure and attain best results for the readers.

Apart from the editorial board, the designing team has also invested a significant amount of their time in understanding the subject and creating the most relevant covers. They scrutinized every image to scout for the most suitable representation of the subject and create an appropriate cover for the book.

The publishing team has been an ardent support to the editorial, designing and production team. Their endless efforts to recruit the best for this project, has resulted in the accomplishment of this book. They are a veteran in the field of academics and their pool of knowledge is as vast as their experience in printing. Their expertise and guidance has proved useful at every step. Their uncompromising quality standards have made this book an exceptional effort. Their encouragement from time to time has been an inspiration for everyone.

The publisher and the editorial board hope that this book will prove to be a valuable piece of knowledge for researchers, students, practitioners and scholars across the globe.

List of Contributors

José Gerardo Carneiro
Department of Biochemistry and Molecular Biology, Federal University of Ceará, s/n Humberto Monte Avenue, Pici Campus, 60455-760 Fortaleza, Brazil
Federal Institute of Education, Science and Technology of Ceará, Armando Sales Louzada Street, 62580-000 Acaraú, Brazil

Ticiana de Brito Lima Holanda, Ana Luíza Gomes Quinderé, Annyta Fernandes Frota, Vitória Virgínia Magalhães Soares, Rayane Siqueira de Sousa, Norma Maria Barros Benevides and Manuela Araújo Carneiro
Department of Biochemistry and Molecular Biology, Federal University of Ceará, s/n Humberto Monte Avenue, Pici Campus, 60455-760 Fortaleza, Brazil

Dainesy Santos Martins and Antoniella Souza Gomes Duarte
Department of Morphoology, Faculty of Medicine, Federal University of Ceará, s/n Delmiro de Farias Street, Porangabuçu Campus, 60416-030 Fortaleza, Brazil

Gerdien A. H. Korte-Bouws, Floor van Heesch, Koen G. C. Westphal, Lisa M. J. Ankersmit and Edwin M. van Oosten
Division of Pharmacology, Utrecht Institute for Pharmaceutical Sciences (UIPS), Utrecht University, Faculty of Science, Universiteitsweg 99, 3584 CG Utrecht, The Netherlands

S. Mechiel Korte
Division of Pharmacology, Utrecht Institute for Pharmaceutical Sciences (UIPS), Utrecht University, Faculty of Science, Universiteitsweg 99, 3584 CG Utrecht, The Netherlands
Department of Biopsychology, Faculty of Psychology, Ruhr-Universität Bochum, Universitätsstraße 150, D-44780 Bochum, Germany

Onur Güntürkün
Department of Biopsychology, Faculty of Psychology, Ruhr-Universität Bochum, Universitätsstraße 150, D-44780 Bochum, Germany

José J. Jarero-Basulto, Yadira Gasca-Martínez, Martha C. Rivera-Cervantes and Alfredo I. Feria-Velasco
Cellular Neurobiology Laboratory, Cell and Molecular Biology Department, CUCBA, University of Guadalajara, 45220 Zapopan, Jalisco, Mexico

Mónica E. Ureña-Guerrero
Neurotransmission Biology Laboratory, Cell and Molecular Biology Department, CUCBA, University of Guadalajara, 45220 Zapopan, Jalisco, Mexico

Carlos Beas-Zarate
Development and Neural Regeneration Laboratory, Cell and Molecular Biology Department, CUCBA, University of Guadalajara, 45220 Zapopan, Jalisco, Mexico

Othman Al Musaimi and Danah Al Shaer ID
College of Health Sciences, University of KwaZulu-Natal, Durban 4000, South Africa; School of Chemistry, University of KwaZulu-Natal, Durban 4001, South Africa

Fernando Albericio
School of Chemistry, University of KwaZulu-Natal, Durban 4001, South Africa
CIBER-BBN, Networking Centre on Bioengineering, Biomaterials and Nanomedicine, University of Barcelona, 08028 Barcelona, Spain
Department of Organic Chemistry, University of Barcelona, 08028 Barcelona, Spain

Beatriz G. de la Torre
KRISP, College of Health Sciences, University of KwaZulu-Natal, Durban 4001, South Africa

Sally Miller, Alex Ciesielski, Ken Mackie and Alex Straiker
The Gill Center for Biomolecular Science, The Department of Psychological and Brain Sciences, Indiana University, Bloomington, IN 47405, USA

Shashank Kulkarni, Spyros P. Nikas and Alexandros Makriyannis
Center for Drug Discovery, Departments of Chemistry and Chemical Biology and Pharmaceutical Sciences, Northeastern University, Boston, MA 02115, USA

Jaume Folch
Departament de Bioquímica i Biotecnologia, Facultat de Medicina i Ciències de la Salut, Universitat Rovirai Virgili, 43201 Reus, Spain
Biomedical ResearchNetworking Centre in Neurodegenerative Diseases (CIBERNED), 28031 Madrid, Spain

Miren Ettcheto and Oriol Busquets
Departament de Bioquímica i Biotecnologia, Facultat deMedicina i Ciències de la Salut, Universitat Rovirai Virgili, 43201 Reus, Spain

Biomedical ResearchNetworking Centre in Neuro-degenerative Diseases (CIBERNED), 28031Madrid, Spain
Departament de Farmacologia, Toxicologia i Química Terapèutica, Facultat de Farmàcia i Ciències de l'Alimentació, Universitat de Barcelona, Av. Joan XXIII 27/31, E-08028 Barcelona, Spain
Institut de Neurociències, Universitat de Barcelona, E-08028 Barcelona, Spain

Antoni Camins
Biomedical ResearchNetworking Centre in Neuro-degenerative Diseases (CIBERNED), 28031Madrid, Spain
Departament de Farmacologia, Toxicologia i Química Terapèutica, Facultat de Farmàcia i Ciències de l'Alimentació, Universitat de Barcelona, Av. Joan XXIII 27/31, E-08028 Barcelona, Spain Institut de Neurociències, Universitat de Barcelona, E-08028 Barcelona, Spain

Elena Sánchez-López
Biomedical Research Networking Centre in Neurodegenerative Diseases (CIBERNED), 28031 Madrid, Spain
Unitat de Farmàcia, Tecnologia Farmacèutica i Fisico-química, Facultat de Farmàciai Ciències de Institute of Nanoscience and Nanotechnology (IN2UB), University of Barcelona, Barcelona E-08028, Spain

Carme Auladell and Ester Verdaguer
Biomedical Research Networking Centre in Neurodegenerative Diseases (CIBERNED), 28031 Madrid, Spain
Institut de Neurociències, Universitat de Barcelona, E-08028 Barcelona, Spain
Departament de Biologia Cel_lular, Fisiologia i Immunologia, Facultat de Biologia, Universitat de Barcelona, E-08028 Barcelona, Spain

Rubén D. Castro-Torres
Biomedical Research Networking Centre in Neurodegenerative Diseases (CIBERNED), 28031 Madrid, Spain
Departament de Farmacologia, Toxicologia i Química Terapèutica, Facultat de Farmàcia i Ciències de l'Alimentació, Universitat de Barcelona, Av. Joan XXIII 27/31, E-08028 Barcelona, Spain
Institut de Neurociències, Universitat de Barcelona, E-08028 Barcelona, Spain
Departament de Biologia Cel_lular, Fisiologia i Immunologia, Facultat de Biologia, Universitat de Barcelona, E-08028 Barcelona, Spain
Laboratorio de Regeneración y Desarrollo Neural, Instituto de Neurobiología, Departamento de Biología Celular y Molecular, Centro Universitario de Ciencias Biológicas y Agropecuarias, Universidad de Guadalajara, Zapopan 44600, Mexico

Saghar Rabiei Poor
Departament de Farmacologia, Toxicologia i Química Terapèutica, Facultat de Farmàcia i Ciències de l'Alimentació, Universitat de Barcelona, Av. Joan XXIII 27/31, E-08028 Barcelona, Spain

Patricia R. Manzine
Departament de Farmacologia, Toxicologia i Química Terapèutica, Facultat de Farmàcia i Ciències de l'Alimentació, Universitat de Barcelona, Av. Joan XXIII 27/31, E-08028 Barcelona, Spain
Department of Gerontology, Federal University of São Carlos (UFSCar), São Carlos 13565-905, Brazil

María Luisa García
Unitat de Farmàcia, Tecnologia Farmacèutica i Fisico-química, Facultat de Farmàcia i Ciències de l'Alimentació, Universitat de Barcelona, E-08028 Barcelona, Spain
Institute of Nanoscience and Nanotechnology (IN2UB), University of Barcelona, Barcelona E-08028, Spain

Carlos Beas-Zarate
Laboratorio de Regeneración y Desarrollo Neural, Instituto de Neurobiología, Departamento de Biología Celular y Molecular, Centro Universitario de Ciencias Biológicas y Agropecuarias, Universidad de Guadalajara, Zapopan 44600, Mexico

Jordi Olloquequi
Instituto de Ciencias Biomédicas, Facultad de Ciencias de la Salud, Universidad Autónoma de Chile, Talca 3460000, Chile

Eka Ginanjar
Department of Internal Medicine, Faculty of Medicine, University of Indonesia/Dr Cipto Mangunkusumo Hospital, Jakarta 10430, Indonesia

Lilik Indrawati and Ina S. Timan
Department of Clinical Pathology, Faculty of Medicine, University of Indonesia/Dr Cipto Mangunkusumo Hospital, Jakarta 10430, Indonesia

Iswari Setianingsih and Alida Harahap
Eijkman Institute for Molecular Biology, Jakarta 10430, Indonesia

Djumhana Atmakusumah
Division of Hematology and Medical Oncology, Department of Internal Medicine, Faculty of Medicine, University of Indonesia/Dr Cipto Mangunkusumo Hospital, Jakarta 10430, Indonesia

Joannes J. M. Marx
Department of Medical Microbiology, University Medical Centre Utrecht, Heidelberglaan 100, Utrecht 3584 CX, The Netherlands

Won Hyung Choi
Marine Bio Research and Education Center, Kunsan National University, 558 Daehak-ro, Gunsan-si, Jeollabuk-do 54150, Korea

In Ah Lee
Department of Chemistry, College of Natural Science, Kunsan National University, 558 Daehak-ro, Gunsan-si, Jeollabuk-do 54150, Korea

Lillian Mørch Jørgensen
Optimed, Clinical Research Centre, Copenhagen University Hospital Hvidovre, Kettegård Alle 30, Department 056, 2650 Hvidovre, Denmark

Morten Baltzer Houlind, Mia Aakjær and Charlotte Treldal
Optimed, Clinical Research Centre, Copenhagen University Hospital Hvidovre, Kettegård Alle 30, Department 056, 2650 Hvidovre, Denmark
The Capital Region Pharmacy, Marielundvej 25, 2730 Herlev, Denmark
Section of Pharmacotherapy, Department of Drug Design and Pharmacology, University of Copenhagen, Universitetsparken 2, 2100 København Ø, Denmark

Janne Petersen
Optimed, Clinical Research Centre, Copenhagen University Hospital Hvidovre, Kettegård Alle 30, Department 056, 2650 Hvidovre, Denmark
Section of Biostatistics, Department of Public Health, University of Copenhagen, Øster Farimagsgade 5, Enterance B, 2nd floor, 1014 København, Denmark

Ove Andersen
Optimed, Clinical Research Centre, Copenhagen University Hospital Hvidovre, Kettegård Alle 30, Department 056, 2650 Hvidovre, Denmark
Emergency Department, Copenhagen University Hospital Hvidovre, Kettegård Alle 30, Department 436, 2650 Hvidovre, Denmark

Lona Louring Christrup
Section of Pharmacotherapy, Department of Drug Design and Pharmacology, University of Copenhagen, Universitetsparken 2, 2100 København Ø, Denmark

Kristian Kjær Petersen
Center for Sensory-Motor Interaction (SMI), Department of Health Science and Technology, Faculty of Medicine, Aalborg University, Fredrik Bajers Vej 7, building A2-206, 9220 Aalborg Ø, Denmark

Henrik Palm
Orthopedic Department, Copenhagen University Hospital Bispebjerg, Bispebjerg Bakke 2400 København, Denmark

Boshuai Mu and Simon M. Ametamey
Center of Radiopharmaceutical Sciences of ETH, PSI and USZ, Department of Chemistry and Applied Biosciences, Swiss Federal Institute of Technology, Vladimir-Prelog-Weg 4, 8093 Zurich, Switzerland

Linjing Mu and Roger Schibli
Center of Radiopharmaceutical Sciences of ETH, PSI and USZ, Department of Chemistry and Applied Biosciences, Swiss Federal Institute of Technology, Vladimir-Prelog-Weg 4, 8093 Zurich, Switzerland
Department of Nuclear Medicine, University Hospital Zurich, Ramistrasse 101, 8003 Zurich, Switzerland

Selena Milicevic Sephton
Center of Radiopharmaceutical Sciences of ETH, PSI and USZ, Department of Chemistry and Applied Biosciences, Swiss Federal Institute of Technology, Vladimir-Prelog-Weg 4, 8093 Zurich, Switzerland
Department of Nuclear Medicine, University Hospital Zurich, Ramistrasse 101, 8003 Zurich, Switzerland
Molecular Imaging Chemistry Laboratory, Wolfson Brain Imaging Centre, Department of Clinical Neurosciences, University of Cambridge, Box 65 Cambridge Biomedical Campus, Cambridge CB2 0QQ, UK

Christelle Marminon and Zouhair Bouaziz D
Faculté de Pharmacie—ISPB, EA 4446 Bioactive Molecules and Medicinal Chemistry, SFR Santé Lyon-Est CNRS UMS3453—INSERM US7, Université de Lyon, Université Claude Bernard Lyon 1, Avenue Rockefeller, F-69373 Lyon CEDEX 8, France

Abdelhamid Nacereddine
Faculté de Pharmacie—ISPB, EA 4446 Bioactive Molecules and Medicinal Chemistry, SFR Santé Lyon-Est CNRS UMS3453—INSERM US7, Université de Lyon, Université Claude Bernard Lyon 1, 8 Avenue Rockefeller, F-69373 Lyon CEDEX 8, France

Andre Bollacke, Joachim Jose and Marc Le Borgne
Institute of Pharmaceutical and Medicinal Chemistry, PharmaCampus, Westfälische Wilhelms-Universität Münster, Corrensstr. 48, 48149 Münster, Germany

Ferenc Fenyvesi and Ildikó Katalin Bácskay
Department of Pharmaceutical Technology, Faculty of Pharmacy, University of Debrecen, Nagyerdei körút 98, H-4032 Debrecen, Hungary

Eszter Róka
Department of Pharmaceutical Technology, Faculty of Pharmacy, University of Debrecen, Nagyerdei körút 98, H-4032 Debrecen, Hungary

CSAp, Institut de Chimie et Biochimie Moléculaires et Supramoléculaires, Bâtiment Raulin, Université de Lyon, Université Lyon 1, 43 Bd du 11 novembre 1918, 69622 Villeurbanne CEDEX, France

Florent Perret
CSAp, Institut de Chimie et Biochimie Moléculaires et Supramoléculaires, Bâtiment Raulin, Université de Lyon, Université Lyon 1, 43 Bd du 11 novembre 1918, 69622 Villeurbanne CEDEX, France

David Alsina, Rosa Purroy, Joaquim Ros and Jordi Tamarit
Departament de Ciències Mèdiques Bàsiques, IRBLleida, Universitat de Lleida, 25198 Lleida, Spain

Lide Gu, Wanli Yan and Le Liu
College of Marine Life and Fisheries, Huahai Institute of Technology, Lianyungang 222005, China

Mingsheng Lyu
College of Marine Life and Fisheries, Huahai Institute of Technology, Lianyungang 222005, China
Marine Resources Development Institute of Jiangsu, Lianyungang 222005, China
Co-Innovation Center of Jiangsu Marine Bio-industry Technology, Huaihai Institute of Technology, Lianyungang 222005, China

Shujun Wang
Marine Resources Development Institute of Jiangsu, Lianyungang 222005, China

Co-Innovation Center of Jiangsu Marine Bio-industry Technology, Huaihai Institute of Technology, Lianyungang 222005, China

Xu Zhang
Co-Innovation Center of Jiangsu Marine Bio-industry Technology, Huaihai Institute of Technology, Lianyungang 222005, China
Verschuren Centre for Sustainability in Energy and the Environment, Cape Breton University, Sydney, NS B1P 6L2, Canada

Sophie A. Millar, Saoirse E. O'Sullivan and Timothy J. England
Division of Medical Sciences and Graduate Entry Medicine, School of Medicine, University of Nottingham, Derby DE22 3DT, UK

Salahaden R. Sultan
Division of Medical Sciences and Graduate Entry Medicine, School of Medicine, University of Nottingham, Derby DE22 3DT, UK
Faculty of Applied Medical Sciences, King Abdulaziz University, Jeddah 21589, Saudi Arabia

Henrike Horn, Beatrice Böhme, Laura Dietrich and Marco Koch
Institute of Anatomy, Medical Faculty, University of Leipzig, 04103 Leipzig, Germany

Index

www.ingramcontent.com/pod-product-compliance
Lightning Source LLC
Chambersburg PA
CBHW080511200326
41458CB00012B/4164